Vestibular Schwannoma: Evidence-based Treatment

Guest Editors

FRED F. TELISCHI, MEE, MD
JACQUES J. MORCOS, MD, FRCS (Eng.), FRCS (Ed)

OTOLARYNGOLOGIC CLINICS OF NORTH AMERICA

www.oto.theclinics.com

April 2012 • Volume 45 • Number 2

SAUNDERS an imprint of ELSEVIER, Inc.

W.B. SAUNDERS COMPANY
A Division of Elsevier Inc.

1600 John F. Kennedy Boulevard • Suite 1800 • Philadelphia, Pennsylvania 19103-2899

http://www.theclinics.com

OTOLARYNGOLOGIC CLINICS OF NORTH AMERICA Volume 45, Number 2
April 2012 ISSN 0030-6665, ISBN-13: 978-1-4557-1115-4

Editor: Joanne Husovski

Otolaryngologic Clinics of North America (ISSN 0030-6665) is published bimonthly by Elsevier, Inc., 360 Park Avenue South, New York, NY 10010-1710. Months of issue are February, April, June, August, October, and December. Business and Editorial Offices: 1600 John F. Kennedy Blvd., Suite 1800, Philadelphia, PA 19103-2899. Customer Service Office: 6277 Sea Harbor Drive, Orlando, FL 32887-4800. Periodicals postage paid at New York, NY and additional mailing offices. Subscription prices is $335.00 per year (US individuals), $628.00 per year (US institutions), $161.00 per year (US student/resident), $442.00 per year (Canadian individuals), $789.00 per year (Canadian institutions), $496.00 per year (international individuals), $789.00 per year (international institutions), $248.00 per year (international & Canadian student/resident). Foreign air speed delivery is included in all *Clinics'* subscription prices. All prices are subject to change without notice. **POSTMASTER:** Send address changes to *Otolaryngologic Clinics of North America*, Elsevier Health Sciences Division, Subscription Customer Service, 3251 Riverport Lane, Maryland Heights, MO 63043. **Telephone: 1-800-654-2452 (U.S. and Canada); 314-447-8871 (outside U.S. and Canada). Fax: 314-447-8029. E-mail: journalscustomerservice-usa@elsevier.com (for print support); journalsonlinesupport-usa@elsevier.com (for online support).**

Reprints. For copies of 100 or more of articles in this publication, please contact the Commercial Reprints Department, Elsevier Inc., 360 Park Avenue South, New York, NY 10010-1710. Tel.: 212-633-3812; Fax: 212-462-1935; E-mail: reprints@elsevier.com.

Otolaryngologic Clinics of North America is also published in Spanish by McGraw-Hill Interamericana Editores S.A., P.O. Box 5-237, 06500 Mexico D.F., Mexico.

Otolaryngologic Clinics of North America is covered in *MEDLINE/PubMed (Index Medicus), Current Contents/Clinical Medicine, Excerpta Medica, BIOSIS, Science Citation Index,* and *ISI/BIOMED.*

Printed and bound by CPI Group (UK) Ltd, Croydon, CR0 4YY

Transferred to Digital Print 2012

Contributors

GUEST EDITORS

FRED F. TELISCHI, MEE, MD, FACS
Chairman of Otolaryngology and Professor, Neurological Surgery and Biomedical Engineering, Department of Otolaryngology, Miami, Florida

JACQUES J. MORCOS, MD, FRCS (Eng.), FRCS (Ed)
Professor of Clinical Neurosurgery and Otolaryngology, Department of Neurological Surgery, Lois Pope Life Center, Miami, Florida

Foreword by DERALD E. BRACKMANN, MD
Clinical Professor of Otolaryngology – Head and Neck Surgery and Neurological Surgery, University of Southern California School of Medicine; Associate, House Ear Clinic, Board of Directors, House Ear Institute, Los Angeles, California

AUTHORS

MOISÉS A. ARRIAGA, MD, MBA, FACS
Clinical Professor of Otolaryngology and Neurosurgery, Director of Otology and Neurotology, Director, LSU Health Sciences Center New Orleans, Hearing and Balance Center, Our Lady of the Lake Regional Medical Center, Baton Rouge, Louisiana

SIMON ANGELI, MD
Professor of Clinical Otolaryngology, Neurotological Skull Base Surgery, Department of Otolaryngology, University of Miami Miller School of Medicine; University of Miami Ear Institute, Miami, Florida

FRED G. BARKER II, MD
Associate Visiting Neurosurgeon, Department of Neurosurgery, Massachusetts General Hospital; Associate Professor of Surgery (Neurosurgery), Department of Surgery, Harvard Medical School, Boston, Massachusetts

DERALD E. BRACKMANN, MD
Clinical Professor of Otolaryngology – Head and Neck Surgery and Neurological Surgery, University of Southern California School of Medicine; Associate, House Ear Clinic, Board of Directors, House Ear Institute, Los Angeles, California

KEVIN BROWN, MD, PhD
Assistant Professor, Department of Otorhinolaryngology-Head & Neck Surgery, Weill Cornell Medical College, New York, New York

PER CAYE-THOMASEN, MD, DMC
Department of Oto-Rhino-Laryngology, Head and Neck Surgery, Rigshospitalet, Faculty of Health Sciences, University of Copenhagen, Copenhagen, Denmark

ROBERTO A. CUEVA, MD, FACS
Kaiser Permanente Medical Center, Department of Head and Neck Surgery, San Diego; Clinical Professor, Voluntary, University of California, San Diego, California

COLIN L.W. DRISCOLL, MD
Professor, Departments of Otolaryngology and Neurologic Surgery, Mayo Clinic and Mayo Foundation, Rochester, Minnesota

MOHAMED SAMY ELHAMMADY, MD
Department of Neurological Surgery, University of Miami, School of Medicine, Miami, Florida

ROBERT L. FOOTE, MD
Professor, Department of Radiation Oncology, Mayo Clinic and Mayo Foundation, Rochester, Minnesota

GERARD J. GIANOLI, MD, FACS
The Ear and Balance Institute, Baton Rouge, Louisiana

JOHN G. GOLFINOS, MD
Professor and Chair, Departments of Neurosurgery; Department of Otolaryngology, New York University, New York, New York

SELENA E. HEMAN-ACKAH, MD, MBA
Neurotology Fellow, Department of Otolaryngology, New York University, New York, New York

MICHAEL HOA, MD
Clinical Fellow, House Clinic, House Research Institute, Los Angeles, California

ROBERT S. HONG, MD, PhD
Fellow, Michigan Ear Institute, Farmington Hills, Michigan

JACK M. KARTUSH, MD
President, Michigan Ear Institute, Farmington Hills; Clinical Professor, Wayne State University, Detroit; Chief Medical Officer, Biotronic, Ann Arbor, Michigan

CHURL-SU KWON, MBBS, MPH
Post-doctoral Fellow, Department of Neurosurgery, Massachusetts General Hospital, Boston, Massachusetts

JAMES LIN, MD
Assistant Professor of Otolaryngology, LSU Health Sciences Center New Orleans, Hearing and Balance Center, Our Lady of the Lake Regional Medical Center, Baton Rouge, Louisiana

MICHAEL J. LINK, MD
Professor, Departments of Neurologic Surgery and Otolaryngology, Mayo Clinic and Mayo Foundation, Rochester, Minnesota

JACQUES J. MORCOS, MD, FRCS (Eng.), FRCS (Ed)
Professor of Clinical Neurosurgery and Otolaryngology, Department of Neurological Surgery, Lois Pope Life Center, Miami, Florida

RÉMY NOUDEL, MD
Service de neurochirurgie, CHU Nord, Marseille Cedex, France

DANIEL R. PIEPER, MD, FACS
Michigan Head and Spine Institute, Novi, Michigan; Associate Professor of Neurosurgery, Oakland University/William Beaumont School of Medicine, Rochester; Director Skull Base Surgery; Director of Gamma Knife, William Beaumont Hospital, Royal Oak, Michigan

SCOTT R. PLOTKIN, MD, PhD
Department of Neurology and Cancer Center, Massachusetts General Hospital, Boston, Massachusetts

BRUCE E. POLLOCK, MD
Professor, Departments of Neurologic Surgery and Radiation Oncology, Mayo Clinic and Mayo Foundation, Rochester, Minnesota

JEAN RÉGIS, MD, PhD
Service de neurochirurgie fonctionnelle et stéréotaxique, CHU la Timone, Marseille, France

JOHN S. RHEE, MD, MPH
Professor and Chairman, Department of Otolaryngology and Communication Sciences, Medical College of Wisconsin, Milwaukee, Wisconsin

PIERRE-HUGUES ROCHE, MD
Service de neurochirurgie, CHU Nord, Marseille Cedex, France

J. THOMAS ROLAND Jr, MD
Professor and Chair, Departments of Otolaryngology; Department of Neurosurgery, New York University, New York, New York

KELLI L. RUDMAN, MD
Resident, Department of Otolaryngology and Communication Sciences, Medical College of Wisconsin, Milwaukee, Wisconsin

MICHAEL C. SCHUBERT, PhD, PT
Associate Professor, Department of Otolaryngology Head and Neck Surgery, Johns Hopkins University, Baltimore, Maryland

SAMUEL H. SELESNICK, MD, FACS
Professor and Vice Chairman, Department of Otolaryngology-Head & Neck Surgery; Professor of Otolaryngology in Neurological Surgery; Professor of Otolaryngology in Neurology, Weill Cornell Medical College, New York, New York

SAMEER A. SHETH, MD, PhD
Chief Resident, Department of Neurosurgery, Massachusetts General Hospital, Boston, Massachusetts

WILLIAM H. SLATTERY III, MD
Associate, House Clinic, Scientist, House Research Institute; Clinical Professor, University Southern California, Los Angeles, California

HILLARY A. SNAPP, AuD
Assistant Professor, Department of Otolaryngology, University of Miami, Miami, Florida

JAMES S. SOILEAU, MD
The Ear and Balance Institute, Baton Rouge, Louisiana

SVEN-ERIC STANGERUP, MD
Department of Oto-Rhino-Laryngology, Head and Neck Surgery, Rigshospitalet, Faculty of Health Sciences, University of Copenhagen, Copenhagen, Denmark

EMILY Z. STUCKEN, MD
Resident, Department of Otolaryngology-Head & Neck Surgery, New York Presbyterian Hospital – Cornell and Columbia, New York, New York

FRED F. TELISCHI, MEE, MD, FACS
Chairman of Otolaryngology and Professor, Neurological Surgery and Biomedical Engineering, Department of Otolaryngology, Miami, Florida

ANNA R. TERRY, MD, MPH
Resident, Department of Neurosurgery, Massachusetts General Hospital, Boston, Massachusetts

JUDY B. VITUCCI
Executive Director, Acoustic Neuroma Association, Cumming, Georgia

Contents

> This article describes various epidemiologic trends for vestibular schwannomas over the last 35 years, including a brief note on terminology. Additionally, it provides information on the natural history of tumor growth and hearing level following the diagnosis of a vestibular schwannoma. A treatment strategy based on the natural history of tumor growth and hearing also is discussed.

> In the past century, significant advances have been made in understanding the clinical features of acoustic neuromas. Furthermore, rapid technological advances have led to the development of sensitive, rapid, and relatively noninvasive diagnostic modalities, which has allowed for earlier discovery of acoustic neuromas and has reduced the average tumor size at time of diagnosis. The ultimate result has been improved clinical outcomes after surgery and radiotherapy.

> This article is a concise clinical review of preoperative, intraoperative, and postoperative auditory evaluation of patients with acoustic neuroma. The author describes behavioral audiometry, auditory brainstem response, and otoacoustic emissions for preoperative evaluation; auditory brainstem and direct eighth-nerve intraoperative monitoring for intraoperative evaluation; and touches on postoperative auditory assessment.

> This article focuses on the facial nerve with additional comments on the recurrent laryngeal nerve as a proxy for the lower cranial nerves. Methods, advantages and disadvantages, and techniques are listed. The article addresses the anatomy of the facial nerve, discusses neurophysiologic

testing, the role of electroneurography in preoperative, intraoperative, and postoperative testing, and presents 7 steps to set up for and perform facial nerve monitoring. Details are provided on interpretation of testing, and the pitfalls of interpretation are discussed. Studies are reviewed presenting outcomes of testing.

approaches in patients with vestibular schwannoma. Treatment of small and large tumors is discussed, along with cystic tumors and NF2-associated VS. Repeating SRS for vestibular schwannoma is also mentioned.

To describe the incidence and the course of complications after the radiosurgical treatment of vestibular schwannomas, the authors reviewed their own experience and reviewed the literature. Failure is described in less than 3% of cases, and this had to be distinguished from transient enlargement of tumor volume. In case of failure, microsurgical resection or another radiosurgical procedure should be discussed. The risk of radio-induced tumorigenesis is not clearly established with single-dose radiosurgical technique. Incidence and management of potential complications should be explained at the time of decision making in the management of vestibular schwannomas.

This review describes the indications and techniques for the retrosigmoid approach for vestibular schwannoma, as performed by the skull base surgery group at the University of Miami. The authors present background of the retrosigmoid approach, surgical steps, and essential "technical pearls" to address complication avoidance, resulting from their expertise with this surgery.

This article presents a comprehensive review of the translabyrinthine surgical approach for vestibular schwannoma. Additionally, it addresses the traditional labyrinthectomy and identifies a time-efficient version. Indications and outcomes of the approach are presented, along with detailed procedural technique from opening incision through closure. Complications and management of complications are discussed in detail, as well as postoperative patient care.

This article discusses the indications, surgical technique, results, and complications of middle fossa craniotomy (MFC) for vestibular schwannoma surgery, focusing on issues such as serviceable hearing, tumor characteristics, and patient-specific factors that help determine options for therapy. MFC is suitable for intracanalicular vestibular schwannomas that extend less than 1 cm into the cerebellopontine angle in patients with good hearing. With the expanding use of modern imaging, many small tumors are being identified in patients with no or minimal symptoms. Patients with these tumors have three therapy options: (1) stereotactic radiotherapy, (2) microsurgery, and (3) observation (ie, wait-and-scan approach).

This article provides an overview of the technical considerations of endos-copy of the posterolateral skull base and cerebellopontine angle (CPA). Specific areas of focus are on the instrumentation requirements for neuro-endoscopy of the CPA; the learning curve associated with this technique; and a complete description of the surgical techniques necessary to perform the procedure, along with outcomes and results. The article pro-vides a general overview of the endoscopic approach to the CPA. For a variety of pathologies, the emphasis is on performing this technique for acoustic tumors and hearing preservation. Insights as to how the author's practice evolved in its use of neuroendoscopic procedures are provided.

Acoustic neuromas (ANs) are the most common tumors of the cerebello-pontine angle. Although numerous advances have occurred in the opera-tive management of AN and perioperative care leading to a significant decrease in associated morbidity and mortality, there are several charac-teristic complications that accompany microsurgical resection of AN. Understanding the types and rates of complications in association with the various approaches is essential in patient counseling, establishing pa-tient expectations, and ensuring the best patient outcome. In this article, the justification for incomplete surgical resection is discussed. Also, the most common complications of AN microsurgery and the associated man-agement are reviewed.

Vestibular schwannomas (VS) are among the most common benign tu-mors of the central nervous system. Bilateral VS are the hallmark of neuro-fibromatosis type II, commonly leading to complete deafness and cranial nerve deficits as a result of tumor progression or treatment with surgery or radiation. Effective medical therapies are needed to address tumor pro-gression and treatment-related morbidity. This article reviews the standard therapies for VS, summarizes the molecular biology of these tumors, and describes potential targets for chemotherapeutic agents. The article also defines and recommends the use of specific clinical end points in future drug trials, describes previous and current experience with anti-VEGF and anti-EGFR agents, and delineates areas of future research.

Although unilateral hearing loss is often the initial sign of vestibular schwannoma (VS), the pathogenesis of the associated structures within the cerebellopontine angle can result in vestibular, facial, or vascular symptoms. Removal of a VS causes deficits in hearing, balance, and

FORTHCOMING ISSUES

RECENT ISSUES

RELATED INTEREST

Imaging of the Cerebellopontine Angle
Authors: Magge Lakshmi, MD, and Christine M. Glastonbury, MBBS In:
Neuroimaging Clinics of North America, August 2009 (Volume 19, Issue 3) Pages 393–406
Skull Base and Temporal Bone Imaging
Vincent Fook-Hin Chong, MBBS, MBS, FAMS, *Guest Editor*

THE CLINICS ARE NOW AVAILABLE ONLINE!

Access your subscription at:
www.theclinics.com

Foreword

Vestibular Schwannoma (Acoustic Neuroma)

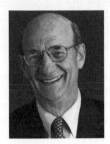

Derald E. Brackmann, MD

It is my privilege and pleasure to write this brief foreword for this volume on acoustic neuromas.

BRIEF RETROSPECTIVE OF ACOUSTIC NEUROMA TREATMENT

Sandifort in 1777 provided the first description of an acoustic neuroma. Sir Charles Balance was the first to remove an acoustic neuroma successfully in 1894. The classical suboccipital approach was used and this remained the standard of care until the early 1960s. There were refinements in diagnosis and treatment with major contributions from first Harvey Cushing and then Walter Dandy, but mortality and morbidity remained high. In 1960 when Dr William House first became interested in acoustic neuromas, a noted Swedish neurosurgeon Olivecrona reported a 4.5% mortality rate for small tumors and a 22.5% mortality rate for large tumors. Virtually all patients had facial paralysis and many also had ataxia. In California, the mortality rate for acoustic neuromas in 1961 was 43.5%.

At this time, rapid advances in audiology and radiology made earlier diagnosis possible. Dr William House was able to diagnose a small acoustic neuroma in a young fireman and referred him to a neurosurgeon for treatment. Faced with the possibility of mortality, the consultant recommended observation. The tumor was rapidly growing and he was operated 2 years later when it became large; he expired during the procedure. This experience prompted Dr William House to explore other management possibilities.

OPERATIVE APPROACHES
Middle Fossa Approach

By this time, Dr House had developed the middle cranial fossa approach for decompression of the internal auditory canal for advanced otosclerosis. Although shown not to be effective for that condition, Bill recognized the possibility of approaching

Otolaryngol Clin N Am 45 (2012) xiii–xv
doi:10.1016/j.otc.2011.12.017
0030-6665/12/$ – see front matter © 2012 Elsevier Inc. All rights reserved.

tumors from the middle fossa and he teamed with a Los Angeles neurosurgeon, Dr John B. Doyle, with the aim of developing a new technique for the removal of acoustic neuromas that would lower morbidity and mortality. The initial plan was to approach the tumor through the middle fossa, identify the facial nerve and trace it back to the posterior fossa, and then remove the remainder of the tumor from the suboccipital route. The first microsurgical removal of an acoustic neuroma was done on February 15, 1961, through a middle fossa craniotomy approach using the Zeiss operating microscope. A partial removal was accomplished. The patient subsequently underwent two suboccipital procedures before dying in 1967.

The initial eight cases were done using the middle cranial fossa approach, which was expanded into the cerebellopontine angle by drilling the labyrinth from above. Only partial removal could be done using this approach. It occurred to Dr House that a more direct route through the mastoid could be a better choice since he and Dr Doyle were destroying the labyrinth from above. Panse in 1904 had approached the CPA through the mastoid. His approach included a radical mastoidectomy and sacrifice of the facial nerve. Cerebrospinal fluid leaks were a major postoperative problem and this approach was greatly criticized by the neurosurgical community and never adopted.

Translabyrinthine Approach

Dr William House performed a series of cadaver dissections to work out a method to expose the CPA through the mastoid. With the aid of a surgical microscope, a dental drill, and suction irrigation, he was able to devise a method to preserve the posterior canal wall, the tympanic membrane, and the facial nerve. The translabyrinthine approach was developed.

In July, 1963, Dr William Hitselberger began to work with Dr House. They began using the translabyrinthine procedure on a routine basis for tumors of all sizes. The first series of 53 patients was published in 1964. Many of those patients underwent subtotal removal. Facial nerve preservation, however, became routine and the mortality rate was greatly reduced. As experience was gained, the percentage of subtotal removal became much less.

The neurosurgical community continued to disagree with the translabyrinthine approach, but slowly over the next several years, a few neurosurgeons became supportive. The first International Symposium on Acoustic Neuromas was organized in 1965. For 5 days leading neurosurgeons, otologists, neurologists, and audiologists attended the meeting and covered a wide range of subjects. This set the stage for early detection of acoustic neuromas and management with microsurgical techniques including the translabyrinthine approach. Over the years, it has become recognized that all three approaches (retrosigmoid, translabyrinthine, and middle fossa) are valuable. The extended middle fossa approach and the transcochlear approach were added to the surgical repertoire to allow management of most tumors in the posterior fossa. The approach is selected depending on the size and location of the tumor as well as the preoperative hearing status and the patient's general condition.

DEVELOPMENTS IN DIAGNOSING AND TREATING ACOUSTIC NEUROMA

Over the years, there have been major advances in audiometry including auditory brainstem response audiometry and imaging techniques, first CT and now MRI with gadolinium, which have greatly aided early diagnosis.

The development of facial nerve monitoring and intraoperative auditory monitoring has played major roles in reducing morbidity. Improvements in surgical microscopes with brilliant illumination have facilitated tumor dissection, as have devices to reduce tumor bulk safely. These devices include the rotary dissector, ultrasonic aspirator, and the laser.

Development of radiosurgery over the past 30 years has also altered greatly the management of acoustic neuromas. The role of radiosurgery is evolving, as is the role of the various techniques. The role of observation in acoustic neuroma management is expanding. As tumors are observed, it is surprising how many remain stable over time.

INSIGHTS FROM Dr BRACKMANN ON ACOUSTIC NEUROMA

The editors asked me to summarize briefly my current management of acoustic neuromas. For patients under age 65 with small tumors and good hearing, I recommend microsurgical removal of the tumor using a middle cranial fossa approach. For small tumors with poor hearing, regardless of age, I recommend observation. If tumors show growth, I recommend treatment. For young patients, I recommend a translabyrinthine removal, whereas for older patients, I recommend gamma knife radiosurgery. I do not recommend radiosurgical treatment for non-growing tumors. For tumors up to 2.5 centimeters with good hearing, I recommend a retrosigmoid approach for younger patients and radiosurgery for older patients with growing tumors. I recommend a translabyrinthine approach for all tumors 3 centimeters or larger, regardless of age or hearing.

It's hard to imagine that advances over the next 50 years will approach those of the past 50 years, but without question, there will be an evolution of management of these lesions. Long-term follow-up of patients treated with radiation will clarify that treatment further. If only growing tumors are treated, the true effectiveness of radiation will be revealed. As adverse effects to radiation are delayed many years, only time will reveal their incidence. Undoubtedly, there will be improvements in surgical techniques as well.

It has been an exciting ride on the acoustic neuroma treatment train over my 40-year career. I wish my young colleagues equal challenges and advances.

Derald E. Brackmann, MD
Otolaryngology Head and Neck Surgery and Neurological Surgery
University of Southern California School of Medicine
House Ear Clinic, House Ear Institute
House Research Institute
2100 West, 3rd Street
Los Angeles, CA 90057, USA

Preface

Vestibular Schwannoma: Evidence-based Treatment

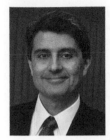 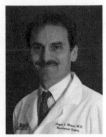

Fred F. Telischi,
MEE, MD

Jacques J. Morcos, MD,
FRCS (Eng.), FRCS (Ed)

Guest Editors

"Advise the patient in front of you as you would your own mother." Too often, conflicts of interest creep into the doctor–patient relationship. Surgeons want to operate and radiotherapists recommend radiation therapy. From recent studies on the natural history of vestibular schwannomas, we have learned that many of these benign tumors remain quiescent for long periods of time. Therefore, more and more patients are being observed with serial imaging and audiometric testing. Longer term studies are demonstrating that radiation therapy and radiosurgery appear to have favorable rates of tumor control. Radiosurgery certification has been offered to surgeons of multiple specialties, reducing the natural bias to recommend the single modality of treatment available from one's original training. Chemotherapy with new anti-angiogenic agents appears promising at least for tumors related to neurofibromatosis type 2. Pilot studies are looking at the possibility of using these medications for sporadic, unilateral tumors.

For this issue, we recruited a group of experts in the field who present particular niches of vestibular schwannoma management with which they are particularly familiar. We have endeavored to communicate the latest, evidenced-based treatment modalities that readers can consider incorporating into their practices. While controversies always will simmer, the contributors labored to present a balanced review of current thought. We are grateful to all of them. Although there are a number of senior practitioners in this field, it was appropriate that Derald Brackmann wrote the introductory piece recounting the recent history of vestibular schwannoma management, given his stature and continuing contributions. Although the editors acknowledge the appropriate appellation of *vestibular schwannoma* for tumors traditionally termed acoustic neuroma, the names are used interchangeably in the manuscript at the discretion of the contributing authors.

Otolaryngol Clin N Am 45 (2012) xvii–xviii
doi:10.1016/j.otc.2012.01.002
0030-6665/12/$ – see front matter © 2012 Elsevier Inc. All rights reserved.

oto.theclinics.com

We hope that you enjoy reading this issue and find something new to add to your knowledge base within this information. In the end, physicians strive to give the best advice, choosing for their patients as they would for their own family members based on their education, experiences, and continued learning. Hopefully the information contained herein will help you answer the frequently asked patient question, *"Doctor, what would you do if you were in my shoes?"*

Fred F. Telischi, MEE, MD
Neurological Surgery and Biomedical Engineering
Department of Otolaryngology
Miami, FL, USA

Jacques J. Morcos, MD, FRCS (Eng.), FRCS (Ed)
Department of Neurological Surgery
Lois Pope Life Center
Miami, FL, USA

E-mail addresses:
ftelischi@med.miami.edu (F.F. Telischi)
jmorcos@med.miami.edu (J.J. Morcos)

Epidemiology and Natural History of Vestibular Schwannomas

Sven-Eric Stangerup, MD*, Per Caye-Thomasen, MD, DMC

KEYWORDS

• Acoustic neuroma • Tumour growth • Hearing preservation
• Word recognition scoring • Treatment strategy

This article describes various epidemiologic trends for vestibular schwannomas over the last 35 years and includes a brief note on terminology.

Knowledge of the spontaneous course or natural history of a disease is imperative to evaluate the outcome of various treatments properly. Accordingly, this article provides information on the natural history of tumor growth and hearing level following the diagnosis of a vestibular schwannoma (VS).

Finally, a treatment strategy based on the natural history of tumor growth and hearing is discussed.

TERMINOLOGY OF ACOUSTIC NEUROMA AND VESTIBULAR SCHWANNOMA

The term neuroma was originally applied for this tumor by Virchow, because of the macroscopic appearance and the histologic structure that showed many parallel fibers thought to be axons. Because of the hearing loss associated with these tumors, the origin of the tumor was thought to be the cochlear nerve, whereafter the term acoustic neuroma emerged and was widely used for many years. However, the name is a misnomer, as the cells of origin were identified by Murrey & Stout[1] to be Schwann cells (termed after the German physiologist and histologist Theodor Schwann who originally described the nerve sheath cells in the 1800s). In 1975, Steward and Schuknecht[2] found that the neurilemmal–glial junction was the site of predilection of the tumor. Moreover, the tumor is usually confined to the vestibular component of the eighth cranial nerve, although invasion of the cochlear nerve[3,4] and facial nerve[5] has been described. The term vestibular schwannoma was first recommended by Eldridge and Parry at a consensus meeting in 1992,[5,6] followed by wide acceptance.

Department of Oto-Rhino-Laryngology, Head and Neck Surgery, Rigshospitalet, Faculty of Health Sciences, University of Copenhagen, Blegdamsvej 9, 2100 Copenhagen, Denmark
* Corresponding author.
E-mail address: stangerup@pc.dk

Otolaryngol Clin N Am 45 (2012) 257–268
doi:10.1016/j.otc.2011.12.008
0030-6665/12/$ – see front matter © 2012 Elsevier Inc. All rights reserved.

Based on the finding that the response to the caloric stimulation test was reduced in most cases of VS,[7,8] an assumption was made that the tumor originated from the superior vestibular nerve. However, in a recent prospective study, the tumor originated from the inferior vestibular nerve in more than 90% of the cases.[9]

EPIDEMIOLOGY OF VESTIBULAR SCHWANNOMAS
Incidence

Several centers have reported an increasing number of diagnosed vestibular schwannomas during the last several years. In the period from January 1957 to July 1976 the incidence of VS in Denmark was estimated to be 5.4 vestibular schwannomas per 1 million population per year. This estimate was based on publications from Danish neurosurgical departments.[10,11]

Since 1976, data for all diagnosed VS in Denmark, with a population of 5.4 million people, have been entered prospectively into a national database, which by the end of 2010 includes more than 2500 patients. The data and the results from the observed patients (the wait-and-scan strategy) from this database form the basis for the present epidemiologic results, as well as the results of the natural course of the disease, including growth and hearing data.

Since 1976, the number of diagnosed vestibular schwannomas has been constantly increasing from 7.8 vestibular shwannomas per 1million population per year,[12] until an apparent peak in 2004, with 123 diagnosed tumors (23 vestibular schwannomas per 1 million population per year). From 2004, the incidence decreased to 19 vestibular schwannomas per 1 million population per year in 2008 (**Fig. 1**). Thus, after several decades with an increasing incidence of diagnosed tumors, a peak seems to have been reached. This leveling may reflect an approximation to the true incidence.

The increase in the number of diagnosed vestibular schwannomas has plausibly been caused by several factors, the most important being continuously improving access to continuously improving diagnostic equipment (ie, magnetic resonance imaging [MRI]). Another cause may be heightened symptom awareness among the general population and especially among the elderly, as a longer and healthier lifespan may be expected in developed countries. Better and more widespread audiological

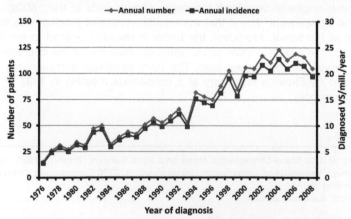

Fig. 1. Annual number of diagnosed vestibular schwannoma and corresponding annual incidence.

testing equipment, as well as the easier access to diagnostic imaging may in addition have heightened the awareness of a possible VS among general practitioners and otolaryngologists.

Tumor Size at Diagnosis

From a mean extrameatal size of about 30 mm in the mid-1970s, the tumor size at diagnosis has decreased continuously over the decades, to a mean size of 10 mm in the most recent period from 2003 to 2008. In the 1970s, no purely intrameatal tumors were diagnosed, whereas the large and giant tumors constituted about 40% of all the tumors. Now, the intrameatal tumors constitute 33% of tumors diagnosed, whereas the large and giant tumors constitute a mere 6% of the diagnosed tumors (**Fig. 2**).

Age at Diagnosis

The age of the patient at the time of diagnosis of the VS has been slowly increasing from 49 years in 1976 to 58 years in 2008 (**Fig. 3**).

Analyzing the diagnostic age distribution throughout the 33-year period, the number of patients aged 40 years or less has remained almost unchanged. Thus, the increasing number of diagnosed VS is primarily constituted by patients belonging to the age group older than 50 years.

In the beginning of the period covered, 81% of the patients were 60 years or younger, and only 4% were older than 70 years. At the end of the period, 59% of the patients were younger than 60 years, and 12% were older than 70 years.

In the age group of 40 years or younger, the mean tumor size at diagnosis was 23 mm. The size decreased with increasing age, and was 13 mm in the group of patients 70 years or older, even though the mean tumor size decreased throughout the period.

NATURAL HISTORY OF VS (GROWTH PATTERN AND HEARING)

The natural history of VS growth is enigmatic. The tumor may grow continuously or only to a certain size, followed by stagnation or even shrinkage. Progressive growth in the cerebellopontine angle will eventually lead to compression of the brain stem and/or the cerebellum, occlusion of the fourth ventricle, and subsequently incarceration.

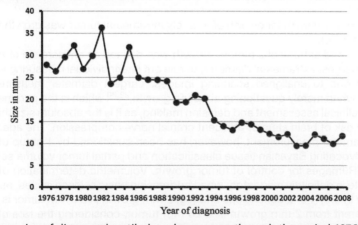

Fig. 2. Mean size of diagnosed vestibular schwannoma through the period 1976 to 2009.

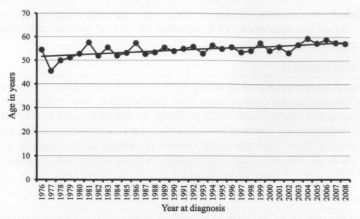

Fig. 3. Mean age at diagnosis of vestibular schwannoma through the period from 1976 to 2009.

The percentage of growing tumors has been reported to vary from 30% to 90%,[13-30] depending at least in part on the length of the observation period. Most of growth observation studies have, however, surveyed a relatively small number of patients and have further been subject to considerable referral bias and patient selection bias, by only including very old patients, patients unwilling to undergo surgery, or patients not eligible for surgery due to significant concurrent disease. The growth and hearing data presented are based on the Danish patients from 1976 to 2008, with a diagnostic tumor size less than 20 mm extrameatal and allocated primarily to observation by wait-and-scan.

Measurement of Tumor Size and Determination of Growth Rate

According to the consensus meeting in Japan in 2003,[31] a tumor should be defined as either purely intrameatal or intra-extrameatal, in case of tumor extension into the cerebello-pontine angle. The size of an intra- and extrameatal tumor is determined by the largest extrameatal diameter, excluding the intrameatal portion.

Determined tumor growth rate may depend on the diagnostic tool (computed tomography [CT] vs MRI),[16] the method of measurement (number or plane of dimensions assessed),[29] and criteria for the determination for growth (number of millimeters).

The present criterium for growth of a purely intrameatal tumor was growth to extrameatal extension.

For intra- and extrameatal tumors, growth was defined as an increase of at least 3 mm in the largest extrameatal diameter, to rule out interindividual measuring variability and error due to unaligned scanning images. Largest diameter measurement is adequate when merely questioning absolute growth,[22,30] which is the parameter relevant for a clinical assessment and decision making, as it is the absolute size that determines the risk of brain stem or adjacent cranial nerve compression. The adequacy of largest diameter measurement, however, has been questioned by 1 group of investigators, advocating Bayesian tissue classification and partial tumor volume segmentation on MR images for control of tumor growth. Volumetric determination of relative growth rate is definitely mandatory when addressing basic science issues, as a tumor may grow in only 1 or 2 dimensions and (eg, 2 mm growth in a 6 mm tumor is dramatically different from 2 mm growth in a 26 mm tumor, considering the rate of cellular proliferation).

Growth of Intrameatal Tumors

Of the intrameatal tumors, 83% remained purely intrameatal during the observation. In 17% of tumors, the intrameatal tumor increased in size to extrameatal extension (**Fig. 4**). Of the tumors that grew over the years of observation the following was noted:

- 64% grew during the first year
- 23% grew during the second year
- 5% grew during the third year
- 8% grew during the fourth year
- No tumor growth occurred after the fifth year of observation (see **Fig. 4**).

The mean annual growth rate was 10.3 mm per year if growth was determined during the first year, compared with 0.9 mm per year during the fourth year.[22,30,32] There were no significant differences in growth between male and female patients or between different age groups.

Growth of Intra-extrameatal Tumors

Of the extrameatal tumors, during the course of observation the following was noted:

- 1% decreased in size.
- 70% remained unchanged.
- 29% increased in size (see **Fig. 4**).

Growth was determined during

- The first year of observation in 62% of tumors
- The second year in 26% of tumors
- The third year in 10% of tumors
- The fourth year in 2% of tumors
- No tumor growth occurred after the fifth year of observation (see **Fig. 4**).

In growing tumors, the mean annual growth rate was relatively high if growth was determined during the first year of observation, compared with later growth determination.

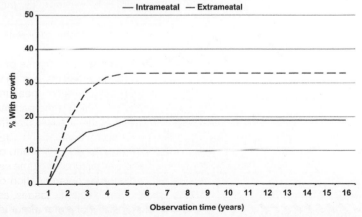

Fig. 4. Nelson-Aalen curve of growth of intrameatal and extrameatal vestibular schwannoma related to length of observation.

There was no significant difference in proportion of patients with growth between male and female patients, age groups, or diagnostic tumor size. Importantly, the growth occurrence or rate is not related to gender or age, which is in agreement with a recent publication addressing potentially predictive parameters for tumor growth.[32]

Spontaneous Change of Hearing Level

The hearing quality may be evaluated by the pure tone hearing and by speech discrimination (SD).

To classify the pure tone hearing, the pure tone average (PTA) is most frequently used. The PTA is calculated as the mean of the hearing level (dB) at the frequencies 500 Hz, 1000 Hz, and 3000 Hz, or 500 Hz, 1000 Hz, 2000 Hz, and 4000 Hz. In the period 1976 through 1978, 9% of the patients had a PTA better than 30 dB at diagnosis. In the period 2006 through 2008, 23% had a PTA better than 30 dB. The mean PTA at diagnosis improved from 70 dB in the beginning of the period to 48 dB at the end of the period (**Fig. 5**).

The SD test is performed in quiet, using word list scoring by phonemes correctly repeated at the most comfortable hearing level. The mean SD at diagnosis improved from 30% in the beginning of the period to 60% at the end of the period (**Fig. 6**).

In the period 1976 through 1978, 21% had SD of 70% or better at diagnosis, which is an accepted category for good hearing. The percentage of patients in this category has gradually increased over the years, to 57% in 2008. The improved hearing at diagnosis is even clearer when considering patients with 100% SD at diagnosis. In 1976, 3% of the patients had modified word recognition scoring (mWRS) class 0, compared with 21% in 2008.

Different hearing classifications systems can be used to evaluate the overall hearing acuity.

THE AMERICAN ACADEMY OF OTOLARYNGOLOGY–HEAD AND NECK SURGERY CLASSIFICATION

The American Academy of Otolaryngology–Head and Neck Surgery (AAO-HNS) classification of the hearing level is as follows[33]:

- Class A: PTA less than 30 dB and SD 70% or greater
- Class B: PTA less than 50 dB and SD 50% or greater

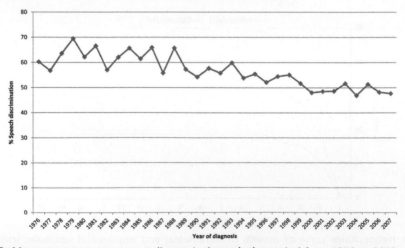

Fig. 5. Mean pure tone average at diagnosis through the period from 1976 to 2008.

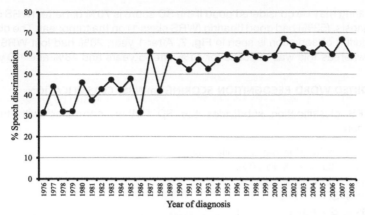

Fig. 6. Mean speech discrimination at diagnosis through the period from 1976 to 2008.

- Class C: PTA greater than 50 dB and SD 50% or greater
- Class D: SD less than 50%

Most authors consider AAO class A for good and preservable hearing.

At diagnosis, 19% of the patients had AAO class A hearing on the tumor ear. The hearing deterioration during observation is seen in **Fig. 7**. After 1 year, 26% had lost class A hearing, whereas this was the case for 45% after 5 years and 54% after 10 years.

THE WORD RECOGNITION SCORING (WRS) CLASSIFICATION

The Word Recognition Scoring classification (WRS)[34,35] has:

Class 1: SD = 100% to 70%
Class 2: SD = 69% to 50%
Class 3: SD = 49% to 1%
Class 4: SD = 0%

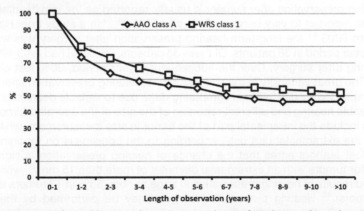

Fig. 7. Preservation of good hearing (American Academy of Otolaryngology class A or modified word recognition scoring class 0/1) during observation for patients with good hearing at diagnosis.

The hearing may be considered good if the SD score is 70% or better (WRS class 1).

At diagnosis, (53%) had good hearing (WRS class 1) on the tumor ear. The change in hearing during observation is seen in **Fig. 7**. After 1 year, 20% had lost WRS class 1 hearing, whereas this was the case for 41% after 5 years and 48% after 10 years.

THE MODIFIED WORD RECOGNITION SCORING (mWRS) CLASSIFICATION

The mWRS classification subdivides the SD further, compared with the WRS classification:

- Class 0 designates patients with 100% speech discrimination
- Class 1: SD = 99% to 70%
- Class 2: SD = 69% to 50%
- Class 3: SD = 49% to 1%
- Class 4: SD = 0%

Good hearing is considered if the speech discrimination score is 70% or better (class 0/1).

The change in hearing over the years in patients with mWRS class 0 hearing at diagnosis (SD = 100%) is seen in **Fig. 7**. After 1 year, 3% had lost class 1 hearing. After 5 years, 12% had lost class 1 hearing, and after 10 years 31% had lost good hearing. In patients with even a minor loss of SD at diagnosis (1% to 10%), 18% had lost good hearing after 1 year; 60% had lost good hearing after 5 years, and only 38% of the patients with SD loss between 1% and 10% maintained good hearing.

Overall, the mean annual speech discrimination loss was 6.6% in patients with WRS class 1 hearing. The discrimination loss per year is not linear, but almost inversely logarithmic. The mean annual SD loss is 10.5% the first year after diagnosis, 7.6% the second, and 5.1% during the fifth year of observation. Looking at the group of patients with 1% to 30% SD at diagnosis, the SD loss is 13.1% the first year after diagnosis, 8.8% the second, and 6.5% in the fifth year of observation. However, remarkably, the annual SD loss is almost constant with 2% to 4% a year in the group of patients with 100% SD at diagnosis.

COMPARISON OF THE SPONTANEOUS COURSE OF HEARING AND ACTIVE TREATMENT

The hearing preservation after surgery is usually reported as the results after 1 year, and this is reported to vary between 24% and 83%.[36–40] In a study from House Ear Clinic from 2003,[41] the long-term hearing preservation after surgery was evaluated over a 5-year period in 38 patients. Of these 38 patients, 23 (61%) had AAO-HNS class A-B hearing after surgery. Over the subsequent 5-year period, 30% lost class A-B hearing. The great variability in the success rate of hearing preservation after surgery may be explained by difficulties in comparing data, due to variable definitions of good or serviceable hearing and different reporting of the size of the operated tumor. Some surgeons include the intrameatal part of the tumor in size measurement, while others measure the extrameatal part only, according to the consensus on reporting tumor size.[31] Most authors agree that the chance of hearing preservation is significantly reduced for tumors with an extrameatal diameter of more than 15 mm,[31] while others have good results of hearing preservation in large tumors (58% in T3 tumors and 29% in T4 tumors).[42] Hearing preservation surgery may be performed by the middle fossa approach, the retrolabyrintine approach, or by the retrosigmoidal approach. Comparing the approaches, it seems that the results are better by the middle fossa approach in small and intrameatal tumors.[43]

The hearing preservation results after radiotherapy is reported to vary between 33% and 79%.[44–47]

During wait & scan, 73% of patients with AAO-HNS class A hearing at diagnosis preserved good hearing after 1 year of observation. According to the WRS classification, 87% of patients with WRS class 1 hearing at diagnosis maintained good hearing. The spontaneous outcome is emphasized further by the mWRS classification, in which 99% of tumor ears with class 0 hearing at diagnosis preserved good hearing after 1 year, whereas 91% of patients preserved good hearing after 5 years of observation, and 68% after 10 years **(Fig. 8)**.[34]

The main clinical implication of the hearing results is that they indicate that it may be possible to identify patients who have a good chance of maintaining good long-term hearing spontaneously, by focusing on the SD at the time of diagnosis. Thus, a small nongrowing tumor with 100% discrimination should be allocated to wait-and-scan, since it is highly likely that the patient will preserve good long-term hearing spontaneously and thus have an outcome superior to radiotherapy or hearing preservation surgery.

A TREATMENT STRATEGY BASED ON THE NATURAL HISTORY OF TUMOR GROWTH AND HEARING

As more primarily small and medium-sized vestibular schwannomas are diagnosed and need to be treated,[18,48,49] the medical community is in need of a treatment strategy based on hard data on the spontaneous course of hearing and the growth pattern of these tumors.

Based on the data presented, the authors' center has adapted and proposed the following strategy for all sporadic, unilateral vestibular schwannomas smaller than 15 to 20 mm extrameatal:

1. Yearly MRI for 5 years
2. Followed by MRI every other year for 4 years
3. Followed by MRI after 5 years
4. After which the observation is terminated, if no growth occurs.

A rigid data interpretation indicates no reason to follow patients for more than 5 years, as tumor growth only occurred within the first 5 years after diagnosis. The

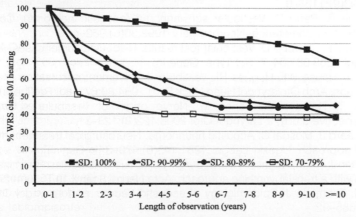

Fig. 8. Preservation of good hearing (modified word recognition scoring class 0/1) during observation related to the different speech discrimination groups at diagnosis.

authors, however, have chosen the aforementioned treatment policy, as only a few tumors have been followed for more than a decade and to be most certain.

If significant growth occurs, active treatment (surgery or radiotherapy) is recommended. Naturally, special considerations may indicate an aberration from this management policy (eg, observation of old patients with large tumors or surgery of small tumor in patients insisting on primary operation. However, unless realistic hearing preservation is intended,[50] or special reasons (eg, patient psychology) prevail, there are no available data indicating or substantiating a reason for active treatment of a non-cystic, nongrowing VS smaller than 15 mm. Although reasonably surmount, both surgery and radiotherapy are associated with risks, and the quality of life of patients appears to be significantly better when their disease is observed.[51]

Primary treatment of tumors larger than 15 to 20 mm is recommended, as further growth extends the tumor diameter into the range associated with a considerable increase in treatment comorbidity (eg, damage to the facial nerve function).[52] Cystic tumors are not eligible for radiotherapy, and primary surgery is recommended, as these tumors may display sudden and dramatic growth, which implicates a poorer surgical outcome.[53] NF-2 associated vestibular schwannomas are treated individually, as these tumors often display a distinct growth pattern[21,54] and often are subject to special consideration.

REFERENCES

1. Murray M, Stout AP. Schwann cell versus fibroblast as origin of specific nerve sheath tumor, observations about normal nerve sheaths and neurilemmomas in vitro. Am J Pathol 1940;16:41–60. Ref Type: Generic.
2. Stewart TJ, Schuknecht HF. Occult schwannomas of the vestibular nerve. Arch Otolaryngol 1975;101:91–5. Ref Type: Generic.
3. Neely JG. Gross and microscopic anatomy of the eighth cranial nerve in relationship to the solitary schwannoma. Laryngoscope 1981;91:1512–31.
4. Marquet JF, Forton GE, Offeciers FE, et al. The solitary schwannoma of the eighth cranial nerve. An immunohistochemical study of the cochlear nerve-tumor interface. Arch Otolaryngol Head Neck Surg 1990;116(9):1023–5.
5. Luetje CM, Whittaker CK, Callaway LA, et al. Histological acoustic tumor involvement of the VIIth nerve and multicentric origin in the VIIIth nerve. Laryngoscope 1983;93(9):1133–9.
6. Eldridge R, Parry D. Vestibular schwannoma (acoustic neuroma). Consensus development conference. Neurosurgery 1992;30(6):962–4.
7. Linthicum F, Churchill D. Vestibular test results in acoustic tumor cases. Arch Otolaryngol 1968;88:604–7. Ref Type: Generic.
8. Pulec J, House WF, Hughes RI. Vestibular involvement and testing in acoustic neuromas. Arch Otolaryngol Head Neck Surg 1964;80:677–81. Ref Type: Generic.
9. Khrais T, Romano G, Sanna M. Nerve origin of vestibular schwannoma: a prospective study. J Laryngol Otol 2008;122(2):128–31.
10. Overgaard J, Mosdal C. Acoustic neurinoma. Neurosurgical treatment by suboccipital approach. Ugeskr Laeger 1981;143(8):470–3 [in Danish].
11. Thomsen J, Tos M, Harmsen A, et al. Surgery of acoustic neuromas. Preliminary experience with a translabyrinthine approach. Acta Neurol Scand 1977;56(4):277–90.
12. Tos M, Thomsen J. Epidemiology of acoustic neuromas. J Laryngol Otol 1984; 98(7):685–92.
13. Bederson JB, von AK, Wichmann WW, et al. Conservative treatment of patients with acoustic tumors. Neurosurgery 1991;28(5):646–50.

14. Charabi S, Tos M, Thomsen J, et al. Vestibular schwannoma growth–long-term results. Acta Otolaryngol Suppl 2000;543:7–10.
15. Deen HG, Ebersold MJ, Harner SG, et al. Conservative management of acoustic neuroma: an outcome study. Neurosurgery 1996;39(2):260–4.
16. Fiirgaard B, Pedersen CB, Lundorf E. The size of acoustic neuromas: CT and MRI. Neuroradiology 1997;39(8):599–601.
17. Hoistad DL, Melnik G, Mamikoglu B, et al. Update on conservative management of acoustic neuroma. Otol Neurotol 2001;22(5):682–5.
18. Jorgensen BG, Pedersen CB. Acoustic neuroma. Follow-up of 78 patients. Clin Otolaryngol Allied Sci 1994;19(6):478–84.
19. Mirz F, Pedersen CB, Fiirgaard B, et al. Incidence and growth pattern of vestibular schwannomas in a Danish county, 1977–98. Acta Otolaryngol Suppl 2000;543: 30–3.
20. Nedzelski JM, Schessel DA, Pfleiderer A, et al. Conservative management of acoustic neuromas. 1992. Neurosurg Clin N Am 2008;19(2):207–16.
21. Ogawa K, Kanzaki J, Ogawa S, et al. The growth rate of acoustic neuromas. Acta Otolaryngol Suppl 1991;487:157–63.
22. Rosenberg SI. Natural history of acoustic neuromas. Laryngoscope 2000;110(4): 497–508.
23. Shin YJ, Fraysse B, Cognard C, et al. Effectiveness of conservative management of acoustic neuromas. Am J Otol 2000;21(6):857–62.
24. Silverstein H, Rosenberg SI, Flanzer JM, et al. An algorithm for the management of acoustic neuromas regarding age, hearing, tumor size, and symptoms. Otolaryngol Head Neck Surg 1993;108(1):1–10.
25. Smouha EE, Yoo M, Mohr K, et al. Conservative management of acoustic neuroma: a meta-analysis and proposed treatment algorithm. Laryngoscope 2005;115(3):450–4.
26. Strasnick B, Glasscock ME III, Haynes D, et al. The natural history of untreated acoustic neuromas. Laryngoscope 1994;104(9):1115–9.
27. Tschudi DC, Linder TE, Fisch U. Conservative management of unilateral acoustic neuromas. Am J Otol 2000;21(5):722–8.
28. Valvassori GE, Guzman M. Growth rate of acoustic neuromas. Am J Otol 1989; 10(3):174–6.
29. Vokurka EA, Herwadkar A, Thacker NA, et al. Using Bayesian tissue classification to improve the accuracy of vestibular schwannoma volume and growth measurement. AJNR Am J Neuroradiol 2002;23(3):459–67.
30. Walsh RM, Bath AP, Bance ML, et al. Comparison of two radiologic methods for measuring the size and growth rate of extracanalicular vestibular schwannomas. Am J Otol 2000;21(5):716–21.
31. Kanzaki J, Tos M, Sanna M, et al. New and modified reporting systems from the consensus meeting on systems for reporting results in vestibular schwannoma. Otol Neurotol 2003;24(4):642–8.
32. Stangerup SE, Caye-Thomasen P, Tos M, et al. The natural history of vestibular schwannoma. Otol Neurotol 2006;27(4):547–52.
33. Committee on Hearing and Equilibrium guidelines for the evaluation of hearing preservation in acoustic neuroma (vestibular schwannoma). American Academy of Otolaryngology-Head and Neck Surgery Foundation, Inc. Otolaryngol Head Neck Surg 1995;113(3):179–80.
34. Stangerup SE, Caye-Thomasen P, Tos M, et al. Change in hearing during 'wait and scan' management of patients with vestibular schwannoma. J Laryngol Otol 2008;122(7):1–9, 673–81.

35. Meyer TA, Canty PA, Wilkinson EP, et al. Small acoustic neuromas: surgical outcomes versus observation or radiation. Otol Neurotol 2006;27(3):380–92.
36. Gardner G, Robertson JH. Hearing preservation in unilateral acoustic neuroma surgery. Ann Otol Rhinol Laryngol 1988;97(1):55–66.
37. Moriyama T, Fukushima T, Asaoka K, et al. Hearing preservation in acoustic neuroma surgery: importance of adhesion between the cochlear nerve and the tumor. J Neurosurg 2002;97(2):337–40.
38. Post KD, Eisenberg MB, Catalano PJ. Hearing preservation in vestibular schwannoma surgery: what factors influence outcome? J Neurosurg 1995; 83(2):191–6.
39. Samii M, Matthies C. Management of 1000 vestibular schwannomas (acoustic neuromas): hearing function in 1000 tumor resections. Neurosurgery 1997; 40(2):248–60.
40. Shelton C. Hearing preservation in acoustic tumor surgery. Otolaryngol Clin North Am 1992;25(3):609–21.
41. Friedman RA, Kesser B, Brackmann DE, et al. Long-term hearing preservation after middle fossa removal of vestibular schwannoma. Otolaryngol Head Neck Surg 2003;129(6):660–5.
42. Matthies C, Samii M. Vestibular schwannomas and auditory function: options in large T3 and T4 tumors? Neurochirurgie 2002;48(6):461–70.
43. Irving RM, Jackler RK, Pitts LH. Hearing preservation in patients undergoing vestibular schwannoma surgery: comparison of middle fossa and retrosigmoid approaches. J Neurosurg 1998;88(5):840–5.
44. Hasegawa T, Kida Y, Kobayashi T, et al. Long-term outcomes in patients with vestibular schwannomas treated using gamma knife surgery: 10-year follow up. J Neurosurg 2005;102(1):10–6.
45. Lunsford LD, Niranjan A, Flickinger JC, et al. Radiosurgery of vestibular schwannomas: summary of experience in 829 cases. J Neurosurg 2005;102:195–9.
46. Myrseth E, Pedersen PH, Moller P, et al. Treatment of vestibular schwannomas. Why, when and how? Acta Neurochir (Wien) 2007;149(7):647–60.
47. Rowe JG, Radatz MW, Walton L, et al. Gamma knife stereotactic radiosurgery for unilateral acoustic neuromas. J Neurol Neurosurg Psychiatry 2003;74(11): 1536–42.
48. Herwadker A, Vokurka EA, Evans DG, et al. Size and growth rate of sporadic vestibular schwannoma: predictive value of information available at presentation. Otol Neurotol 2005;26(1):86–92.
49. Tos M, Stangerup SE, Caye-Thomasen P, et al. What is the real incidence of vestibular schwannoma? Arch Otolaryngol Head Neck Surg 2004;130(2):216–20.
50. Sanna M, Khrais T, Russo A, et al. Hearing preservation surgery in vestibular schwannoma: the hidden truth. Ann Otol Rhinol Laryngol 2004;113(2):156–63.
51. Tos T, Caye-Thomasen P, Stangerup SE, et al. Long-term socio-economic impact of vestibular schwannoma for patients under observation and after surgery. J Laryngol Otol 2003;117(12):955–64.
52. Tos M, Charabi S, Thomsen J. Clinical experience with vestibular schwannomas: epidemiology, symptomatology, diagnosis, and surgical results. Eur Arch Otorhinolaryngol 1998;255(1):1–6.
53. Fundova P, Charabi S, Tos M, et al. Cystic vestibular schwannoma: surgical outcome. J Laryngol Otol 2000;114(12):935–9.
54. Evans DG, Moran A, King A, et al. Incidence of vestibular schwannoma and neurofibromatosis 2 in the North West of England over a 10-year period: higher incidence than previously thought. Otol Neurotol 2005;26(1):93–7.

Clinical and Diagnostic Evaluation of Acoustic Neuromas

Emily Z. Stucken, MD[a], Kevin Brown, MD, PhD[b],
Samuel H. Selesnick, MD[b],*

KEYWORDS

- Acoustic neuroma • Symptoms • Diagnosis • Presentation
- Auditory brainstem response testing • Magnetic resonance imaging

Acoustic neuromas are rare tumors of the vestibular nerve. Although they are benign, their location within the internal auditory canal and growth into the cerebellopontine angle result in significant morbidity and even mortality if left untreated. This location also results in a specific pattern of symptom development, which forms the basis for a modern clinician's ability to accurately diagnose these tumors. The understanding of this symptom progression and appropriate clinical judgment will determine when further diagnostic tests are required to evaluate a patient for this rare tumor.

CLINICAL PROGRESSION OF PATIENTS WITH ACOUSTIC NEUROMAS: PERSPECTIVE

Clinical comprehension of the signs and symptoms of acoustic neuromas has undergone considerable evolution since the diagnosis was first described. In the early 1900s, the diagnosis of acoustic neuromas was based solely on clinical history and physical examination; no further accurate diagnostic modalities were available. Often the diagnosis was established during postmortem examination.[1] In the case of antemortem diagnosis, patients commonly presented with advanced neurologic signs such as papilledema, hydrocephalus, blindness, anosmia, headache, and cerebellar and cranial nerve dysfunction.[1] Since that time great advances have been made in understanding the clinical signs and symptoms of tumors of the cerebellopontine angle, which have allowed the clinician to initiate a diagnostic quest at an earlier time in tumor development.

The authors have nothing to disclose.
a Department of Otolaryngology-Head & Neck Surgery, New York Presbyterian Hospital – Cornell and Columbia, 180 Fort Washington Avenue, HP8-814, New York, NY 10032, USA
b Department of Otolaryngology-Head and Neck Surgery, Weill Cornell Medical College, 1305 York Avenue, 5th Floor, New York, NY 10021, USA
* Corresponding author.
E-mail address: shselesn@med.cornell.edu

Otolaryngol Clin N Am 45 (2012) 269–284
doi:10.1016/j.otc.2011.12.001
0030-6665/12/$ – see front matter © 2012 Elsevier Inc. All rights reserved.

Harvey Cushing, in his series of 30 patients, was the first to describe the progression of symptoms and natural history of acoustic neuromas. In his 1917 publication, he described the following stages of clinical progression:

1. Auditory and labyrinthine dysfunction
2. Occipitofrontal pain
3. Cerebellar ataxia
4. Involvement of adjacent cranial nerves
5. Evidence of increased intracranial pressure
6. Dysphagia and dysarthria
7. Brainstem compression, leading to decreased respiratory drive and death.[2]

With modern advances in diagnostic tools, the evolution of symptoms has been reclassified into 4 stages based on the size and location of the tumor[3]:

1. Intracanalicular
2. Cisternal
3. Brainstem compressive
4. Hydrocephalic.

Each stage can be characterized by different symptoms.

Intracanalicular Stage

This stage involves hearing loss, tinnitus, and vertigo.

Cisternal Stage

Tumor involves the cistern of the cerebellopontine angle. Early growth into the cerebellopontine angle cistern affords the tumor room to grow without significant impingement by local structures. At this stage, auditory symptoms worsen, vertigo transitions into dysequilibrium, and headache may begin. This stage is unique in that there can be considerable tumor growth without, necessarily, a concordant increase in tumor symptoms.

Brainstem Compressive Stage

In this stage, hearing loss and dysequilibrium worsen and the patient may develop trigeminal symptoms.

Hydrocephalic Stage

Tumor growth causes obstruction of the fourth ventricle with associated hydrocephalus, and is accompanied by rapid clinical deterioration associated with generalized headache, facial twitch and weakness, visual loss or diplopia, lower cranial nerve dysfunction, and finally long tract signs and death due to tonsillar herniation.[3]

In a study at The University of California, San Francisco (UCSF), it was determined that the average duration of hearing loss and tinnitus before diagnosis of acoustic neuroma was almost 4 years. Vertigo was generally noted 3.6 years before diagnosis. Headache developed on average 2.2 years before diagnosis, followed by dysequilibrium 1.7 years before diagnosis. Late symptoms, such as trigeminal dysfunction, occurred at 0.9 year before diagnosis and facial nerve dysfunction at 0.6 year before diagnosis.[3] With this understanding of the natural history in mind, the goal of current otolaryngologists is to diagnose acoustic neuromas at the earliest stage, hopefully when a patient presents with only hearing loss, tinnitus, or vertigo, and before progression to more ominous symptoms.

TECHNOLOGICAL ADVANCES OF MODALITIES USED TO DIAGNOSE ACOUSTIC NEUROMAS: ANOTHER PERSPECTIVE

Concurrent with our improved understanding of the presenting symptoms of acoustic neuromas, there have been advances in technology that have allowed identification of tumors in patients for whom a practitioner has clinical suspicion. The twentieth century has seen the development of audiovestibular testing and imaging techniques that have allowed for earlier diagnosis of acoustic neuromas. Earlier tumor discovery has resulted in decreased tumor size at time of diagnosis. Tumors as small as 3 mm are now being discovered, sometimes even before the onset of symptoms, which has greatly reduced the morbidity of treatment for acoustic neuromas.

The first tests described for the detection of acoustic neuromas were rudimentary devices, such as tuning forks, which had low specificity and sensitivity for tumor detection. Since that time, diagnostic tests have greatly improved in sensitivity and specificity. In 1910, Henschen and Towne described a technique of using radiographs to image the petrous pyramid.[4] Cerebral pneumography, which allowed for improved visualization of the cerebellopontine angle, was introduced in 1918.[5] In the 1960s, advances in audiometry and vestibular testing achieved increased sensitivity and specificity for detecting retrocochlear lesions. At the same time radiologic techniques, such as iophendylate myelography and polytomography with contrast myelography, were developed.[5] During the 1970s, computed tomography (CT) was introduced and replaced other radiologic studies as the primary tool for evaluation of acoustic neuromas.[5] Also in the 1970s, auditory brainstem evoked response (ABR) testing was developed.[6] ABR was initially reported to have a sensitivity of 95% to 100% in the detection of tumors of the cerebellopontine angle, although this has been called into question in the modern era of magnetic resonance imaging (MRI).[7] With the development of MRI in the 1980s, diagnostic yields as high as 100% without false-positive or false-negative results have been reported.[7] Considerable attention will be given to the effectiveness of modern diagnostic modalities, such as ABR and MRI, later in this article.

With improvement in diagnostic modalities, tumor size at time of presentation has decreased. This trend was examined by Welling and colleagues,[5] who reviewed the number of tumors measuring greater than 3 cm at the time of diagnosis during 3 different time periods. These investigators found that 48% of tumors diagnosed between 1969 and 1975 were larger than 3 cm. This finding compared with 25% of tumors diagnosed from 1984 to 1985 and 7% of tumors diagnosed from 1988 to 1989. As expected, this has been accompanied by an increase in the number of acoustic neuromas that are diagnosed at a smaller size, particularly as we have entered the MRI era. In 1993, a UCSF study reported that 24% of patients were diagnosed with tumors measuring smaller than 1 cm.[3] This percentage represents a notable increase in previous figures: a study by Matthew and colleagues[8] published in 1978 describes 5% of patients who had tumors smaller than 1 cm at time of diagnosis, and a study from the Mayo Clinic in 1981 reported that 9% of tumors diagnosed at that time were smaller than 1 cm.[9]

The consequence of small tumor size at time of diagnosis is a generalized improvement in postoperative hearing preservation and facial nerve function. Multiple studies have noted a significant correlation between smaller tumor size and improvement in postoperative hearing preservation.[10–14] Improved postoperative outcomes in facial nerve function in patients with smaller tumors have also been described.[15]

CLINICAL EVALUATION: A SYMPTOM-BY-SYMPTOM REVIEW

A retrospective study by Selesnick and colleagues[3] tabulated the presenting symptomatology of patients with acoustic neuromas in the MRI era. These investigators found hearing loss to be the most common symptom, present in 85% of patients; this was also the most frequent initial presenting symptom. This symptom was followed by tinnitus (present in 56% of patients), dysequilibrium (48% of patients), trigeminal nerve dysfunction (20% of patients), vertigo (19% of patients), headache (19% of patients), facial nerve dysfunction (10% of patients), and diplopia (3% of patients). No patient in their study demonstrated long tract signs, lower cranial nerve dysfunction, or visual loss.

Hearing Loss

Hearing loss is traditionally the index symptom in patients presenting with acoustic neuromas in the modern era. Hearing loss is typically gradual in onset and is a unilateral, asymmetric sensorineural loss of hearing.[4,7] A certain number of patients, however, will present with atypical hearing loss or even normal hearing; therefore, clinicians should maintain a high level of suspicion if there are other symptoms or signs suggesting the possibility of an acoustic neuroma.

Sudden hearing loss

Sudden sensorineural hearing loss is a well-described presentation in patients with acoustic neuroma.[3,16–20] Whereas only 1% to 2% of patients who develop sudden sensorineural hearing loss will be found to have an acoustic neuroma, up to 26% of patients with an acoustic neuroma will have experienced sudden hearing loss during their clinical course.[4] Reports of sudden hearing loss as a presentation of acoustic neuroma date back to Cushing's 1917 case series, which featured 2 patients who experienced sudden hearing loss.[2] Since then, an incidence of 3% to 26% has been published in various papers on the subject.[3,16–20] It is therefore imperative to screen patients with sudden sensorineural hearing loss for retrocochlear lesions. Of note, Friedman and colleagues[21] studied outcomes in this cohort of patients in a retrospective review of 45 patients who underwent hearing-preservation operations for acoustic neuromas after presenting with sudden hearing loss. In this study, there was no significant difference in postoperative hearing outcomes in patients who had presented with sudden hearing loss in comparison with those who had presented with progressive hearing loss. Some, but not all, of the patients who presented with sudden hearing loss recovered hearing preoperatively. Some of the patients recovered after treatment with steroids for sudden sensorineural hearing loss whereas others recovered untreated; this had no significant correlation with postoperative hearing outcomes.

Normal hearing and symmetric hearing loss

A subset of patients with acoustic neuromas present with normal hearing or with sensorineural hearing loss that is bilaterally symmetric. This hearing loss has been estimated to occur in 1% to 15% of patients with acoustic neuroma.[7,16,22–29] The most common presenting symptom in this patient population is dysequilibrium.[26,27] Other presenting symptoms include abnormalities of cranial nerves V and VII, routine screening for family members of patients with neurofibromatosis type 2, asymmetric tinnitus, headaches, and as an incidental finding during evaluation for another problem.[27] Lustig and colleagues[27] found this presentation to be more common with small (<1 cm) and medium-sized (1–3 cm) tumors than with large (>3 cm) tumors. Selesnick and Jackler[28] also found that subjectively normal hearing was most frequent in patients with small (<1 cm) tumors. The number of patients with this atypical presentation can be expected to increase with the increasing number of small tumors diagnosed with MRI.

Tinnitus

Tinnitus has been described in 53% to 70% of patients with acoustic neuromas.[3,9,16,22] The classical description is an ipsilateral high-pitched, continuous tinnitus, although it may also present as low-pitched, "whistling, roaring, or pulsatile" tinnitus.[4] Tinnitus is generally accompanied by hearing loss. Few patients with acoustic neuroma will present with isolated tinnitus in the absence of hearing loss.[22,23] Asymmetric tinnitus without hearing loss should raise suspicion of the possibility of retrocochlear pathology. A clinician must take into account the fact that approximately 15% of the population complains of tinnitus.

Vertigo

Vertigo is a sensation of motion that may be characterized by movement of the patient in the surrounding environment or movement of the environment itself. Vertigo tends to occur early in the sequence of symptom development and may spontaneously resolve.[4] The reported incidence varies from 18% to 58% in assorted studies.[3,16,22,23,30] These figures may seem surprisingly low given the origin of acoustic neuromas from the superior and inferior vestibular nerves. This is explained by the body's ability to compensate for vestibular dysfunction by way of the central and contralateral vestibular systems. Because acoustic neuromas show slow growth, there is time to allow for gradual compensation, and many patients do not experience vertigo. The appearance of vertigo may correspond to a period of rapid tumor growth, or a vascular event that leads to an abrupt change in the capabilities of the vestibular system.

Dysequilibrium

Dysequilibrium was present in 48% of patients in the study by Selesnick and colleagues.[3] Dysequilibrium is commonly described as an unsteady or off-balance sensation. Whereas vertigo is an indicator of involvement of the peripheral vestibular symptom, dysequilibrium suggests cerebellar involvement either alone or in combination with peripheral dysfunction. As such, dysequilibrium tends to occur later in the course of tumor growth. Once initiated, cerebellar symptoms, such as dysequilibrium, tend to be continuous and enduring.[3,4]

Trigeminal Nerve Dysfunction

Patients with trigeminal nerve dysfunction may complain of hypesthesia, paresthesia, or pain, most commonly in the malar region. More frequently, patients may be without complaints referable to the trigeminal nerve but will be found on clinical examination to have decreased or absent corneal reflexes.[3] A UCSF study found trigeminal dysfunction in 20% of a series of patients with acoustic neuroma.[3] Earlier studies have cited higher prevalence, from 33% to 71%,[8,16,22,23] which may be attributable to the higher prevalence of larger tumors in earlier studies, because the UCSF data found that the presence of trigeminal dysfunction markedly depended on tumor size. No patient in that study with tumors less than 1 cm in size had trigeminal symptoms, whereas

20% of those with tumors 1 to 3 cm in size and 48% of patients with tumors larger than 3 cm showed trigeminal dysfunction.[3]

Headache

Headache caused by acoustic neuroma is commonly described as dull or of moderate intensity, and gradual in onset. Location can be general, and although there is a predilection for symptoms ipsilateral to the tumor, many patients cannot establish laterality of their headache.[3,4] Reported incidence of this symptom varies from 19% to 85% of patients,[3,16,22,23,30] and has been found to be associated with tumor size.[3] This figure must be taken in the context of the incidence of headache in the general population. Point prevalence of headache has been estimated at 11% in men and 22% in women, with a lifetime prevalence of 69% in men and 88% in women.[31]

Symptoms of Increased Intracranial Pressure

Signs and symptoms of increased intracranial pressure include headache, nausea, vomiting, decreased vision, diplopia, papilledema, anosmia, and obtundation. Although these symptoms were common in early reports,[2,16,22] the incidence has decreased in the modern era. For example, diplopia was a presenting symptom in 66% of Cushing's case series from 1917,[2] but was present in only 3% of patients in a study published in 1993 from UCSF.[3]

Facial Nerve Dysfunction

Facial nerve dysfunction may present as either hyperfunction (facial twitching or spasm) or hypofunction (facial paresis or paralysis.) Estimates of the prevalence of facial nerve dysfunction range from 10% to 18% in the literature.[2,3,9,16,23] These numbers are relatively low given the location of the facial nerve within the internal auditory canal, and likely reflect the resilience of facial nerve fibers to tumor compression. Hyperfunction of the facial nerve may indicate a primary facial nerve tumor.

Lower Cranial Nerve Dysfunction and Long Tract Signs

Symptoms of lower cranial nerve palsies include hoarseness, dysphagia, and dysarthria. These symptoms were more common in older reports (prevalence estimates in the 20%–30% range),[22,23] but are rarely reported in the modern era.[3] Long tract signs such as hyperreflexia, hemiparesis, and hemiplegia represent advanced disease, and are mainly described in the historical literature.[16,22,23] It is rare for patients currently to present with such advanced symptoms.[3]

Asymptomatic Tumors

Acoustic neuromas may be diagnosed incidentally after a patient undergoes MRI evaluation for an unrelated problem. Two such patients were described in the 1993 series from UCSF.[3] Selesnick and colleagues later described 4 cases of incidentally discovered acoustic neuromas, but did not find any cases in a prospective study of patients undergoing gadolinium-enhanced MRI for diagnoses other than acoustic neuroma or sensorineural hearing loss.[32] As MRI technology continues to evolve and become more accessible, it is likely that this class of patients will increase in number. Of note, some patients who have had an incidental discovery of acoustic neuromas may, in fact, not be asymptomatic. On questioning, these patients may have recognized, for example, a long-standing hearing loss that they have attributed to some other cause, and so have not sought the care of a physician.

AUDIOLOGIC EVALUATION
Pure Tone Audiogram

After obtaining a clinical history and performing a physical examination, the first diagnostic test generally performed is a pure tone audiogram with speech reception thresholds and speech discrimination analysis. Johnson[33] performed a retrospective review of audiologic testing in 500 patients with acoustic neuromas. Pure tone thresholds in this group ranged from 5 to 130 dB (no response), with a mean pure tone threshold of 66.5 dB. Sixteen percent of patients had a complete loss of hearing in the involved ear that precluded classification of the audiometric pattern. In patients who had adequate hearing to obtain pure tone audiograms, pure tone loss was classified into 4 groups: high tone loss, flat, trough-shaped, and low tone loss. Sixty-five percent of patients were found to have high-frequency hearing loss, followed by flat type loss in 22% of patients.[33]

Poor speech discrimination, particularly when out of proportion to pure tone threshold responses, has traditionally been an indicator of retrocochlear pathology.[4] This finding was corroborated by Johnson's study,[33] in which 24% of patients with testable hearing had 0% speech discrimination. Overall, 44% of patients with testable hearing were able to achieve a speech discrimination score of 62% or more, whereas the remaining 56% had speech discrimination scores of 60% or less. The correlation between acoustic neuroma and poor speech discrimination was less impressive in a study by Hirsch and Anderson,[18] which found that only 45% of patients with acoustic neuromas had abnormal speech discrimination.

Impedance Testing

The acoustic reflex is analyzed in impedance testing, and represents the contraction of the stapedius muscle in response to a high-intensity sound. The absence of the acoustic reflex and reflex decay (decay of 50% of a tone administered at 10 dB over threshold) have been associated with retrocochlear lesions.[4] Reports of the sensitivity of acoustic reflex testing vary widely, ranging from 21% to 90%.[18,33,34] The sensitivity of reflex decay ranges from 36% to 100% in the literature.[18,33,34] For these reasons, data from impedance testing are poor indicators of the presence of an acoustic neuroma. An advantage of this test over other audiometric tests in the basic testing battery is that the acoustic reflex is involuntary and, thus, measurements obtained are not subjective.

Auditory Brainstem Response Testing

ABR testing, also known as brainstem auditory evoked response (BAER) testing, is a recording of the synchronized response of neurons in the lower auditory pathways in response to a stimulus. ABR was first described by Sohmer and Feinmesser[35] in 1967, followed shortly thereafter by Jewett and colleagues[36] in 1970. The clinical applications of ABR were expanded on by Selters and Brackmann[37] in 1977, at which point ABR became an established tool to screen patients for acoustic neuromas. ABR involves generating a stimulus and recording the evoked response. The most commonly used stimulus is a 100-microsecond click. This rapid and brief stimulus results in many auditory nerve fibers firing nearly synchronously, occurring in the first 10 milliseconds after the stimulus is presented. The response is recorded from scalp electrodes and is displayed as a predictable series of peaks. These peaks are labeled waves I through V. Waves I and V are the largest and most reliable responses obtained from the click stimulus. Wave I represents response activity from the cochlear nerve, whereas wave V represents the response from neurons of the inferior colliculus. The peak amplitudes and latencies are recorded and interaural comparisons can be drawn. The most reliable latency measurement in the diagnosis of acoustic neuroma is the interaural wave I to V latency difference, known as IT5.[4] This latency is compared between the normal ear and the test ear. A latency difference of 0.2 milliseconds or greater generally signifies an abnormal result.

ABR testing became a key component in the diagnosis of acoustic neuromas shortly after its introduction. ABR is a noninvasive, rapidly administered, and painless test that is well tolerated by patients and is not affected by attention, sedation, or anesthesia. A notable shortcoming of the technique is the inability to obtain accurate results when a patient's hearing threshold is greater than 80 dB at 4 kHz. Initial reports of sensitivity in diagnosing acoustic neuromas were excellent. Early publications cited sensitivity figures of 93% to 100% in diagnosing acoustic neuromas, with a specificity of 90%.[7,9,19,26,34,38] Such high figures were called into question after the introduction of MRI, which allowed for detection of smaller tumors than had been identified by previous radiologic modalities. In the MRI era, new studies have shown the sensitivity of ABR in detecting acoustic neuromas to be 63% to 95%.[1,6,39–42] A common thread in these studies has been the inability of ABR to diagnose small tumors with high sensitivity. Gordon and Cohen[39] performed a prospective study of 105 patients with surgically proved acoustic neuromas who underwent preoperative ABRs. These investigators found that 100% of patients with tumors larger than 2 cm had abnormal ABRs, but only 69% of patients with tumors smaller than 1 cm had an abnormal ABR. Schmidt and colleagues[41] performed a retrospective review of 58 patients with acoustic neuromas who had undergone both ABR and MRI. Although overall sensitivity for ABR in detecting acoustic neuromas was 90%, sensitivity decreased with tumor size and was as low as 58% in tumors measuring 1 cm or smaller. A similar study was performed by Zappia and colleagues,[42] who examined 111 patients with acoustic neuroma who underwent preoperative ABR and MRI. These investigators found ABR to be 95% sensitive overall for recognizing acoustic neuromas; again, sensitivity was related to tumor size, with 100% sensitivity in tumors larger than 2 cm and only 89% sensitivity for tumors measuring 1 cm or less. In a retrospective series by Wilson and colleagues,[6] ABR was found to have an overall sensitivity of 85%; sensitivity decreased to 67% in intracanalicular tumors. Hashimoto and colleagues[43] found a 22% false-negative rate for ABR in a study of 20 small acoustic neuromas with extra-meatal size of less than 15 mm.

STACKED ABR

With the discovery that ABR is not as sensitive as was originally believed, particularly in the case of small tumors, a shift began to occur away from reliance on ABR as a diagnostic modality for acoustic neuromas. A new ABR technique known as stacked ABR, however, has improved sensitivity. Investigators of stacked ABR propose that in standard ABR, a subset of high-frequency fibers dominates the peak wave-V latency. Don and colleagues[44] are of the opinion that small tumors often do not affect a sufficient number of these dominant cochlear nerve fibers to produce aberrancies in the ABR reading, thus affording false-negative results. This lack of effect on the wave-V latency is not only due to the size of a tumor, but also depends on the location of the tumor with respect to the cochleotopic organization of the eighth cranial nerve. This theory explains why there is not a linear relationship between tumor size and ABR result; the effect of the tumor on surrounding structures depends on both size and tumor location. These investigators proposed that stacked ABR is more sensitive than standard ABR measures because it represents an assessment of essentially all of the eighth-nerve fibers rather than just a subset, and thus does not so much depend on tumor size and location.[44,45]

Several publications by Don and colleagues[44] have demonstrated an improved ability of stacked ABR to detect small and intracanalicular tumors. A 1997 publication described a series of 25 acoustic neuromas and found that 5 small (1 cm or less), intra-canalicular tumors were missed by standard ABR but were detected by stacked ABR. In 2005, Don and colleagues[45] published a series of 54 patients with tumors that either measured 1 cm or less or were undetected by standard ABR methods. Each of these patients was tested with stacked ABR. This series demonstrated 95% sensitivity and 88% specificity; sensitivity was increased to 100% when parameters were set to provide 50% specificity. The group advocates that the improved sensitivity with the technique of stacked ABR will necessitate fewer MRIs to be performed.

VESTIBULAR TESTING
Electronystagmography

Before the advent of ABR, electronystagmography (ENG) was regularly used as part of the testing battery to screen for acoustic neuromas. Typical findings in patients with acoustic neuromas include ipsilateral reduced vestibular caloric responses as well as spontaneous nystagmus to the contralateral side of the tumor. Larger tumors may also display failure of fixation suppression, bilateral slowing of optokinetic nystagmus, abnormal saccadic pursuit, and bilateral horizontal-gaze nystagmus.[4] With the development of ABR and later, MRI, it was found that sensitivity with ENG was not high enough to be clinically useful.[5,18] Of note, ENG tests the horizontal semi-circular canals that are innervated by the superior vestibular nerve, so that small tumors arising from the inferior vestibular nerve may be missed. Linthicum and colleagues[46] cite ENG results in a series of patients with acoustic neuromas; ENG was abnormal in 98% of cases with tumors arising from the superior vestibular nerve and in 60% of cases with tumors arising from the inferior vestibular nerve. Modified ENG techniques have been developed to assess inferior vestibular nerve lesions; however, their utility has been overshadowed by the presence of more sensitive imaging techniques, such as MRI.[46]

IMAGING

Radiologic imaging was first used to detect acoustic neuromas in 1910 by Henschen, who evaluated erosion of the porus acusticus on plain film radiographs.[4] Despite this promising application of radiographs, sensitivity was very poor, reflected by Cushing's lament in 1917 that "even in advanced cases, there is apt to be little demonstrable difference between the pori interni of the affected and unaffected side."[2] In his series, Cushing found that only 37% of patients with acoustic neuromas demonstrated enlargement of the porus acusticus on radiograph. In 1918, Dandy introduced cerebral pneumography in an attempt to improve visualization of the cerebellopontine angle.[5] This attempt was followed by iophendylate myelograms and polytomography with contrast myelography, which improved diagnostic capabilities within the posterior cranial fossa until the introduction of CT by Hounsfield in the 1970s.[5]

Computed Tomography

At the time of their development, CT scanners were able to detect acoustic tumors as small as 2.0 cm, but often missed smaller tumors.[5] The development of CT with air or CO_2 cisternography improved the sensitivity of detecting small and intracanalicular tumors; however, diagnostic precision was still lacking.[1,7,47] In 1984, Barrs and colleagues[48] published a series of false-positive results using CT with gas cisternography. In their series, several unnecessary surgical explorations were performed in which no tumor was found. The study cites a false-positive rate of up to 22% with this technique. Moreover, CT cisternography was a very painful and time-consuming procedure, and not without risk.

Magnetic Resonance Imaging

MRI was introduced in the 1980s and was found to be at least as effective at diagnosing acoustic neuromas as CT with iodinated contrast or gas cisternography, and was better tolerated.[49] Diagnostic yields as high as 100% without false-positive or false-negative results were reported.[7] Gadolinium enhancement was introduced in 1987 and became the gold standard for diagnosis of acoustic neuromas, displaying improved sensitivity, particularly for small tumors. As described by Jackler and colleagues,[50] gadolinium enhancement permitted identification of small tumors that were not evident on unenhanced scans, and allowed for differentiation of residual/recurrent tumor from scar tissue in postoperative patients. Gadolinium enhancement also provided a more reliable estimate of depth of tumor penetration into the internal auditory canal, which allowed for improved surgical planning, particularly an improved ability to properly select patients for hearing-conservation surgery.

Imaging Characteristics

MRI with gadolinium may detect tumors as small as 3 mm.[51] On MRI, acoustic neuromas most often appear to be centered on the internal auditory canal and mainly enlarge the internal auditory canal rather than cause bony erosion or hyperostosis. These neuromas generally have a spherical or ovoid shape, and form an acute bone-tumor angle. Acoustic neuromas are isointense or hypointense on both T1 and T2 MRI, and demonstrate marked enhancement with gadolinium.[52]

SPECIAL CONSIDERATIONS WITH MRI FOR ACOUSTIC NEUROMA

Although MRI with gadolinium has achieved the highest sensitivity and specificity for detection of acoustic neuromas, several practical aspects must be considered when determining who should undergo MRI evaluation. MRI does not involve radiation exposure. The use of gadolinium is relatively safe; gadolinium is excreted unchanged by the kidneys, and allergies to gadolinium are far less frequent than those to iodinated contrast material.[50] A gadolinium-enhanced MRI of the internal auditory canals and brain routinely costs up to $2500, and some areas have limited availability of scanners. Patient claustrophobia within the typical closed MRI scanner is not uncommon, and this can often be overcome by scanning in an open MRI unit. Some patients are limited by a body habitus that precludes their entry into MRI units. Patients with implanted ferromagnetic prostheses or fragments are unable to enter an MRI unit.

MODIFIED MRI TECHNIQUES FOR ACOUSTIC NEUROMA

In response to concerns about the cost of routine screening for acoustic neuromas with gadolinium, several new techniques in MRI have been developed that provide focused imaging of the internal auditory canal and cerebellopontine angle at a lower cost. Heavily T2-saturated fast spin-echo MRI is a technique that provides a focused study without the need for intravenous contrast administration. This technique is less affected than traditional MRI by the diverse tissue interfaces in the region of the temporal bone, allowing for the acquisition of high-resolution images of the inner ear, internal auditory canal, and cerebellopontine angle. The technique uses dual

3-inch phased-array temporomandibular joint receiver coils centered over the external meatus to provide a limited but high-quality image of this region. Of note, because fast spin-echo MRI is a focused examination, it may not identify subtle meningeal disorders and inflammatory intralabyrinthine lesions if other routine MRI sequences are not obtained.[53] Shelton and colleagues[54] published a retrospective study comparing fast spin-echo MRI with the current gold standard of gadolinium-enhanced MRI. These investigators performed a blinded review of the imaging results of 25 patients with acoustic neuromas and 25 control patients, all of whom underwent both enhanced conventional spin-echo MR imaging and unenhanced fast spin-echo MR imaging of the cerebellopontine angle/internal auditory canal region. Acoustic neuromas were correctly diagnosed in 98% of the fast spin-echo images and in 100% of the enhanced conventional spin-echo images; there was no significant difference in the sensitivity and specificity of the two examinations. Acquisition time for fast spin-echo images was 8 minutes. The estimated cost of the test in Utah in 1996 was $350 to $400, including both technical and professional charges.[53,54] Marx and colleagues[55] performed a similar review of 25 patients (50 ears) in whom there was clinical suspicion of acoustic neuroma. All patients underwent both unenhanced fast spin-echo MRI and traditional gadolinium-enhanced MRI. Results demonstrated a sensitivity of 100% and specificity of 100%. Naganawa and colleagues[56] reported their use of unenhanced fast spin-echo MRI in detecting acoustic neuromas. In their hands, fast spin-echo MRI was found to have 100% sensitivity and 99.5% specificity.

Hermans and colleagues[57] described a different modification of MRI known as 3-dimensional Fourier transform-constructive interference in steady state (3DFT-CISS). This protocol is also performed without the use of intravenous contrast agent, reducing the scan time and cost of the examination. In their study, the group describes 89% to 94% sensitivity and 94% to 97% specificity in diagnosing acoustic neuromas compared with the reference of contrast-enhanced T1-weighted spin-echo MRI images. Stuckey and colleagues[58] published a series using this technique in which the sensitivity was 97.2%, with a specificity of 95.8%.

COST-EFFECTIVENESS OF DIAGNOSTIC MODALITIES

Although gadolinium-enhanced MRI remains the current gold standard in the diagnosis of acoustic neuromas, the significant cost of this examination precludes its unrestricted use. The ideal screening tool would have optimal sensitivity and specificity and be widely available at a low cost. As noted in a publication by Murphy and Selesnick,[59] the most sensitive diagnostic modality (MRI) is cost-prohibitive in some societies, so the choice of diagnostic modality remains a philosophic and macroeconomic decision as much as a technological one. Current estimates place the cost of MRI scanning at up to $2500; however, test results are generally definitive. Although ABR testing is significantly less expensive ($250–$500), one must take into account the cost of repeat ABRs and additional follow-up examinations when MRI is not performed.

Several investigators have attempted to formulate a cost-effective strategy for the diagnosis of acoustic neuromas through decision-tree analysis. These publications have mainly addressed the role of ABR and MRI in screening for acoustic neuromas. Cheng and colleagues[60] performed a retrospective comparison between diagnostic pathways. In their traditional diagnostic strategy, patients who were found on audiologic evaluation to have asymmetric sensorineural hearing loss underwent an ABR, and ABR was followed by an MRI only in the event of abnormal ABR results. This was compared with a strategy in which all patients found to have asymmetric sensorineural hearing loss underwent MRI directly. These investigators found cost savings of $119 per patient by performing ABR as a primary screening tool for acoustic neuroma, thus reducing the number of MRI scans performed. This strategy does not take into account the cost of missed tumors because it assumes that a normal ABR excludes retrocochlear pathology.

Another approach that has been studied stratifies patients into risk groups to evaluate the most cost-effective approach for each group. Welling and colleagues[5] assigned probabilities to patients for harboring acoustic neuromas based on clinical symptom complexes. In their evaluation, these investigators advocate the use of ABR screening in low-probability patients. All others should proceed directly to MRI imaging. A similar technique was used by Robinette and colleagues,[61] who found that screening with ABR before proceeding to MRI resulted in cost savings for patients in the low-risk or intermediate-risk groups for having acoustic neuromas. This saving was reversed in patients in the high-risk group, in whom it was more cost-effective to undergo MRI alone. Again, this strategy does not take into account missed tumors because it assumes that a normal ABR excludes retrocochlear pathology.

Several other studies examining cost-effectiveness have recommended proceeding directly to MRI based on clinical suspicion and audiometry results. Robson and colleagues[62] studied differences in costs between initial evaluation with ABR and caloric testing versus MRI as the primary screening procedure. These investigators found a cost saving by bypassing audiovestibular testing and proceeding directly with MRI, and concluded that MRI can be a cost-effective and accurate single screening procedure for acoustic neuromas. Ravi and Wells[63] also conclude that the routine use of MRI for the detection of acoustic neuromas is cost-effective and more effective than the use of conventional testing.

Studies that have compared the cost-effectiveness of modified MRI techniques with ABR as an initial screening tool have uniformly found MRI to be more cost-effective. Daniels and colleagues[64] performed a cost analysis in patients with sudden sensorineural hearing loss, comparing a routine evaluation that included ABR with screening with fast spin-echo MRI, and found a 54% reduction in screening costs with fast spin-echo MRI alone. Carrier and colleagues[65] compared the cost of focused enhanced MRI with abbreviated sequencing with primary screening with ABRs, and found focused MRI to be more cost-effective. In a systematic review of the subject, Fortnum and colleagues[66] recommended noncontrast T2-weighted MRI as the initial screening tool to evaluate for acoustic neuroma, rather than ABR or gadolinium-enhanced MRI. Doyle[67] published a literature review in which she recommended patients to undergo low-cost MRI as the primary screening modality. Doyle described a role for ABR in patients in whom MRI is contraindicated because of ferromagnetic implants or excessive obesity, and in patients who are poor surgical candidates whose life span is unlikely to be altered by the discovery of a small acoustic neuroma but in whom a large tumor must be ruled out. The third use described is a preoperative ABR to predict the likelihood of success with hearing-preservation surgery.[67]

SUMMARY

From the early descriptions of acoustic neuromas to the modern era, great advances have been made in understanding the clinical features of this rare tumor. Furthermore, rapid technological changes in the past century have led to the development of sensitive, rapid, and relatively noninvasive diagnostic modalities, which has allowed for earlier discovery of acoustic neuromas and has significantly reduced the average tumor size at time of diagnosis. The result has been improved clinical outcomes after surgery and radiotherapy. Although the current gold standard for acoustic neuroma detection remains gadolinium-enhanced MRI, new techniques, such as stacked ABR and modified MRI, are adding to the array of cost-effective diagnostic tools becoming available to the clinician.

REFERENCES

1. Cueva RA. Auditory brainstem response versus magnetic resonance imaging for the evaluation of asymmetric sensorineural hearing loss. Laryngoscope 2004; 114(10):1686–92.
2. Cushing H. Tumors of the nervus acusticus and the syndrome of the cerebello-pontine angle. Philadelphia: WB Saunders; 1917.
3. Selesnick SH, Jackler RK, Pitts LW. The changing clinical presentation of acoustic tumors in the MRI era. Laryngoscope 1993;103(4 Pt 1):431–6.
4. Selesnick SH, Jackler RK. Clinical manifestations and audiologic diagnosis of acoustic neuromas. Otolaryngol Clin North Am 1992;25(3):521–51.
5. Welling DB, Glasscock ME 3rd, Woods CI, et al. Acoustic neuroma: a cost-effective approach. Otolaryngol Head Neck Surg 1990;103(3):364–70.
6. Wilson DF, Hodgson RS, Gustafson MF, et al. The sensitivity of auditory brainstem response testing in small acoustic neuromas. Laryngoscope 1992;102(9):961–4.
7. Brackmann DE, Kwartler JA. A review of acoustic tumors: 1983-1988. Am J Otol 1990;11(3):216–32.
8. Mathew GD, Facer GW, Suh KW, et al. Symptoms, findings, and methods of diagnosis in patients with acoustic neuroma. Laryngoscope 1978;88(12):1893–903, 1921.
9. Harner SG, Laws ER Jr. Diagnosis of acoustic neurinoma. Neurosurgery 1981; 9(4):373–9.
10. Cohen NL, Lewis WS, Ransohoff J. Hearing preservation in cerebellopontine angle tumor surgery: the NYU experience 1974-1991. Am J Otol 1993;14(5): 423–33.
11. Nadol JB Jr, Chiong CM, Ojemann RG, et al. Preservation of hearing and facial nerve function in resection of acoustic neuroma. Laryngoscope 1992;102(10): 1153–8.
12. Glasscock ME 3rd, Hays JW, Minor LB, et al. Preservation of hearing in surgery for acoustic neuromas. J Neurosurg 1993;78(6):864–70.
13. Josey AF, Glasscock ME 3rd, Jackson CG. Preservation of hearing in acoustic tumor surgery: audiologic indicators. Ann Otol Rhinol Laryngol 1988;97(6 Pt 1): 626–30.
14. Shelton C, Brackmann DE, House WF, et al. Acoustic tumor surgery. Prognostic factors in hearing conversation. Arch Otolaryngol Head Neck Surg 1989; 115(10):1213–6.
15. Wiegand DA, Ojemann RG, Fickel V. Surgical treatment of acoustic neuroma (vestibular schwannoma) in the United States: report from the acoustic neuroma registry. Laryngoscope 1996;106(1 Pt 1):58–66.
16. Edwards CH, Paterson JH. A review of the symptoms and signs of acoustic neurofibromata. Brain 1951;74(2):144–90.
17. Higgs WA. Sudden deafness as the presenting symptom of acoustic neurinoma. Arch Otolaryngol 1973;98(2):73–6.
18. Hirsch A, Anderson H. Audiologic test results in 96 patients with tumours affecting the eighth nerve. A clinical study with emphasis on the early audiological diagnosis. Acta Otolaryngol Suppl 1980;369:1–26.

19. Pensak ML, Glasscock ME 3rd, Josey AF, et al. Sudden hearing loss and cerebellopontine angle tumors. Laryngoscope 1985;95(10):1188–93.
20. Sataloff RT, Davies B, Myers DL. Acoustic neuromas presenting as sudden deafness. Am J Otol 1985;6(4):349–52.
21. Friedman RA, Kesser BW, Slattery WH 3rd, et al. Hearing preservation in patients with vestibular schwannomas with sudden sensorineural hearing loss. Otolaryngol Head Neck Surg 2001;125(5):544–51.
22. Erickson LS, Sorenson GD, McGavran MH. A review of 140 acoustic neurinomas (neurilemmoma). Laryngoscope 1965;75:601–27.
23. Pool JL, Pava AA. The early diagnosis and treatment of acoustic nerve tumors. Springfield (IL): Charles C Thomas; 1957.
24. Thomsen J, Tos M. Acoustic neuroma: clinical aspects, audiovestibular assessment, diagnostic delay, and growth rate. Am J Otol 1990;11(1):12–9.
25. Beck HJ, Beatty CW, Harner SG, et al. Acoustic neuromas with normal pure tone hearing levels. Otolaryngol Head Neck Surg 1986;94(1):96–103.
26. Roland PS, Glasscock ME 3rd, Bojrab DI, et al. Normal hearing in patients with acoustic neuroma. South Med J 1987;80(2):166–9.
27. Lustig LR, Rifkin S, Jackler RK, et al. Acoustic neuromas presenting with normal or symmetrical hearing: factors associated with diagnosis and outcome. Am J Otol 1998;19(2):212–8.
28. Selesnick SH, Jackler RK. Atypical hearing loss in acoustic neuroma patients. Laryngoscope 1993;103(4 Pt 1):437–41.
29. Saleh EA, Aristegui M, Naguib MB, et al. Normal hearing in acoustic neuroma patients: a critical evaluation. Am J Otol 1996;17(1):127–32.
30. Olsen A, Horrax G. The symptomatology of acoustic tumors with special reference to atypical features. J Neurosurg 1944;1:371–8.
31. Rasmussen BK, Jensen R, Schroll M, et al. Epidemiology of headache in a general population—a prevalence study. J Clin Epidemiol 1991;44(11):1147–57.
32. Selesnick SH, Deora M, Drotman MB, et al. Incidental discovery of acoustic neuromas. Otolaryngol Head Neck Surg 1999;120(6):815–8.
33. Johnson EW. Results of auditory tests in acoustic neuroma patients. In: House WF, Luetje CM, editors. Acoustic tumors, vol. 1. Baltimore (MD): University Park Press; 1979. p. 209–24.
34. Moffat DA, Hardy DG, Baguley DM. Strategy and benefits of acoustic neuroma searching. J Laryngol Otol 1989;103(1):51–9.
35. Sohmer H, Feinmesser M. Cochlear action potentials recorded from the external ear in man. Ann Otol Rhinol Laryngol 1967;76(2):427–35.
36. Jewett DL, Romano MN, Williston JS. Human auditory evoked potentials: possible brain stem components detected on the scalp. Science 1970;167(924):1517–8.
37. Selters WA, Brackmann DE. Acoustic tumor detection with brain stem electric response audiometry. Arch Otolaryngol 1977;103(4):181–7.
38. Flood LM, Brammer RE, Graham MD, et al. Pitfalls in the diagnosis of acoustic neuroma. Clin Otolaryngol Allied Sci 1984;9(3):165–70.
39. Gordon ML, Cohen NL. Efficacy of auditory brainstem response as a screening test for small acoustic neuromas. Am J Otol 1995;16(2):136–9.
40. Ruckenstein MJ, Cueva RA, Morrison DH, et al. A prospective study of ABR and MRI in the screening for vestibular schwannomas. Am J Otol 1996;17(2):317–20.
41. Schmidt RJ, Sataloff RT, Newman J, et al. The sensitivity of auditory brainstem response testing for the diagnosis of acoustic neuromas. Arch Otolaryngol Head Neck Surg 2001;127(1):19–22.

42. Zappia JJ, O'Connor CA, Wiet RJ, et al. Rethinking the use of auditory brainstem response in acoustic neuroma screening. Laryngoscope 1997;107(10):1388–92.
43. Hashimoto S, Kawase T, Furukawa K, et al. Strategy for the diagnosis of small acoustic neuromas. Acta Otolaryngol Suppl 1991;481:567–9.
44. Don M, Masuda A, Nelson R, et al. Successful detection of small acoustic tumors using the stacked derived-band auditory brain stem response amplitude. Am J Otol 1997;18(5):608–21 [discussion: 682–85].
45. Don M, Kwong B, Tanaka C, et al. The stacked ABR: a sensitive and specific screening tool for detecting small acoustic tumors. Audiol Neurootol 2005; 10(5):274–90.
46. Linthicum FH Jr, Waldorf R, Luxford WM, et al. Infrared/video ENG recording of eye movements to evaluate the inferior vestibular nerve using the minimal caloric test. Otolaryngol Head Neck Surg 1988;98(3):207–10.
47. Clark WC, Acker JD, Robertson JH, et al. Neuroradiological detection of small and intracanalicular acoustic tumors: an emphasis on CO_2 contrast-enhanced computed tomographic cisternography. Neurosurgery 1982;11(6):733–8.
48. Barrs DM, Luxford WM, Becker TS, et al. Computed tomography with gas cisternography for detection of small acoustic tumors. A study of five false-positive results. Arch Otolaryngol 1984;110(8):535–7.
49. Lhuillier FM, Doyon DL, Halimi PM, et al. Magnetic resonance imaging of acoustic neuromas: pitfalls and differential diagnosis. Neuroradiology 1992; 34(2):144–9.
50. Jackler RK, Shapiro MS, Dillon WP, et al. Gadolinium-DTPA enhanced magnetic resonance imaging in acoustic neuroma diagnosis and management. Otolaryngol Head Neck Surg 1990;102(6):670–7.
51. Press GA, Hesselink JR. MR imaging of cerebellopontine angle and internal auditory canal lesions at 1.5 T. AJR Am J Roentgenol 1988;150(6):1371–81.
52. Lo WM. Tumors of the temporal bone and cerebellopontine angle. In: Som PT, Bergeron RT, editors. Head and neck imaging. St Louis (MO): Mosby; 1991.
53. Allen RW, Harnsberger HR, Shelton C, et al. Low-cost high-resolution fast spin-echo MR of acoustic schwannoma: an alternative to enhanced conventional spin-echo MR? AJNR Am J Neuroradiol 1996;17(7):1205–10.
54. Shelton C, Harnsberger HR, Allen R, et al. Fast spin echo magnetic resonance imaging: clinical application in screening for acoustic neuroma. Otolaryngol Head Neck Surg 1996;114(1):71–6.
55. Marx SV, Langman AW, Crane RC. Accuracy of fast spin echo magnetic resonance imaging in the diagnosis of vestibular schwannoma. Am J Otolaryngol 1999;20(4):211–6.
56. Naganawa S, Ito T, Fukatsu H, et al. MR imaging of the inner ear: comparison of a three-dimensional fast spin-echo sequence with use of a dedicated quadrature-surface coil with a gadolinium-enhanced spoiled gradient-recalled sequence. Radiology 1998;208(3):679–85.
57. Hermans R, Van der Goten A, De Foer B, et al. MRI screening for acoustic neuroma without gadolinium: value of 3DFT-CISS sequence. Neuroradiology 1997;39(8):593–8.
58. Stuckey SL, Harris AJ, Mannolini SM. Detection of acoustic schwannoma: use of constructive interference in the steady state three-dimensional MR. AJNR Am J Neuroradiol 1996;17(7):1219–25.
59. Murphy MR, Selesnick SH. Cost-effective diagnosis of acoustic neuromas: a philosophical, macroeconomic, and technological decision. Otolaryngol Head Neck Surg 2002;127(4):253–9.

60. Cheng G, Smith R, Tan AK. Cost comparison of auditory brainstem response versus magnetic resonance imaging screening of acoustic neuroma. J Otolaryngol 2003;32(6):394–9.

61. Robinette MS, Bauch CD, Olsen WO, et al. Auditory brainstem response and magnetic resonance imaging for acoustic neuromas: costs by prevalence. Arch Otolaryngol Head Neck Surg 2000;126(8):963–6.

62. Robson AK, Leighton SE, Anslow P, et al. MRI as a single screening procedure for acoustic neuroma: a cost effective protocol. J R Soc Med 1993;86(8):455–7.

63. Ravi KV, Wells SC. A cost effective screening protocol for vestibular schwannoma in the late 90s. J Laryngol Otol 1996;110(12):1129–32.

64. Daniels RL, Shelton C, Harnsberger HR. Ultra high resolution nonenhanced fast spin echo magnetic resonance imaging: cost-effective screening for acoustic neuroma in patients with sudden sensorineural hearing loss. Otolaryngol Head Neck Surg 1998;119(4):364–9.

65. Carrier DA, Arriaga MA. Cost-effective evaluation of asymmetric sensorineural hearing loss with focused magnetic resonance imaging. Otolaryngol Head Neck Surg 1997;116(6 Pt 1):567–74.

66. Fortnum H, O'Neill C, Taylor R, et al. The role of magnetic resonance imaging in the identification of suspected acoustic neuroma: a systematic review of clinical and cost effectiveness and natural history. Health Technol Assess 2009;13(18): iii–iiv, ix–xi, 1–154.

67. Doyle KJ. Is there still a role for auditory brainstem response audiometry in the diagnosis of acoustic neuroma? Arch Otolaryngol Head Neck Surg 1999; 125(2):232–4.

Preoperative, Intraoperative, and Postoperative Auditory Evaluation of Patients with Acoustic Neuroma

Roberto A. Cueva, MD[a,b]

KEYWORDS

- Acoustic neuroma • Preoperative auditory evaluation
- Postoperative auditory evaluation • Intraoperative monitoring for acoustic neuroma
- Audiometry • Neurotology

PREOPERATIVE EVALUATION OF ACOUSTIC NEUROMA
Behavioral Audiometry

Because patients with acoustic neuroma (AN) typically present with unilateral sensorineural (SNHL) hearing loss as their most common presenting symptom, most of them would already have had behavioral audiometry. This test evaluates the entirety of the auditory system, including the tympanic membrane/middle ear, cochlea, cochlear nerve, dorsal and ventral cochlear nuclei, trapezoid body and its nucleus, superior olivary nuclei, lateral lemniscus and its nuclei, inferior colliculus, medial geniculate body, auditory radiations via the posterior limb of the internal capsule, and finally the auditory cortex in the transverse gyri of Heschl. For the purpose of this section, the focus is on tests that may be done as part of the preoperative assessment of a patient with AN. Pure tone auditory thresholds and speech discrimination score (SDS) are the most important factors in preoperative decision making. Even patients with relatively poor pure tone thresholds would remain candidates for attempted hearing-preservation surgery if their SDS were good enough to allow successful amplification. Traditionally the 50/50 rule is used as a guideline in this decision making; that is, a patient with hearing equal to or better than 50 dB pure tone average (PTA) and better than 50% SDS may be considered for hearing-preservation surgery. This also, of course, depends on tumor size because the likelihood of hearing preservation is inversely proportional to increasing tumor size.

[a] Kaiser Permanente Medical Center, Department of Head and Neck Surgery, 5893 Copley Drive, San Diego, CA, USA
[b] University of California, San Diego, CA, USA
E-mail address: roberto.a.cueva@kp.org

Otolaryngol Clin N Am 45 (2012) 285–290
doi:10.1016/j.otc.2011.12.002
0030-6665/12/$ – see front matter © 2012 Elsevier Inc. All rights reserved.

Auditory Brainstem Response

Some investigators advocate the use of auditory brainstem response (ABR) testing as a way to prognosticate chances for hearing preservation.[1] In the absence of a good-quality ABR, some surgeons would advise translabyrinthine surgery because there would be no ABR signal to monitor during attempted hearing-preservation surgery. On the other hand, those surgeons who routinely use direct eighth-nerve monitoring (DENM) during surgery have found that a cochlear nerve action potential (CNAP) is routinely recorded even when preoperative ABR is poor or absent.[2] Therefore, ABR is thought to be of little utility for preoperative assessment by surgeons using DENM because it does not influence their decision to attempt hearing preservation or their ability to monitor hearing intraoperatively.

ABR is a far-field technique for monitoring sound-evoked electrical activity in the auditory system from the cochlea/cochlear nerve through the brainstem. Because signal amplitude is negatively affected by increasing distance from the source of the neuronal activity, ABR has relatively small amplitudes on the order of tenths of a microvolt. In addition, averaging of hundreds to thousands of stimulus/response events is necessary to separate the desired signal from the random background electrical activity of the brain. Given the necessity of averaging many stimulus/response events, obtaining an ABR can take from 2 to 5 minutes. Pure tone thresholds less than 70 dB at 2 kHz and more are usually required to achieve an interpretable ABR. In patients with hearing worse than this, waveforms III through V may be of poor quality or absent. However, poor-quality or absent ABR waveforms do not preclude attempted hearing preservation during surgery because DNEM is often useful in this setting. Since the identification of ABR as a reliable tool in the assessment of the auditory system, a significant amount of research has endeavored to identify the location of the neural generators for the waveforms.

Animal studies investigating ABR, primarily in cats, were conducted in the mid- to late 1970s.[3–5] Correlation of ABR waveforms with their neural generators in humans was investigated in the mid-1970s and continued into the 1990s by studies looking at ABR abnormalities related to known lesions of the central nervous system[6–8] and studies using intracranially recorded auditory responses during surgery.[9–11] Based on these investigations, generally accepted neural generators for ABR waves I and II have been established. However, the precise identity of the neural generators for waves III, IV, and V remains unclear because of conflicting reports from various laboratories. **Fig. 1** demonstrates a normal ABR with the waveforms labeled with Roman numerals I through V. **Table 1** indicates the first 5 ABR waveforms, their typical latencies, and their proposed neural generators.[12–14] The most important waveforms regarding preoperative and intraoperative assessment of the auditory system in patients with ANs are I, III, and V. These waveforms correlate with the functional status of anatomic structures from the cochlea to the inferior colliculus. If these waveforms are present preoperatively then reasonable cochlear nerve integrity can be assumed. Likewise, if these waveforms are present at the conclusion of acoustic tumor surgery, the likelihood of hearing preservation is good.

Otoacoustic Emissions

Otoacoustic emissions (OAEs) in their different variations (distortion product OAE and transient-evoked OAE) can differentiate cochlear from noncochlear hearing losses and, thus, may be useful in a retrocochlear screening test battery.[15] Although the expected pattern would be one of poor hearing and intact OAEs, it was somewhat surprising to discover that more than half of ANs had reduced cochlear function as

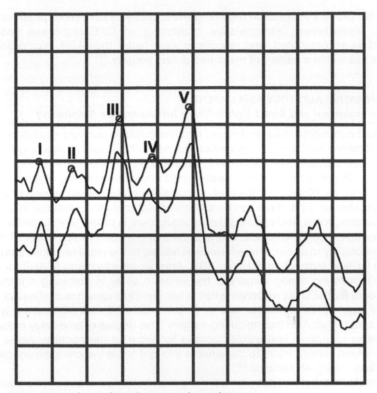

Fig. 1. ABR tracing with numbered waves I through V.

measured by OAEs. It has been shown that OAEs can be preserved in the setting of severe cochlear nerve dysfunction.[16] Some tumors result in abnormally large OAE, presumably because of loss of efferent suppressions from tumor compression of the eighth cranial nerve. Intraoperative assessment of the auditory system is related to acoustic tumors because they are a measure of cochlear (outer hair cell) function

Table 1		
Proposed neural generators of ABR waveforms		
Waveforms	**Proposed Neural Generators**	**Latency (ms)**
I	Cochlear nerve: modiolus/IAC	1.7 ± 0.15
II	Cochlear nerve: proximal CPA portion	2.8 ± 0.17
III	Cochlear nucleus	3.9 ± 0.19
IV	Superior olive/lateral lemniscus	5.1 ± 0.24
V	Terminal fibers of lateral lemniscus into inferior colliculus	5.7 ± 0.25

Abbreviations: CPA, cerebellopontine angle; IAC, internal auditory canal.
Data from Latency values adapted from Martin WH, Pratt H, Schwegler JW. The origin of the human auditory brain-stem response wave II. Electroencephalogr Clin Neurophysiol 1995;96:357–70; and Grundy BL, Jannetta PJ, Procopio PT, et al. Intraoperative monitoring of brain-stem auditory evoked potentials. J Neurosurg 1982;57:674–81.

and do not provide information regarding the auditory system more proximal to the cochlea. Nevertheless, intraoperative monitoring of OAE responses has been successfully accomplished, and responses were faster than ABR, suggesting their potential use within a battery of measures during surgery.[17]

INTRAOPERATIVE AUDITORY ASSESSMENT
Auditory Brainstem and Direct Eighth-Nerve Intraoperative Monitoring

The 2 most commonly used techniques for intraoperative auditory monitoring during AN resection are ABR and DENM. Because of early challenges maintaining electrode placement on the cochlear nerve during DENM, the technique fell into disfavor. This resulted in ABR becoming the most widely used auditory monitoring technique during AN surgery in the 1980s.[18,19] However, the operating room poses several challenges to ABR monitoring. First, there can be a tremendous amount of electrical interference in the operating room, and ensuring that all equipment is properly grounded is necessary to minimize 60-Hz electrical interference that may overwhelm the ABR tracing. This susceptibility to electrical interference is related to the small response amplitudes found in far-field techniques, such as ABR. Another disadvantage of ABR for intraoperative monitoring during surgery is the inherent delay in obtaining a tracing. To compensate for the small response amplitudes, literally thousands of stimulus repetitions are required. At a stimulus rate of 11 per second, 2 to 3 minutes are typically needed to obtain an ABR tracing during surgery. This degree of time delay in the operative setting can allow irreversible damage to occur to the cochlear nerve or the cochlear blood supply. Injury to the latter is thought to be the predominant cause of hearing loss during AN removal.[20]

The development of an electrode achieving more reliable and atraumatic positioning on the cochlear nerve in the late 1990s stimulated resurgence in the use of DENM.[21,22] To perform DENM, the scalp electrode setup is the same as for performing ABR. The difference is that once the cochlear nerve is exposed, an electrode is placed on the cochlear nerve, preferably proximal to the area of tumor involvement. Because the electrode is placed directly on the nerve of interest, this is a near-field monitoring technique and therefore response amplitudes are much stronger than ABR reducing (but not eliminating) susceptibility to electrical interference. Typical CNAP responses are from 1 to 50 μV. Furthermore, because response amplitudes are larger, less averaging is needed to generate a reliable CNAP. DENM requires on average less than 20 stimulus/response events to record a CNAP. This translates to about 1 to 2 seconds to generate a CNAP, resulting in near instantaneous intraoperative feedback during AN surgery. Such rapid feedback regarding the integrity of the cochlea and cochlear nerve during tumor dissection allows for interruption of surgical maneuvers that may be placing undue stress on the nerve or cochlear blood supply. As mentioned earlier, studies have indicated that the CNAP, recorded from the proximal portion of the cochlear nerve, corresponds to wave II of the ABR.[11]

In both ABR and DENM, the first sign of stress on the cochlear nerve or cochlear blood supply is a prolongation of the waveform latencies. Should further deterioration in function occur, response amplitudes begin to diminish. An exception to this can occur during DENM, when a drop in amplitude without a significant change in latency can occur if the area where the electrode is contacting the cochlear nerve is bathed in excess blood or cerebrospinal fluid (CSF). Blood in the area of the electrode/nerve interface appears to affect the CNAP recording more than CSF does. Preservation of CNAP at the conclusion of tumor removal is highly correlated with preservation of hearing. It is not uncommon to see CNAP amplitudes improve after tumor removal.

The absence of a CNAP at the conclusion of tumor removal is likewise correlated with loss of hearing. Sometimes, however, hearing may be preserved despite an absent CNAP. This is likely caused by transient spasm of the internal auditory artery. The presence of good ABR waveforms is also highly correlated with hearing preservation, but the absence of a good ABR does not particularly predict hearing loss.

POSTOPERATIVE AUDITORY ASSESSMENT

Initial assessment of patients' hearing after resection of their AN is often performed with a tuning fork or whisper test in the operated ear with the contralateral ear canal occluded by a finger. This action can be easily performed at the bedside once the patient has recovered from general anesthetic. More formal evaluation of auditory function is performed using behavioral audiometry. The current reporting standards for postoperative auditory function (American Academy of Otolaryngology—Head and Neck Surgery, Gardner-Robinson) tend to overweigh PTA in determining "class of hearing." It is becoming increasingly recognized that the SDS is, by far, more important in a patient's ability to successfully use his or her postoperative hearing. It is obvious that if the SDS is preserved at a good level but PTA declines, amplification can successfully rehabilitate the loss. If, however, PTA is preserved but SDS is poor, amplification is less useful.

REFERENCES

1. Brackmann DE, Owens RM, Friedman RA, et al. Prognostic factors for hearing preservation in vestibular schwannoma surgery. Am J Otol 2000;21(3):417–24.
2. Jackson L, Roberson J. Acoustic neuroma surgery: use of cochlear nerve action potential monitoring for hearing preservation. Am J Otol 2000;21:249–59.
3. Buchwald JS, Huang CM. Far field acoustic response: origins in the cat. Science 1975;189:382–4.
4. Achor LJ, Starr A. Auditory brain stem responses in the cat I. Intracranial and extracranial recordings. Electroencephalogr Clin Neurophysiol 1980;48:154–73.
5. Achor LJ, Starr A. Auditory brain stem responses in the cat. II. Effects of lesions. Electroencephalogr Clin Neurophysiol 1980;48:174–90.
6. Stockard JJ, Stockard JE, Sharbrough FW. Detection and localization of occult lesions with brainstem auditory responses. Mayo Clin Proc 1977;52:761–9.
7. Starr A, Hamilton AE. Correlation between confirmed sites of neurological lesions and abnormalities of far-field auditory brainstem responses. Electroencephalogr Clin Neurophysiol 1976;41:595–608.
8. Stockard JJ, Rossiter VS. Clinical and pathologic correlates of brain stem auditory response abnormalities. Neurology 1977;27:316–25.
9. Moller AR, Jannetta P, Bennett M, et al. Intracranially recorded responses from the human auditory nerve: new insights into the origin of the brain stem evoked potentials (BSEPs). Electroencephalogr Clin Neurophysiol 1981;52:18–27.
10. Moller AR, Jannetta PJ, Moller MB. Neural generators of the brainstem evoked potentials. Results from human intracranial recordings. Ann Otol Rhinol Laryngol 1981;90:591–6.
11. Martin WH, Pratt H, Schwegler JW. The origin of the human auditory brain-stem response wave II. Electroencephalogr Clin Neurophysiol 1995;96:357–70.
12. Grundy BL, Jannetta PJ, Procopio PT, et al. Intraoperative monitoring of brainstem auditory evoked potentials. J Neurosurg 1982;57:674–81.

13. Moller AR, Janetta PJ, Sekhar LN. Contributions from the auditory nerve to the brain-stem auditory evoked potentials (BAEPs): results of intracranial recording in man. Electroencephalogr Clin Neurophysiol 1988;71:198–211.

14. Sabo DL, Durrant JD, Curtin H, et al. Correlations of neuro-anatomical measures to brainstem auditory evoked potential latencies. Ear Hear 1992;18:213–22.

15. Telischi FF. An objective method of analyzing cochlear versus noncochlear patterns of distortion product otoacoustic emissions in patients with acoustic neuromas. Laryngoscope 2000;110(4):553–62.

16. Cacace AT, Parnes SM, Lovely TJ, et al. The disconnected ear: phenomenological effects of a large acoustic tumor. Ear Hear 1994;15(4):287–98.

17. Morawski K, Namyslowski G, Lisowska G, et al. Intraoperative monitoring of cochlear function using distortion product otoacoustic emissions (DPOAE) in patients with cerebellopontine angle tumors. Otol Neurotol 2004;25(5):818–25.

18. Kveton J. The efficacy of brainstem auditory evoked potentials in acoustic tumor surgery. Laryngoscope 1990;100:1171–3.

19. Battista R, Wiet R, Paauwe L. Evaluation of three intraoperative auditory monitoring techniques in acoustic neuroma surgery. Am J Otol 2000;21:244–8.

20. Cueva RA, Thedinger BA, Harris JP, et al. Electrical promontory stimulation in patients with intact cochlear nerve and anacusis following acoustic neuroma surgery. Laryngoscope 1992;102(11):1220–4.

21. Cueva RA, Morris GF, Prioleau GR. Direct cochlear nerve monitoring: first report on a new, atraumatic, self-retaining electrode. Am J Otol 1998;19(2):202–7.

22. Danner CJ, Mastrodimos B, Cueva RA. A comparison of direct eighth nerve monitoring and ABR in hearing preservation surgery for vestibular schwannoma. Otol Neurotol 2004;25(5):826–32.

Acoustic Neuroma Neurophysiologic Correlates:

Facial and Recurrent Laryngeal Nerves Before, During, and After Surgery

Robert S. Hong, MD, PhD[a], Jack M. Kartush, MD[a,b,c],*

KEYWORDS

- Facial nerve • Otolaryngologic surgery • Recurrent laryngeal nerve • Cranial nerve
- Vestibular schwannoma • Neurophysiology • EMG • Intraoperative monitoring
- Electroneurography

THE FACIAL NERVE

One of the primary concerns of the surgeon during resection of an acoustic neuroma (vestibular schwannoma) is injury to the facial nerve. The facial nerve takes a long, winding course from the brainstem into the temporal bone and out to the muscles of facial expression. Any segment of the facial nerve from brainstem to stylomastoid foramen may be injured during the course of surgery, leading to postoperative facial weakness, with potentially devastating functional and social consequences for the patient. The inherent complexity of facial nerve anatomy, made more difficult in the context of a tumor that can stretch the nerve and distort adjacent structures, has prompted methods to minimize facial nerve injury during tumor surgery. Although adoption of the operating microscope and transtemporal surgical approaches have been helpful, it was not until routine use of intraoperative electromyographic facial nerve monitoring that dramatic reductions of postoperative facial palsy were realized. Before monitoring, many publications reported on the anatomic preservation rate of the facial nerve. However, anatomically intact nerves that have undergone trauma from stretching and ischemia may be nonfunctional, which is the only parameter of interest to both patient and surgeon. Facial monitoring helps locate the nerve and provides real-time feedback to the surgeon about its neurophysiologic status. Many studies have shown improved postoperative facial nerve outcomes with its use[1–5]

[a] Michigan Ear Institute, 30055 Northwestern Highway, Suite 101, Farmington Hills, MI 48334, USA
[b] Wayne State University, Detroit, MI, USA
[c] Biotronic, Ann Arbor, MI, USA
* Corresponding author. Michigan Ear Institute, 30055 Northwestern Highway, Suite 101, Farmington Hills, MI 48334.
E-mail address: jkartush@comcast.net

Otolaryngol Clin N Am 45 (2012) 291–306
doi:10.1016/j.otc.2011.12.003
0030-6665/12/$ – see front matter © 2012 Elsevier Inc. All rights reserved.

oto.theclinics.com

and its cost-effectiveness.[6] The efficacy of monitoring for routine use during vestibular schwannoma surgery seems clear, with its use being advised by the National Institutes of Health.[7]

Neurophysiology

Neurophysiologic testing of the facial nerve plays an important role throughout the workup and treatment of vestibular schwannomas. Electroneurography (ENoG) may be used to determine the preoperative status of the facial nerve. Electromyography (EMG) is used during surgery to monitor for injury to the nerve. Both of these tests rely on measurements of the compound muscle action potential (CMAP) generated by the muscles of facial expression. Monitoring the CMAP allows a response that is an order of magnitude larger than if a nerve action potential was recorded because of the amplifying effect of the muscle response.

Depolarization of the facial nerve may occur following a mechanical or electrical stimulus, resulting in the generation of a nerve action potential. The nerve action potential is transmitted distally along the facial nerve until it reaches the motor end plates, where it is translated into motor unit potentials emanating from the corresponding muscle fibers. When summed, these motor unit potentials result in the measured CMAP, which reflects the activity of the muscles of facial expression. When the facial nerve is injured, information about the extent of injury can be obtained by examining the CMAP. With respect to electrically evoked CMAPs, the response differs depending on the site of nerve stimulation and extent of injury. When an electrical stimulus is applied proximal to the site of injury, nerves suffering from mild to moderate trauma exhibit reductions in amplitude and prolonged latency. Increasing injury requires an increasing amount of current to elicit a response. Although some nerves may be transected or crushed, many surgically induced injuries are a combination of physiologic conduction block (neuropraxia) and physically injured neural elements (axonotmesis or neurotmesis). An accurate assessment requires stimulation proximal to the anticipated site of injury. When an electrical stimulus is applied distal to the injury in the acute setting, the nerve and muscle still respond, because progressive distal degeneration of the axon (wallerian degeneration) following severe nerve injury takes 48 to 72 hours to reach the nerve ending.

ENoG

ENoG can be used for preoperative assessment of the patient with a vestibular schwannoma to establish the presence of preexisting subclinical facial nerve dysfunction.[8,9] To perform ENoG:

- The electrical stimulus is applied transcutaneously at the main nerve trunk near the stylomastoid foramen
- The CMAP is measured via surface recording electrodes placed at the nasolabial crease to assess orbicularis oris function in response to stimulation
- The relevant metric is comparison of the peak-to-peak amplitude of the CMAP at a supramaximal stimulus between the side with the tumor and the, presumably normal, contralateral side.

Interpretation of ENoG

Like electronystagmography, there are normal, expected variations from side to side and from person to person. Therefore, there must be at least a 30% difference between the 2 sides before it can be regarded as evidence of facial nerve dysfunction on the side with the smaller amplitude.[8–10] Care must be taken in the interpretation of

ENoG results, because operator error can result in poor test-retest reliability. In particular, ENoG testing requires training and experience for it to be accurate, including the use of an optimized lead placement strategy instead of standardized placement.[11–13]

ENoG before surgery is useful for multiple reasons. Patients with clinically normal facial function may have subclinical neuropathy. With this knowledge, the surgeon can better counsel the patient with severe preoperative ENoG abnormalities who may be at higher risk of postoperative facial paralysis. Reasons for severe preoperative ENoG abnormalities include:

1. An acoustic tumor being more infiltrative or compressive than typical tumors
2. The presence of another type of tumor that may have a higher risk of facial palsy (eg, facial neuroma).

Preoperative counseling in these circumstances can include a greater emphasis on treatment of facial palsy, subtotal resection, or decompression in lieu of resection. Residual tumor can be followed or treated with stereotactic radiosurgery. Preoperative facial nerve dysfunction can influence intraoperative facial nerve monitoring, making such monitoring less effective because the nerve is often in a hyperexcitable state.[14] ENoG allows the surgeon and monitoring neurophysiologist to be prepared for this possibility.

In contrast, ENoG is not typically helpful in the postoperative setting, even in the case of a delayed facial palsy following surgery. ENoG may be helpful in the context of a complete postoperative facial paralysis to determine when facial nerve decompression is indicated, in the same way that it used for patients with Bell palsy, in which edema at the meatal foramen (the narrowest point of the fallopian canal) is posited to be the epicenter of neural injury. However, abnormal postoperative ENoG does not pinpoint the meatal foramen as the epicenter of injury after it has undergone sustained surgical dissection over a broad segment of the nerve during tumor resection. Thus, the usefulness of surgical reexploration to decompress the nerve after an abnormal electroneurogram is unclear, because there may be multiple causes for facial nerve injury. Our practice is to routinely decompress the meatal foramen during the initial translabyrinthine and middle cranial fossa approaches for vestibular schwannoma to minimize this potential mechanism of postoperative nerve injury.[15] In addition, with a postoperative facial palsy, we institute therapy with steroids and antivirals, because viral reactivation is another potential cause of postoperative facial nerve weakness.[16]

Intraoperative Facial Nerve Monitoring

Facial nerve monitoring is routinely used in surgery for acoustic tumors because:

1. It aids in the early identification of the facial nerve
2. It detects nerve injury during dissection
3. It provides a means for assessing nerve function after dissection is complete.

Intraoperative monitoring should be used only as an adjunct to surgical judgment in the assessment of the facial nerve. False-positives and false-negatives can occur with monitoring, so a knowledgeable surgeon and monitoring team are essential because "poor monitoring is worse than no monitoring."[8,9] Operating with poor monitoring is comparable with using a malfunctioning minesweeper: if it cannot be relied on, it is best not used at all. If the monitoring results are not consistent with the surgeon's assessment of anatomy, tumor, and the perceived position and status of the nerve, the surgeon should proceed with caution and may even choose to reject the monitoring information if it contradicts these parameters.

Numerous facial nerve monitoring systems are in use today. Most systems are EMG based, such as the Medtronic Nerve Integrity Monitor (NIM) (Jacksonville, FL, USA) and the Neurosign system (Carmarthenshire, UK). However, the Silverstein Facial Nerve Monitor (Medical Electronics Co., Stillwater, MN, USA) uses a motion pressure detector attached to the cheek. Several studies have suggested that EMG-based systems are more sensitive than motion detection systems for facial nerve monitoring, and thus should be considered the monitor of choice for vestibular schwannoma surgery.[2,17] False-positives have been reported with motion detection systems, such as stimulation of the trigeminal nerve resulting in contraction of mastication muscles that can trigger the motion detector, leading to an inaccurate impression of facial nerve stimulation.[18] In contrast, the primary limitation of EMG-based systems is that facial nerve monitoring is disabled during the use of electrocautery, which causes a high-intensity electrical artifact that obscures the true EMG signal. Future generations of commercial facial nerve monitoring systems will address the issue of monitoring during cautery, especially during bipolar cauterization, which is more localized than unipolar cauterization in terms of current spread and interference with EMG monitoring. Research is underway examining other potential avenues for facial nerve monitoring, including use of transcranial magnetic stimulation,[19] optical stimulation,[20] and video monitoring.[21] Numerous multi-modality neurophysiologic monitoring devices are also available for facial nerve monitoring, but because they are intended to perform many other functions, these devices can be complex and require in-depth training before they can be safely used.

Training issues in intraoperative facial nerve monitoring
The successful use of intraoperative facial nerve monitoring requires that the surgeon is trained to understand and interpret the physiologic responses.[22] Furthermore, if the surgeon also takes on the responsibility of the electrode and device setup, specific training in the technical aspects of monitoring is required. Meticulous attention to detail must be paid to anesthesia, the monitoring device, and the electrodes to ensure accurate results. At our institution, the surgeon performs intraoperative monitoring in conjunction with a technologist who has received special training and certification (Certification in Neurophysiologic Intraoperative Monitoring [CNIM]). However, at many institutions, surgeons perform the technical setup. Although this is an appropriate model, many staff physicians have had little or no monitoring training other than a cursory introduction by a sales representative. In academic institutions, monitoring setup is often performed by residents whose only training is cursory, word-of-mouth advice by other residents who themselves typically lack an understanding of the technical aspects of monitoring.

Our review of medicolegal cases, as well as quizzing many residents from around the country, often confirms a lack of monitoring training. Staff surgeons come to rely on the residents, assuming a higher level of knowledge than may be present. To improve monitoring and enhance patient safety, we suggest that a written protocol be established for monitoring at each institution, and that a written curriculum with competency testing be required for all individuals performing monitoring. Furthermore, routine, rather than sporadic, use of facial nerve monitoring during operations in which the nerve potentially is at risk results in staff who are familiar with proper techniques and troubleshooting.

Setup and technique for facial nerve monitoring
Several steps are necessary to reliably perform EMG-based facial nerve monitoring.

Step 1. Ensure that the anesthesiologist avoids the use of long-acting muscle relaxants. Short-acting muscle relaxants such as succinylcholine are typically acceptable for induction, except in the rare case of the patient with pseudocholinesterase deficiency, in whom this drug is broken down slowly and thus experiences prolonged paralysis.

Step 2. Be wary about local anesthesia (eg, lidocaine or marcaine), which can chemically induce a temporary facial paresis, rendering monitoring useless. Most are aware that the injection must avoid the facial nerve at the stylomastoid foramen near the mastoid tip, which is particularly important in children for whom the mastoid tip may be poorly developed. Less well known but of great importance is that care must also be taken to avoid local anesthesia entering the middle ear, which is surprisingly common during chronic ear surgery when injecting the ear canal in the presence of a tympanic membrane perforation.

Step 3. Place electrodes carefully. Intramuscular needle electrodes are inserted in a paired manner at the nasolabial groove (orbicularis oris) and near the eyebrow (orbicularis oculi) on the side to be monitored (**Fig. 1**). Care is taken to direct the electrodes away from the ocular globe to avoid inadvertent trauma to the eye. Our experience over the decades has shown that there is no need to risk ocular injury by placing the needle electrodes inferior to the eyebrow. Two additional electrodes are placed subcutaneously in a distal location such as over the sternum or the ipsilateral shoulder, one serving as a ground for the recording channels and the other as a return for the monopolar nerve stimulator. **Fig. 1** shows the ground and anode electrodes placed on the forehead, a location we had used for many years and is used in many centers today. In more recent years, we place these electrodes on the sternum which appears to result in less cautery artifact. Consistency is important to reduce errors. We routinely color code electrodes: blue for eyes, red for lips, green for ground, white for anode, and black for cathode. Our mnemonic for this, which many have adopted internationally, is Blue Eyes, Red Lips, Green Ground. The cathode is used for stimulation rather than the anode because cathodal stimulation is more effective.

Step 4. After the electrodes are connected to the nerve monitor, check the impedances of the different electrode pairs. The independent electrode impedance should be less than 5 kohm, whereas interelectrode impedance should be less than 2 kohm. If the impedance is too high, this suggests that the needle electrodes may be poorly positioned or faulty; the electrodes should be repositioned or replaced and then retested.

Step 5. Perform a "tap test" to check the integrity from the electrode to the recording device. Tapping the skin over each pair of facial recording electrodes should elicit a visual signal on the oscilloscope as well as a concurrent acoustic signal from the loudspeaker. It is important that facial nerve monitors represent responses not just visually on an oscilloscope but also acoustically so the surgeon receives real-time feedback. The surgeon cannot continually observe the oscilloscope and operate. For those who only rely on a technician watching the screen, if the technician looks away for a moment during a lengthy case, an important response can be missed. Conversely, devices that only have an audible response with no oscilloscope lose the opportunity to differentiate some forms of artifact from true responses. Multimodality monitoring increases the need to have a technical assistant. Other increasingly

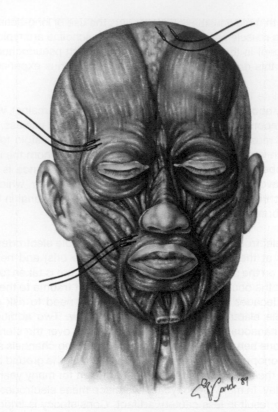

Fig. 1. EMG recording montage used for 2-channel facial nerve monitoring. Paired electrodes are placed subcutaneously at the nasolabial groove (orbicularis oris) and near the eyebrow (orbicularis oculi) on the side to be monitored. Ground and anodal return electrodes can be placed high on the forehead (as shown) or, more commonly today, near the sternum (not shown). (*From* Kartush JM. Electroneurography and intraoperative facial monitoring in contemporary neurotology. Otolaryngol Head Neck Surg 1989;101:501; with permission.)

common modalities include laryngeal monitoring, auditory brainstem recording, somatosensory recording, and transcranial motor evoked potentials.

One common misunderstanding about the tap test is that hearing a response means that everything is working perfectly. This is not the case. Performing a tap test on a paralyzed face also creates a response, because tapping adjacent to an inserted electrode elicits an electrical artifact, not a true CMAP. The tap test has benefit in that it checks whether the connections from the recording electrodes to the oscilloscope and loudspeaker are intact, but it provides no information regarding the stimulating side of the system or about the functional state of the facial nerve or muscles. Thus, the setup is not finished after obtaining a positive tap test, but should also include the final 2 steps (described later).

Step 6. After incision and soft tissue exposure, check for current flow using a nerve stimulator. Touching the stimulator to soft tissue or wet bone should result in near 100% conduction of current from the stimulator to the monitor. Most devices display the returned current visually. Others may present an audible tone (eg, warble) or digital voice confirmation (eg, stimulus) that is distinct from a true response tone (eg, beep). The volume of the nerve monitor should be adjusted from the start to ensure that the surgeon can hear it over the ambient sounds in the operating room (eg, the drill, suction, laser, babble).

Step 7. Stimulate the nerve at an early point in the surgery before any significant manipulation of the nerve is performed. Placing the nerve stimulator near the porus acousticus, the root entry zone, or the second genu of the facial nerve after entry into the mastoid antrum during surgical exposure triggers a CMAP that is detected by the facial nerve monitor. The distance from the nerve and the amount of intervening tissues determines the current setting. Even though a normal facial nerve responds to 0.05 mA in the cerebellopontine angle, if the surgeon has 0.5 cm of intervening soft tissue or a few millimeters of bone, the current may need to be temporarily turned up to 1 to 2 mA before a baseline, far-field response can be obtained by volume conduction of the current through intervening tissue. Once a confirmatory baseline response is obtained, we reduce the current intensity to lower levels based on how distal we are from the nerve. In 30 years of using such mapping techniques with modern current settings (eg, pulse durations ~100 microseconds at ~5 Hz), we have observed no detrimental effect to the nerve. Conversely, those who neglect to routinely obtain a baseline response before nerve dissection risk monitoring with a system that may be faulty due to set up errors, persistent muscle relaxants or chemical paralysis from lidocaine.

See **Box 1** for a summary of steps for facial nerve monitoring.

Interpretation of intraoperative facial nerve EMG monitoring
The surgeon must be knowledgeable not only in anatomy but in the pertinent neurophysiology to make proper use of monitoring. Even flawlessly accrued information conveyed to a surgeon is of little value if the data cannot be interpreted and surgical maneuvers implemented based on the information. Electromyographic responses can:

1. Occur because of trauma or other nonelectric stimuli, or
2. Be electrically triggered.

Continuous free-running EMG Responses caused by trauma or other nonelectric stimuli are detected during continuous free-running EMG, which monitors for CMAPs

---

Box 1
Facial nerve monitoring set up

1. Ensure that the anesthesiologist avoids the use of long-acting muscle relaxants

2. Be wary about local anesthesia (eg, lidocaine or marcaine), which can chemically induce a temporary facial paresis, rendering monitoring useless

3. Place electrodes carefully

4. After the electrodes are connected to the nerve monitor, check the impedances of the different electrode pairs

5. Perform a tap test to check the integrity from the electrode to the recording device

6. After incision and soft tissue exposure, check for current flow using a nerve stimulator

7. Stimulate the nerve at an early point in the surgery before any significant manipulation of the nerve is performed

in response to any type of nerve irritation. Two types of CMAP activity have been categorized, depending on the type of irritation[23]:

1. A burst potential, which consists of a single polyphasic response caused by near-simultaneous activation of multiple motor units (**Fig. 2**)

This is typically observed following direct contact of the nerve with surgical instruments. The response is fatigable with repeated contact with the nerve. In addition, the response is accompanied by a synchronous sound produced by the loudspeaker to provide the surgeon direct feedback.

2. A train potential, which consists of multiple asynchronous responses from different motor units, lasting anywhere from seconds to minutes (**Fig. 3**).

This potential is accompanied by a sound from the loudspeaker described as that of popping corn or an airplane engine. It may be caused by mechanical injury (pressure or stretch) to the nerve from prolonged dissection or retraction, with a greater intensity and longer duration of the potential corresponding with an increased degree of injury. To minimize nerve injury, the surgeon typically stops dissection and removes/relaxes the retractors in response to a prolonged train and waits for the EMG to return to baseline, which may take several minutes. Occasionally, one channel has prolonged train activity and the other channel does not. Many devices allow 1 channel to be silenced in these circumstances but the surgeon should frequently return to check the silenced channel and unmute it as soon as possible to avoid missing relevant feedback.

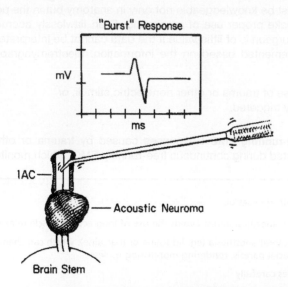

Fig. 2. Burst potential. The burst potential is one type of facial EMG response, often elicited by mechanical contact of surgical instruments with the facial nerve. IAC, internal auditory canal. (*From* Kartush JM. Electroneurography and intraoperative facial monitoring in contemporary neurotology. Otolaryngol Head Neck Surg 1989;101:499; with permission.)

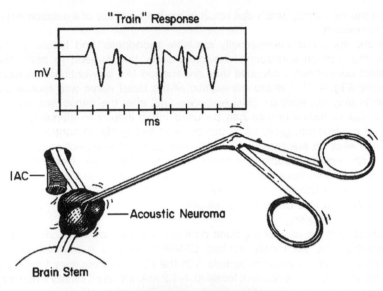

MECHANICAL STIMULATION

Pressure or Traction

Fig. 3. Train potential. The train potential is a second type of facial EMG response, often caused by mechanical/ischemic injury (pressure or stretch) to the nerve from dissection or retraction. (*From* Kartush JM. Electroneurography and intraoperative facial monitoring in contemporary neurotology. Otolaryngol Head Neck Surg 1989;101:500; with permission.)

Another cause of train potentials is thermal injury to the nerve, secondary to use of the laser or electrocautery. The EMG response may occur in a delayed manner following a thermal insult, particularly with electrocautery, because the monitor is disabled due to of the electrical artifact created by the cautery. Severe cautery injury may result in electrical silence without train EMG potentials. Therefore, if cautery injury is suspected, the nerve should be electrically stimulated as soon as possible to determine whether or not the nerve has been injured. Transmission of vibrations from the drill along adjacent bone to the nerve may also trigger a brief train potential, with the largest potentials observed when the drill is directly over the nerve. Other causes of train potentials include temperature irritation from hot or cold irrigation, osmotic irritation from hypertonic saline, and lightening of general anesthesia resulting in facial muscle fasciculations. Simply aspirating cerebrospinal fluid (CSF) from around the nerve in the cerebellopontine angle may result in a temperature change, going from a warm body temperature to as cool as the operating room. This temperature change may trigger a train potential. Although it does not indicate trauma, the surgeon should be aware of it in the differential interpretation of train potentials.

Stimulus-triggered EMG The second manner in which intraoperative facial nerve monitoring is used is via a stimulus-triggered EMG. The nerve can be stimulated with either monopolar or bipolar stimulators, each having its own distinct advantages and disadvantages. Furthermore, because of the presence of CSF and blood in the field, some degree of electrical insulation along the stimulator's shaft is required to reduce current shunting away and causing false-negative errors. High-quality insulation is needed, particularly on probes that have a flexible tip. Bending the tip creates stress on the insulation, which can result in inadvertent loss of insulation fragments within the cranium.

There are numerous commercially available monopolar and bipolar probes. In contrast, the Kartush stimulating dissectors allow the surgeon to both stimulate and dissect concurrently, because they are shaped like conventional microsurgical instruments (**Fig. 4**).[11,12] Sharp transection of the facial nerve with routine surgical instruments may not elicit an EMG response until after the transection has already occurred. Conventional probes can be used intermittently to stimulate the nerve but do not prevent iatrogenic injury unless used frequently. In contrast, stimulating instruments elicit an electrically evoked CMAP during the dissection to provide the surgeon with ongoing feedback on nerve location and integrity. Commercially available stimulating drills have become available as well, although there is little data on their efficacy. Alternatively, as suggested by Silverstein and White years ago, current can be connected to a drill using an alligator clip. The surgeon however should be aware of current shunting.[24]

In contrast with the click of the burst potential and the popping corn sound of the train potential, the electrically evoked CMAP results in a machine-gun sound composed of precisely timed potentials with the stimulus frequency typically set to approximately 5 Hz. Higher current levels (0.4–1.2 mA) are used initially when mapping out the approximate location of the facial nerve with a stimulating instrument. Lower current levels (0.05–0.2 mA) are subsequently used for more precise localization of the nerve and during dissection of the final small tumor remnants. If a nerve is severely injured or transected, stimulation proximal to the site of injury does not evoke a CMAP. However, stimulation distal to the injury evokes a CMAP because, even for the most severe injuries, wallerian degeneration progresses slowly for 48 to 72 hours. Thus, it is important at the end of the case to stimulate the facial nerve at the most proximal extent of the dissection to show that the nerve is intact throughout the surgical field.

False-positive errors can occur with stimulus-triggered EMG. One example is a phenomenon called (current jump), wherein stimulation of a structure near the facial nerve results in stimulation of the nerve itself through volume conduction of current, leading to incorrect identification of that structure as the facial nerve (**Fig. 5**). This error

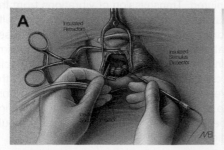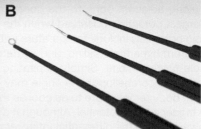

Fig. 4. Use of Kartush stimulating dissectors. (*A*) This set of specialized surgical instruments allows for *simultaneous* dissection and stimulation around motor nerves. They are also useful in spine and brainstem surgery. (*B*) Close-up view of the Kartush Stimulating Instruments (Neurosign, The Magstim Company, Whitland, Carmarthenshire, United Kingdom), with several different configurations to allow for meticulous dissection in a variety of situations. (*From* [*A*] Kartush JM, LaRouere MJ, Graham MD, et al. Intraoperative cranial nerve monitoring during posterior skull base surgery. Skull Base Surg 1991;1:88, with permission; and [*B*] Copyright © Kartush JM, MD.)

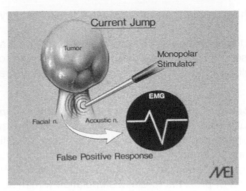

Fig. 5. Current jump. Monopolar stimulation of a structure (such as the acoustic nerve) near the facial nerve can result in a false-positive response if the current jumps via volume conduction to the nearby facial nerve. This jump tends to occur at higher current levels and can be minimized by using lower current levels or bipolar stimulators. (Copyright © Kartush JM, MD.)

can be minimized by using lower current levels when stimulating near the nerve, or by switching to a bipolar stimulator, which has a narrower field of current spread. Bipolar stimulators are superior when discrete differentiation of nerve from adjacent tissue is required, whereas monopolar stimulation is optimal when mapping the general location of the nerve.

False-negative errors can also occur with stimulated EMG. Such errors may be secondary to current shunting away from the nerve into adjacent fluid or soft tissue, resulting in inadequate current to depolarize the nerve despite the probe being close to the nerve (**Fig. 6**). Other causes not directly related to the surgical field include neuromuscular blockade paralysis of the nerve and incorrect setup of the nerve monitor. Repeated stimulation of the facial nerve at appropriate current levels (as

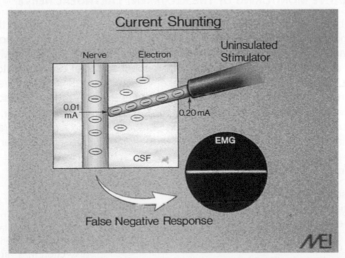

Fig. 6. Current shunting. False-negative responses can occur with current shunting if CSF, blood, or soft tissue shunts current from the nerve stimulator away from the facial nerve. (Copyright © Kartush JM, MD.)

described earlier with stimulating dissectors) does not result in nerve fatigue and false-negatives.

Failure to respond to stimulation can be caused by an anatomically disrupted nerve, but can also be caused by lesser levels of trauma. Thus, failure to respond to stimulation cannot by itself be used as a determinant to resect and graft an unresponsive nerve segment.

Outcomes of intraoperative monitoring for vestibular schwannoma

The use of intraoperative monitoring for vestibular schwannoma surgery has resulted in improved facial nerve outcomes.[25] Several studies have specifically examined the correlation between intraoperative facial nerve monitoring findings and postoperative facial nerve outcomes. Lower final stimulus thresholds, higher CMAP response amplitudes, and lower ratios of proximal to distal stimulation thresholds have been correlated to better postoperative facial nerve outcomes.[26] Recently, Prell and colleagues[27] found that a real-time CMAP measure of train potential time (specifically, the A train, which is one type of this potential) is relevant to facial nerve outcomes. Specifically, they recommended that, if the total accumulated A train potential time was greater than 2.5 seconds, consideration should be given to limiting further dissection, because postoperative facial nerve weakness was more likely.

One of the greatest benefits of facial nerve monitoring is the ability to use it for behavioral modification of surgical technique. If a certain dissection method is leading to repeated CMAPs, the surgeon should consider a different surgical strategy to address the tumor. In particular, monitoring has shown the benefits of sharp rather than blunt dissection when the nerve is clearly delineated visually or by electric stimulation.

If monitoring leads to a high suspicion for intraoperative facial nerve injury, consideration may be given for use of intravenous hydroxyethyl starch and/or nimodipine. These compounds may have a vasoactive and neuroprotective effect on the nerve with potentially better postoperative facial nerve outcomes.[28]

INTRAOPERATIVE MONITORING OF THE RECURRENT LARYNGEAL NERVE

When vestibular schwannomas are large and extend significantly toward the jugular foramen, monitoring of the recurrent laryngeal nerve (RLN) should be considered. Similar to facial nerve monitoring, RLN monitoring is also based on the EMG. Therefore, many of the principles discussed with respect to facial nerve monitoring also apply to RLN monitoring. For example, local anesthesia near the nerve should be avoided, which, in the context of the RLN, includes the use of topical viscous lidocaine by the anesthesiologist during intubation. However, as noted later, because RLN monitoring is typically performed using adjacent surface electrodes rather than intramuscular needle electrodes, there is reduced accuracy and greater chances for error.

Three primary methods have been used to record laryngeal responses:

1. Intramuscular needle electrodes
2. Fiberoptic scopes to look for vocal cord movement
3. Surface electrodes along an endotracheal tube.

The first method uses intramuscular needle electrodes placed into the laryngeal musculature either via direct laryngoscopy or percutaneously through the cricothyroid membrane.[29] However, the endolaryngeal method is infrequently performed today because the electrodes are difficult to place accurately (particularly for those outside the field of otolaryngology, who have little experience with direct laryngoscopy). In addition, the use of needle electrodes placed by either technique may cause trauma, bleeding, or infection to the vocal cords. Endotracheal tube balloons have been inadvertently punctured. Furthermore, the electrodes may become displaced during surgery without the surgeon noticing.

The second method to monitor the RLN is the use of fiberoptic scopes to look for vocal cord movement. However, similar to early attempts at visual monitoring of the facial musculature, they do not detect small responses and cannot be observed continuously throughout a surgical procedure.

These limitations have led to the use of surface electrodes along an endotracheal tube, which is the third and most common modality to monitor the RLN, because of their relative ease of use. Laryngeal surface recording electrodes may be manufactured attached to an endotracheal tube (eg, NIM EMG endotracheal tube, Medtronic, Jacksonville, FL, USA), or they may be applied onto any desired endotracheal tube using stick-on surface electrodes (eg, Neurosign, Carmarthenshire, UK; IOM Solutions, Ventura, CA, USA.). By carrying them along with the endotracheal tube, their positioning at the vocal cords is no longer dependent on a surgeon also trained in laryngeal endoscopy. Nevertheless, the tube must be precisely placed during intubation such that the electrodes are at the level of the true vocal cords to allow recording of the laryngeal musculature CMAP. Head rotation or extension may displace the tube and, therefore, reassessment of the tube position with a laryngoscope, fiberoptic scope, or device such as the GlideScope (Verathon Medical, Bothell, WA, USA) should be considered.

Although surface electrode technology is currently the most popular modality for monitoring the RLN, it also has several inherent weaknesses:

- Surface electrodes lack the sensitivity and stability of intramuscular needle electrodes.
- Suboptimal positioning of surface electrodes may impair the ability to detect laryngeal responses, and may also lead to erroneous recording of EMG activity from the adjacent pharyngeal musculature (false-positives), particularly at high levels of stimulation. Poor positioning may occur during intubation or head positioning because of the electrodes being too deep, too shallow, or malrotated.
- With respect to the stick-on electrodes (which are taped on the endotracheal tube about 1–2 cm above the cuff), the electrodes may become displaced, especially during longer surgeries as the adhesive become less adherent in the moist environment of the larynx. To minimize this, if the anesthesiologist prefers to use a standard lubricant on the tube (not lidocaine), it should be applied carefully *after* the electrode has been attached to the dry tube.
- The endotracheal tube size influences the positioning of the electrodes. If the tube is too small in diameter, this may result in marginal contact with the glottic inlet. Conversely, if the diameter of the endotracheal tube is too large, it may result in mechanical trauma to the larynx. As of this writing, Medtronic does not offer half sizes of its NIM endotracheal tubes in the United States, which reduces the opportunity for optimizing the electrode-to-vocal-cord fit. In contrast, stick-on electrodes can be used with any inexpensive endotracheal tube of the anesthesiologist's preference.
- Another caveat clinicians should be aware of regarding the NIM EMG endotracheal tube relates to the wire reinforcement within the tube. Surgeons and anesthesia providers alike should read the Medtronic package insert to maximize

safety and efficacy of this product. Although this reinforcement provides a generally desired increase in rigidity during intubation, the wire can also become
kinked or unraveled, leading to airway obstruction. To date, the internal stiffening
wire have been covered by a thin layer of silicon within the lumen of the endotracheal tube, rather than being integrated in the harder Silastic. Common types of
instrumentation of the tube (such as with a tube exchanger or suctioning with
a catheter) can lead to unraveling of the wire within the tube, leading to buildup
of clot/mucus, with resultant airway obstruction (**Fig. 7**).[30] Similarly, the patient
may inadvertently bite on the tube, resulting in the wire kinking toward the lumen
and not reexpanding, which may also lead to airway obstruction. Thus, to minimize these airway risks (1) a bite block should be used, and (2) suctioning or other
intraluminal manipulations of the NIM tube should be avoided.

• As with facial nerve monitoring, EMG monitoring of the RLN with all types of
recording electrodes is disabled during the use of electrocautery because the
stimulus-ignore period is programmed to disregard the electrical artifact generated by cautery. Thus, thermal nerve injury that occurs during the use of cautery
may not be detected until after the injury has already occurred. To assess for
potential injury, a nerve stimulator can be placed on the vagus or RLN to document an EMG response. If no response is obtained, an option during thyroid
surgery to rule out a false-negative error is finger palpation of the posterior cri-
coarytenoid (PCA) muscle; palpable contraction of the PCA with no signal on
EMG points to a malfunctioning monitoring setup. However, this false-negative
check is not feasible during vestibular schwannoma surgery. Instead, just as in
facial nerve monitoring, baseline stimulation should be performed as early as
possible using moderate-level mapping currents before there is a chance that
the nerve may be traumatized. Stimulation should be repeated before and after
any particularly risky tumor maneuver to ensure appropriate function of the monitoring system and to detect at the earliest possible time the maneuver that may
have resulted in nerve injury.

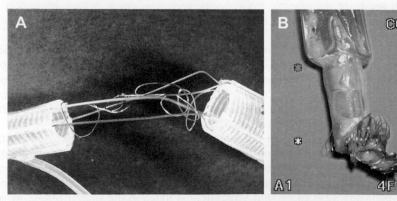

Fig. 7. Airway issues of NIM EMG endotracheal tube. (*A*) Use of instrumentation (eg, suction
catheter) can lead to unraveling of the wires within the endotracheal tube and potential
airway compromise. (*B*) A second example of airway obstruction with the NIM endotracheal
tube, secondary to fibrin clot/mucus buildup on the exposed wires within the lumen of the
tube. (*From* [*A*] Evanina EY, Hanisak JL. Case study involving suctioning of an electromyographic endotracheal tube. AANA J 2005;73:112; with permission; and [*B*] Copyright
© Kartush JM, MD.)

- None of the laryngeal electrodes described are intended for use after surgery, nor are they MRI compatible. When prolonged intubation after surgery is required, all laryngeal electrode devices must be exchanged for a regular endotracheal tube at the end of the procedure. However, an internal tube exchanger should be avoided if possible with the NIM tube because of the risk of wire delamination discussed previously.

SUMMARY

Surface recording of laryngeal responses can reduce the risk of vagal nerve injury during skull base surgery but surgeons and their monitoring personnel must be cognizant of the additional pitfalls of this evolving modality. Although intramuscular facial nerve monitoring is more accurate and reliable at this time, it is incumbent on the surgeon to understand both the technical and interpretive aspects of monitoring to optimize accuracy and patient safety.

REFERENCES

1. Harner SG, Daube JR, Ebersold MJ, et al. Improved preservation of facial nerve function with use of electrical monitoring during removal of acoustic neuromas. Mayo Clin Proc 1987;62:92–102.
2. Dickins J, Graham SS. A comparison of facial nerve monitoring systems in cerebellopontine angle surgery. Am J Otol 1991;12:1–6.
3. Kwartler JA, Luxford WM, Atkins J, et al. Facial nerve monitoring in acoustic tumor surgery. Otolaryngol Head Neck Surg 1991;104:814–7.
4. Silverstein H, Rosenberg SI, Flanzer J, et al. Intraoperative facial nerve monitoring in acoustic neuroma surgery. Am J Otol 1993;14:524–32.
5. Magluilo G, Petti R, Vingolo GM, et al. Facial nerve monitoring in skull base surgery. J Laryngol Otol 1994;108:557–9.
6. Wilson L, Lin E, Lalwani A. Cost-effectiveness of intraoperative facial nerve monitoring in middle ear or mastoid surgery. Laryngoscope 2003;113:1736–45.
7. National Institutes of Health (NIH). Acoustic neuroma. NIH Consens Statement 1991;9:1–24. Available at: http://consensus.nih.gov/1991/1991AcousticNeuroma 087html.htm. Accessed October 22, 2010.
8. Kartush JM. Electroneurography and intraoperative facial monitoring in contemporary neurotology. Otolaryngol Head Neck Surg 1989;101:496–503.
9. Kartush J. President's inaugural address: Poor monitoring is worse than no monitoring. American Society of Neurophysiologic Monitoring, first annual meeting. Novi, 1989.
10. Sittel C, Guntinas-Lichius O, Strepel M, et al. Variability of repeated facial nerve electroneurography in healthy subjects. Laryngoscope 1998;108:1177–80.
11. Kartush JM, Lilly DJ, Kemink JL. Facial electroneurography: clinical and experimental investigations. Otolaryngol Head Neck Surg 1985;93:516–23.
12. Kartush JM, Niparko JK, Bledsoe SC, et al. Intraoperative facial nerve monitoring: a comparison of stimulating electrodes. Laryngoscope 1985;95:1536–40.
13. Kartush JM, LaRouere MJ, Graham MD, et al. Intraoperative cranial nerve monitoring during posterior skull base surgery. Skull Base Surg 1991;1:85–92.
14. Holland NR. Intraoperative electromyography. J Clin Neurophysiol 2002;19:444–53.
15. Sargent EW, Kartush JM, Graham MD. Meatal facial nerve decompression in acoustic neuroma resection. Am J Otol 1995;16:457–64.

16. Gianoli G, Kartush J. Delayed facial palsy after acoustic tumor resection: the role of viral reactivation. Am J Otol 1996;17:625–9.
17. Bendet E, Rosenberg SI, Willcox TO, et al. Intraoperative facial nerve monitoring: a comparison between electromyography and mechanical-pressure monitoring techniques. Am J Otol 1999;20:793–9.
18. Sugita K, Kobayashi S. Technical and instrumental improvements in the surgical management of acoustic neurinomas. J Neurosurg 1982;57:747–52.
19. Akagami R, Dong CC, Westerberg BD. Localized transcranial electrical motor evoked potentials for monitoring cranial nerves in cranial base surgery. Neurosurgery 2005;57:78–85.
20. Teudt IU, Nevel AE, Izzo AD, et al. Optical stimulation of the facial nerve: a new monitoring technique? Laryngoscope 2007;117:1641–7.
21. De Seta E, Bertoli G, Seta DD, et al. New development in intraoperative video monitoring of facial nerve: a pilot study. Otol Neurotol 2010;31:1498–502.
22. Kartush JM, Bouchard KR. Intraoperative facial nerve monitoring: otology, neurotology and skull base surgery. In: Kartush JM, Bouschard KR, editors. Neuromonitoring in otology and head and neck surgery. New York: Raven Press; 1992. p. 99–120.
23. Prass RL, Luders H. Acoustic (loudspeaker) facial electromyographic monitoring: part 1. Neurosurgery 1986;19:392–400.
24. Silverstein H, White D. Continuous electrical stimulation as a helpful adjunct during intraoperative facial nerve monitoring. Skull Base Surgery 1991;1(2): 127–31.
25. Kartush JM, Lundy L. Facial nerve outcomes in acoustic neuroma surgery. Otolaryngol Clin North Am 1992;25:623–47.
26. Yousef AS, Downes AE. Intraoperative neurophysiological monitoring in vestibular schwannoma surgery: advances and clinical implications. Neurosurg Focus 2009;27:E9.
27. Prell J, Rachinger J, Scheller C, et al. A real-time monitoring system for the facial nerve. Neurosurgery 2010;66:1064–73.
28. Scheller C, Richter HP, Engelhardt M, et al. The influence of prophylactic vasoactive treatment on cochlear and facial nerve functions after vestibular schwannoma surgery: a prospective and open-label randomized pilot study. Neurosurgery 2007;61:92–8.
29. Beck DL, Maves MD. Recurrent laryngeal nerve monitoring during thyroid surgery. In: Kartush JM, Bouschard KR, editors. Neuromonitoring in otology and head and neck surgery. New York: Raven Press; 1992. p. 151–62.
30. Evanina EY, Hanisak JL. Case study involving suctioning of an electromyographic endotracheal tube. AANA J 2005;73:111–3.

Acoustic Neuroma Neurophysiologic Correlates:
Vestibular-Preoperative, Intraoperative, and Postoperative

Gerard J. Gianoli, MD*, James S. Soileau, MD

KEYWORDS

• Vestibular schwannoma • Acoustic neuroma • Vestibular loss • Dizziness
• Dysequilibrium • Vestibular testing • Electronystagmography • Rotational chair
• Vestibular evoked myogenic potentials • Posturography

Key Abbreviations: ACOUSTIC NEUROMA NEUROPHYSIOLOGIC CORRELATES	
AN	Acoustic neuroma
BPPV	Benign paroxysmal positional vertigo
CDP	Computerized dynamic posturography
CPA	Cerebellopontine angle
ENG	Electronystagmography
IAC	Internal auditory canal
IVN	Inferior vestibular nerve
SVN	Superior divisions of the vestibular nerve
SOT	Sensory organization test
VEMP	Vestibular evoked myogenic potentials
oVEMP	Ocular vestibular evoked myogenic potentials

Acoustic neuroma (AN) is a misnomer for the benign tumor discussed in this article, because it does not originate from the acoustic nerve and is not a neuroma. AN is a benign tumor arising from the Schwann cells of the vestibular nerve, more appropriately called a vestibular schwannoma. Consequently, the vestibular nerve is always involved with AN and there is virtually always some vestibular system pathology secondary to AN development. Although by far the most common presenting complaints in AN patients are hearing loss and tinnitus, this disorder is primarily one of the vestibular system, specifically the vestibular nerve. It is important to keep this in mind even though most patients do not complain of vestibular symptoms before intervention. However, vestibular complaints are common among patients after intervention.[1]

The Ear and Balance Institute, 17050 Medical Center Drive, Suite # 315, Baton Rouge, LA 70816, USA
* Corresponding author.
E-mail address: ggianoli@gmail.com

Otolaryngol Clin N Am 45 (2012) 307–314
doi:10.1016/j.otc.2011.12.004
0030-6665/12/$ – see front matter © 2012 Elsevier Inc. All rights reserved.

Because intervention for AN by nature results in loss of vestibular function beyond the damage already inflicted by the tumor, it behooves the surgeon to have some knowledge of the preoperative status of the vestibular system because this can, on occasion, affect the treatment mode. Intraoperatively, the origin of the AN from either the inferior (IVN) or superior divisions of the vestibular nerve (SVN) can have some prognostic importance regarding hearing preservation and possible residual vestibular function. Postoperatively, in terms of morbidity from AN treatment, balance dysfunction is one of the most common consequences.[1]

As already mentioned, the AN arises from the Schwann cells surrounding the vestibular division of the eighth cranial nerve. Specifically, it has been proposed that ANs arise at the transition zone of the central myelin and peripheral myelin sheaths, known as the Obersteiner-Redlich zone. This location is also in the same vicinity as the vestibular (Scarpa) ganglion. It should be noted that although this region appears to be the most common site of AN origin, the site of this zone is variable and there are many examples of AN arising distal to this region as well. In any event, the vast majority of ANs appear to arise from within the medial portion of the internal auditory canal (IAC), with only a small minority originating in the lateral end of the IAC. Even fewer appear to originate at the porus acusticus or in the cerebellopontine angle (CPA) cistern itself. There is a small proportion that even arises within the vestibular end organ. AN can arise from either the IVN or SVN, giving somewhat differing functional vestibular pathology.

AN growth results in compression of the surrounding structures. Presumably the resulting compression of the associated vestibular nerve, and/or its blood supply, results in primary neural dysfunction; as already mentioned, it is rare for direct end-organ involvement. However, the degree of compression, or whether compression of the associated nerve occurs at all, is dependent on the size of the tumor and its location. Medially based AN, especially if there is minimal or no IAC component, will tend to have less impact on function, whereas laterally based tumors will tend to have more profound effects on vestibular function. Such effects are likely attributable to the limited degree of expansion for IAC tumors because of their bony confines, compared with the relatively larger area for expansion within the CPA for a medially based AN. This difference explains the incongruity of a large medial tumor with no significant vestibular loss in contrast to a small IAC tumor that may demonstrate near total loss of vestibular function.

Of course, at its outset a small tumor may cause no neural compression and cause no dysfunction, and the patient will be asymptomatic. As the tumor grows and causes surrounding compression, dysfunction occurs as the associated structures are compressed. The 4 anatomic stages of AN growth are:

1. Intracanalicular
2. Cisternal
3. Brainstem compressive
4. Hydrocephalic

In direct opposition to what one may expect, the worst vestibular symptoms are typically seen at the intracanalicular stage. During this stage, as the vestibular nerve is being progressively destroyed the patients may be asymptomatic or may have episodic vertigo suggestive of a peripheral vestibular disorder. As further growth occurs, the vertigo diminishes and the vestibular symptoms usually subside. Later, as the cisternal phase progresses and the brainstem compressive phase begins, onset of dysequilibrium occurs and signs of central vestibular dysfunction arise. The dysequilibrium worsens as the hydrocephalic stage of growth takes place.

Although the primary means of vestibular dysfunction caused by AN appears to be neural compression, distinct end-organ effects have been demonstrated. Specifically, histopathology of the inner ear in some AN patients has demonstrated endolymphatic hydrops, and eosinophilic proteinaceous precipitate in the perilymphatic and endolymphatic spaces. In addition, there is degeneration of other inner ear structures, including hair cells, the stria vascularis, and the spiral ligament.[2] This process may possibly explain how a minority of patients with small AN present with episodic vertigo.

PREOPERATIVE VESTIBULAR TESTING

Vestibular testing has been used in the past as a screening procedure for AN. Although vestibular testing will frequently be abnormal in AN patients, there is a lack of sensitivity or specificity for the purpose of diagnostic screening tests. For vestibular testing to demonstrate an abnormality in an AN case, the tumor must be of adequate size to compromise either the blood supply (to the vestibular nerve or end organ) or the nerve itself to a sufficient degree so as to reduce the vestibular function on the side affected. In addition, the degree of vestibular loss must be sufficient to appear significant on vestibular testing; it must be borne in mind that the state of vestibular testing is such that minor differences in vestibular test responses are often considered insignificant. Consequently, small tumors may not have attained adequate size to result in vestibular loss, thus resulting in false-negative outcomes for vestibular testing as a screening device. By contrast, although vestibular test abnormalities are often the rule among AN patients, abnormalities on vestibular studies are a common finding among a host of other vestibular disorders, resulting in a relatively low degree of specificity in a large screening population. However, this does not mean that vestibular testing in AN patients is without merit.

The values of preoperative vestibular testing are mainly to help distinguish the nerve of origin for the AN, to establish a baseline function in not just the tumor ear but also the contralateral ear, and as a means to help prognosticate about functional postoperative vestibular status. The vestibular-nerve origin has more than just academic significance. SVN tumors have a better prognosis for hearing preservation than IVN tumors. Differentiation between IVN-based and SVN-based tumors can help determine whether a surgical approach to hearing preservation may or may not be warranted. Establishing normal vestibular function in the non-AN ear is important for postoperative rehabilitation. Severely diminished or absent vestibular function in the non-AN ear may warrant a more conservative approach to maintaining vestibular function in the AN ear.

Electronystagmography

Electronystagmography (ENG) has been the most studied vestibular test battery among AN patients, and its most useful subtest is the bithermal caloric test. On caloric testing, the vast majority of AN patients will demonstrate reduced or absent response on the affected side.[3] Because the caloric test is a test of the horizontal semicircular canal function and the SVN, tumors arising from the SVN have a higher rate of reduced caloric response than tumors arising from the IVN. Of course, once tumors of the IVN attain sufficient size they could compromise the adjacent SVN. In addition, the larger the tumor is the more likely that the caloric response will be diminished. As alluded to earlier, this is not a good screening test for AN, but from a practical standpoint a large AN without a corresponding hypoactive caloric response would lead one to suspect that the pathology may be something else, such as a meningioma.

As one would expect, spontaneous nystagmus frequently accompanies AN. Most typically, it is a nystagmus of the paretic type from the loss of unilateral vestibular function. However, other types of nystagmus can also be seen. As the AN grows and causes central compression, signs of brainstem and cerebellar dysfunction may manifest with Bruns nystagmus.[4] Bruns nystagmus is a combination of a gaze-evoked nystagmus from cerebellar compression and a paretic nystagmus from unilateral deafferentation. The resulting nystagmus is an asymmetric one with slow, large-amplitude beats of nystagmus looking to the side of the AN and fast, small-amplitude nystagmus when gaze is directed away from the side of the AN. As the tumor continues to grow, causing bilateral cerebellar compression, a more pure gaze-evoked nystagmus may predominate. Alternatively, with brainstem compression and increased intracranial pressure, vertical down-beat or up-beat nystagmus may be present.

Other abnormalities may be seen on ENG, including positional nystagmus, which can be seen with tumors of all sizes, and central findings that are virtually exclusive to the larger tumors presenting with compressive features. Among the central findings seen with larger tumors are impaired fixation suppression, optokinetic and smooth-pursuit abnormalities, and the aforementioned gaze-evoked nystagmus and vertical nystagmus.

Rotational Studies

Similar to ENG, rotational studies lack both specificity and sensitivity as a means for making the diagnosis of AN[5]; however, rotational chair studies are frequently abnormal, particularly when the tumor has grown in sufficient size to compromise the SVN.[6] Tumors arising from the IVN that are small and do not compromise the SVN should have no identifiable abnormality on rotational chair testing, because this is a test of the horizontal semicircular canal and the corresponding SVN. There is some evidence to suggest that high-frequency, vestibular autorotation testing in the vertical plane may identify vestibular abnormalities in this subgroup of AN patients.[7] When abnormalities are identified, the findings typically reflect evidence of a unilateral vestibular deficit with varying evidence of central compensation. In general, gain reduction is seen, especially if there is a concomitant caloric hypofunction. However, in some of the large tumors an increase in gain may be seen, representing central vestibular dysfunction, which is the inability to suppress vestibular eye movements. Asymmetry tending to the side of the AN is most characteristically seen, but eye asymmetry may occasionally go to the non-AN side.

Computerized Dynamic Posturography

Within the standard vestibular test battery, computerized dynamic posturography (CDP) probably is the least sensitive to identification of AN. However, it is not unusual to see reduced scores among AN patients on CDP. There seems to be a general correlation between the size of the AN and outcomes on sensory organization test condition 5 (SOT 5), with larger tumors resulting in poorer performance.[8] It has also been suggested that CDP may be a means to help identify AN of IVN origin as opposed to SVN origin.[9] CDP is a measure of the vestibulospinal reflex arc, but is more sensitive to end-organ components innervated by the IVN and is relatively less sensitive to the SVN-innervated components. Consequently, one would expect to see more frequent CDP abnormalities (SOT 5) among patients with IVN-based tumors than among those with SVN-based tumors. However, in practice this is not so straightforward and has not yet been definitively shown in study. This finding may possibly be explained by the slow growth of AN and concomitant central compensation/adaptation, resulting in somewhat better performance for some patients with IVN tumors and the eventual compromise of the IVN by tumors arising from the SVN.

Vestibular Evoked Myogenic Potentials

Vestibular evoked myogenic potentials (VEMP) is a testing technique that has recently made the transition from the research laboratory to the clinical laboratory, due to its popularity in the evaluation of patients with superior semicircular canal dehiscence. VEMP is a means of measuring otolithic function. Delivery of sound stimuli to the ear results in stimulation of the otolithic organ, which initiates reflex muscular contraction that can be measured and quantified for sensitivity, latency, and amplitude. The 2 most common methods are the cVEMP (cervical) with measurement of the sternocleidomastoid muscle and the oVEMP (ocular), which measures extraocular muscle contraction.

The generally accepted view at present is that the saccule may be more amenable to air-conducted sound stimuli, whereas the utricle is more sensitive to bone-conducted sound stimuli.[10] Because of this differential sensitivity to stimuli, the otolithic organs can be assessed separately for responsiveness. Consequently, the use of bone-conducted VEMP and air-conducted VEMP may be useful for distinguishing between IVN and SVN tumor origins. Air-conducted VEMP would be expected to more frequently demonstrate a deficit in IVN-based tumors, whereas bone-conducted VEMP would be more likely to demonstrate abnormalities in SVN-based tumors. Of course, the issue found with other distinguishing vestibular tests arises here as well. Once a tumor is of sufficient size, whether it arises from the SVN or the IVN, it has a tendency to compromise both divisions of the vestibular nerve. Therefore, the differential utility of this test is most useful with the smaller tumors.

INTRAOPERATIVE

There is no commonly used means or rationale for intraoperative vestibular nerve monitoring. A few studies, comparing total vestibular nerve resection with preservation of one branch, have demonstrated no significant difference in vestibular/balance outcomes. However, the distinction of AN arising from the IVN or the SVN has importance with regard to hearing preservation. The IVN lies in the inferior compartment of the IAC, adjacent to the cochlear nerve. Consequently, IVN tumors have a higher probability than SVN tumors of cochlear nerve invasion. Similarly, because of the IVN location, surgical dissection of an IVN tumor would more likely disrupt cochlear nerve blood supply to SVN tumors than would dissection of an SVN tumor. Because of these anatomic differences, AN patients who present for possible hearing-preservation surgery generally have a more favorable prognosis when vestibular studies suggest SVN origin for the tumor (absent/reduced caloric response, reduced gain on rotational studies, present air-conducted VEMP, and normal SOT 5 on CDP) than when vestibular studies suggest an IVN origin for the AN (normal caloric response, normal gain on rotational studies, present bone-conducted VEMP, and abnormal SOT 5 on CDP).

POSTOPERATIVE

Vestibular function is virtually always altered postoperatively. The surgical disruption of the vestibular nerve changes the patient's vestibular situation dramatically. Preoperatively, ANs grow slowly and cause a very slow decline in vestibular function. Consequently, central compensation likely occurs as the tumor grows, and most patients do not therefore encounter any significant vestibular symptoms. Postoperatively, the loss of residual vestibular function is sudden. In the case of a large AN that has destroyed most or all of vestibular function preoperatively, there is little or no change in vestibular function after surgical resection. In the case of the small AN that has had little decline in vestibular function preoperatively, surgical resection results in a dramatic change in vestibular function. This process explains the paradoxic phenomenon of patients with a large AN having generally less vertigo immediately after surgery than those with a small AN.

The postoperative vestibular affliction is a total unilateral loss of function in most cases. In the vast majority of cases, central compensation proceeds to the point of essentially normal daily function.[11] Of course, when a patient has only one functioning vestibular end organ there will always be some situations that provoke symptoms of dysequilibrium. These situations are typically novel ones whereby central compensation has not occurred, and with high-velocity movement toward the lesioned ear. In addition, patients who have attained complete central compensation can have recurrent symptoms of dysequilibrium when central decompensation occurs. This decompensation is often brought about during times of extreme fatigue, severe physical stress, and severe emotional stress.

For a minority of patients, central compensation does not occur and postoperative dysequilibrium will persist. The cause for this uncompensated vestibulopathy usually falls into 1 of 3 categories:

1. Central vestibular abnormality
2. Incomplete deafferentation with fluctuating vestibular function in the surgical ear
3. Unrecognized fluctuating vestibulopathy in the nonsurgical ear

Of course, it is certainly possible for more than one of these conditions to exist as well.

Central Vestibular Abnormalities

Central vestibular abnormalities are typically seen with the large AN that has progressed to the point of brainstem or cerebellar compression. Postoperatively, these patients will demonstrate central vestibular test abnormalities in addition to unilateral vestibular deafferentation. The existence of central vestibular abnormalities is the differentiating test finding for this group of patients. Vertical nystagmus, gaze nystagmus, impaired fixation suppression, and optokinetic and smooth-pursuit abnormalities can be seen on ENG. Rotational studies typically demonstrate reduced gain (peripheral loss finding), but may demonstrate an increased gain (central finding) in the rare case where the SVN is preserved. CDP does not help in differentiating these patients from the others, but does help in identifying multisystem balance dysfunction, which can complicate the postoperative AN dysequilibrium picture.

Incomplete Deafferentation

The scenario of incomplete deafferentation with fluctuating vestibular function in the surgical ear requires preservation of one branch of the vestibular nerve and preservation of the vestibular end organ. This situation is seen in hearing-preservation cases using either a middle fossa or retrosigmoid approach for hearing preservation in the typically smaller tumors. There is usually an absence of central vestibular test findings for these patients. The ENG and rotational studies show the picture of unilateral loss of vestibular function with poor compensation, exhibiting paretic spontaneous nystagmus, and unilateral absent caloric response on ENG, with reduced gain and asymmetry on rotational testing. If there has been preservation of the IVN, posterior canal benign paroxysmal positional vertigo (BPPV) may be present, which may cause the continued fluctuation of vestibular stimulation. Similarly, an atypical BPPV (from the horizontal or anterior semicircular canal) may be present with preservation of the SVN. In either of the aforementioned situations, the Dix-Hallpike test likely would be abnormal.

Unrecognized Fluctuating Vestibulopathy

The third scenario, of the unrecognized fluctuating vestibulopathy in the nonsurgical ear, would typically be easiest to recognize when there has been total deafferentation of the AN ear from surgical extirpation in a small or medium AN that had no compression of the brainstem or cerebellum. In this case, as in most cases of dysequilibrium, BPPV must be suspect because of its ubiquity. For absent concomitant BPPV, the test findings one would expect include unilateral absent caloric response in the surgical ear and a hypoactive caloric response in the nonsurgical ear. Spontaneous nystagmus would be present, and rotational studies would demonstrate reduced gain suggestive of bilateral loss of vestibular function.

SUMMARY

AN and vestibular schwannoma are benign tumors that grow from the Schwann cells surrounding the vestibular division of the eighth cranial nerve. Because of their origin, there is virtually always a concomitant vestibular lesion. Depending on the size and location of the AN, there will be a loss of peripheral vestibular function and/or central vestibular dysfunction. Although vestibular testing is frequently abnormal in AN patients, it lacks the sensitivity and specificity for use as a diagnostic screening device. However, vestibular testing is very useful in defining the vestibular abnormality associated with the AN preoperatively and postoperatively, may be helpful in planning surgery for hearing preservation, and is helpful in the diagnosis of postoperative dysequilibrium.

REFERENCES

1. Saman Y, Bamiou DE, Gleeson M. A contemporary review of balance dysfunction following vestibular schwannoma surgery. Laryngoscope 2009;119(11):2085–93.
2. Mahmud MR, Khan AM, Nadol JB. Histopathology of the inner ear in unoperated acoustic neuroma. Ann Otol Rhinol Laryngol 2003;112(11):979–86.
3. Harner SG, Laws ER. Diagnosis of acoustic neurinoma. Neurosurgery 1981;9(4): 373–9.
4. Lloyd SK, Baguley DM, Butler K, et al. Bruns' nystagmus in patients with vestibular schwannoma. Otol Neurotol 2009;30(5):625–8.
5. Moretz WH, Orchik DJ, Shea JJ, et al. Low-frequency harmonic acceleration in the evaluation of patients with intracanalicular and cerebellopontine angle tumors. Otolaryngol Head Neck Surg 1986;95(3 Pt 1):324–32.
6. Olson JE, Wolfe JW, Engelken EJ. Symposium on low-frequency harmonic acceleration, the rotary chair. Responses to low-frequency harmonic acceleration in patients with acoustic neuromas. Laryngoscope 1981;91(8):1270–7.
7. Saadat D, O'Leary DP, Pulec JL, et al. Comparison of vestibular autorotation and caloric testing. Otolaryngol Head Neck Surg 1995;113(3):215–22.
8. Gouveris H, Helling K, Victor A, et al. Comparison of electronystagmography results with dynamic posturography findings in patients with vestibular schwannoma. Acta Otolaryngol 2007;127(8):839–42.

9. Gouveris H, Akkafa S, Lippold R, et al. Influence of nerve of origin and tumor size of vestibular schwannoma on dynamic posturography findings. Acta Otolaryngol 2006;126(12):1281–5.

10. Yang TH, Liu SH, Young YH. Evaluation of guinea pig model for ocular and cervical vestibular-evoked myogenic potentials for vestibular function test. Laryngoscope 2010;120(9):1910–7.

11. Humphriss RL, Baguley DM, Moffat DA. Changes in dizziness handicap after vestibular schwannoma excision. Otol Neurotol 2003;24(4):661–5.

Neurofibromatosis 2

Michael Hoa, MD, William H. Slattery III, MD*

KEYWORDS

- Neurofibromatosis 2 (NF2) • NF2 diagnosis • NF2 imaging • NF2 management
- NF2 surgery

Neurofibromatosis 2 (NF2) is a rare syndrome characterized by:

- Bilateral vestibular schwannomas
- Multiple meningiomas
- Cranial nerve tumors
- Spinal tumors
- Eye abnormalities.

NF2 presents unique challenges to the otologists because hearing loss may be the presenting complaint leading to the diagnosis of the disorder. NF2 is invasive, requiring a multispecialist team approach for the evaluation and treatment of the disorder. The primary impairment is hearing loss resulting from bilateral vestibular schwannomas. NF2 must be differentiated from neurofibromatosis 1 (NF1); although the names are linked, the disease entities are distinctly different. This article reviews the clinical characteristics of NF2 and the current recommendations for evaluation and treatment.

NF2 DIFFERENTIATED FROM NF1

NF1 has distinctly different characteristics from NF2. NF1 and NF2 have been differentiated as completely different genetic diseases based on the chromosome responsible for the disease. NF1 has been localized to chromosome 17 and NF2 to chromosome 22.

NF1 is a multisystem disorder in which some features may be present at birth and others are age-related manifestations. A National Institutes of Health (NIH) Consensus Development Conference identified the following 7 features of the disease, of which 2 or more are required to establish the diagnosis of NF1:

1. Six café au lait spots of 5 mm or more in longest diameter in prepubertal patients and 15 mm in the longest diameter in postpubertal patients.

Funding support: None.
The authors have nothing to disclose.
House Clinic, House Research Institute, 2100 West 3rd Street, Suite 111, Los Angeles, CA 90057, USA
* Corresponding author.
E-mail address: wslattery@hei.org

Otolaryngol Clin N Am 45 (2012) 315–332
doi:10.1016/j.otc.2011.12.005
0030-6665/12/$ – see front matter © 2012 Elsevier Inc. All rights reserved.

2. Two or more neurofibromas of any type or 1 plexiform neurofibroma.
3. Freckling in the axilla or inguinal regions.
4. Optic glioma (optic pathway glioma).
5. Two or more Lisch nodules (iris hamartomas).
6. Distinct osseous lesions, such as sphenoid wing dysplasia or cortical thinning of the cortex of long bones with or without pseudoarthrosis.
7. First-degree relative (parent, sibling, or child) with NF1 according to the above-listed criteria.

Some patients also manifest learning disabilities or language disorders. A careful examination and detailed history of the patient's symptoms help distinguish NF1 and NF2.

CLINICAL CHARACTERISTICS OF NF2
Definition

The NIH Consensus Development Conference also developed guidelines for the diagnosis of NF2. NF2 is distinguished by bilateral vestibular schwannomas with multiple meningiomas, cranial nerve tumors, optic gliomas, and spinal tumors. A definite diagnosis is made based on the presence of bilateral vestibular schwannomas or developing a unilateral vestibular schwannoma by 30 years and a first-degree blood relative with NF2, or the presence of a unilateral vestibular schwannoma and developing at least 2 of the following conditions known to be associated with NF2: meningioma, glioma, schwannoma, or juvenile posterior subcapsular lenticular opacity/juvenile cortical cataract (**Box 1**).[1]

NF2 Clinical Presentation

There may be significant heterogeneity in the presentation of the disease from one individual to the other. Some individuals may have a very mild form of the disease, such as small vestibular schwannomas manifesting in an older individual, whereas some children present with multiple intracranial tumors at a very young age. Despite

---

Box 1
NF2 diagnostic criteria

Confirmed (definite) NF2

Bilateral VS or family history of NF2 (first-degree family relative) *plus*

1. Unilateral VS before 30 years of age *or*

2. Any 2 of the following: meningioma, glioma, schwannoma, or juvenile posterior subcapsular lenticular opacities/juvenile cortical cataract

Presumptive or probable NF2: Should evaluate for NF2

Unilateral VS before 30 years of age *plus* at least 1 of the following: meningioma, glioma, schwannoma, or juvenile posterior subcapsular lenticular opacities/juvenile cortical cataract

Multiple meningiomas (≥2) *plus* unilateral VS before 30 years of age *or* 1 of the following: glioma, schwannoma, or juvenile posterior subcapsular lenticular opacities/juvenile cortical cataract

Abbreviation: VS, vestibular schwannoma.
Adapted from Slattery WH. Neurofibromatosis 2. In: Brackmann DE, Shelton C, Arriaga MA, editors. Otologic surgery. Philadelphia: Elsevier; 2010. p. 691–701; with permission.

the heterogeneity of the disease, the expression of NF2 tends to be very similar within a family.[2]

There is a significant genetic component to the disease with much variability within the parameters of the observed phenotype. Studies have shown that a truncating mutation (nonsense and frame shift) may be linked with a more severe form of NF2.[3,4] The more severe form of NF2 is termed the Wishart form. Individuals with this severe form present with an early onset of the disease with multiple intracranial schwannomas and meningiomas that result in blindness, deafness, paralysis, and possible death by 40 years. Despite the strong genotype-phenotype correlation, individual differences in tumor growth occur within individuals, making it difficult to predict how an individual's tumors will change over time, even when the genotype is known. The milder form of NF2, or the Gardner form, is less debilitating. Schwannomas may remain stable for many years; few meningiomas develop; and patients may not develop symptoms until later in life and often have fewer associated disabilities. The genetic basis of the mild form has not been well characterized. Many of these may be mosaic forms of the disease.[2-10]

Prevalence and Incidence of NF2

The average age of diagnosis of NF2 is 25 years; however, many patients present with symptoms before the diagnosis. There is an average delay in the diagnosis of approximately 7 years.[11] There is no difference in the proportion of men versus women who develop NF2, and no prevalence has been described based on ethnicity. Epidemiologic studies place the incidence of NF2 between 1 in 33,000 live births[3] and 1 in 87,410 live births.[12]

Imaging Studies for NF2

All patients suspected of NF2 should have a high-quality magnetic resonance imaging (MRI) scan performed with thin cuts through the internal auditory canal (IAC). All patients diagnosed with a unilateral vestibular schwannoma should have a dedicated IAC series performed to ensure that there is no tumor on the opposite side. Patients diagnosed with NF2 should have a complete spine series performed to evaluate the spine and stage the disease. Commonly, small spinal tumors may be found in the cauda equina, and occasionally, a large asymptomatic schwannoma or meningioma may be found in the spine that could require treatment. Early treatment of spinal tumors can significantly reduce the morbidity associated with these tumors. Older patients who present with bilateral IAC tumors must be worked up for other carcinomas. It is unusual for patients older than 40 years to present with NF2, although with more sensitive MRI scanning techniques, most of these individuals are being diagnosed at an older age. Metastasis may rarely manifest with bilateral IAC lesions, and carcinoma should be ruled out in any patient older than 40 years who presents with bilateral IAC lesions.

A patient diagnosed with NF2 should have a complete cranial MRI scan with cervical, thoracic, and lumbar spinal imaging, which serves as a baseline. A 6-month follow-up MRI scan is recommended for patients with intracranial tumors. If the tumors exhibit stability, a yearly MRI scan of the intracranial structures is performed. Large tumors in the spine may be monitored with a similar frequency. If no spinal tumors are present, spinal imaging should be performed when the patient becomes symptomatic. Monitoring small-to-medium spinal tumors every 3 years is recommended when these tumors are present. Intracranial imaging is performed on a yearly basis unless studies over several years indicate stability of the tumors.

Box 2	
MRI studies for vestibular schwannoma	
Patient's Status	Imaging Study
Unilateral vestibular schwannoma	IAC
Screening for NF2	IAC
Diagnosis of NF2	AC/Cranial
	Complete Spine Series
	✔ Initial 6 month follow-up
	✔ 12 month scan if stable
	✔ 3 years for small spine tumors

Molecular Genetics of NF2

The NF2 gene was mapped to chromosome 22q12.2 in 1993.[13–15] The NF2 gene located at chromosome 22 codes for a tumor suppressor protein termed Merlin or Schwannomin, which negatively regulates Schwann cell production. The loss of this protein allows overproduction of Schwann cells. The mutation in the NF2 chain predisposes individuals to developing a schwannoma when the second hit occurs to the gene; control of Schwann cells is lost or mutated within the cell. Various types of mutations have been identified, including single-base substitutions, insertions, and deletions.[2,4,16–18] The mild, or Gardner, type of NF2 may be associated with missense mutations, whereas associations between the other mutations and phenotypes are not as clear.[10] The occurrence of NF2 is not restricted to families known to carry the mutation. Frequently, genetic mosaicism occurs, which may not be detected by common mutation analysis techniques.[19] Unilateral vestibular schwannomas may exhibit the same type of genetic markers as NF2.[20] The mutations in unilateral vestibular schwannomas are confined to the affected tumor tissue. In patients with NF2, the mutation is present in all cell types.[19]

Family History of NF2

NF2 is an autosomal dominant disease, and 50% of children of the affected individuals are at risk for developing the disease. Of the patients diagnosed with NF2, 50% present with a family history of NF2 and the other half have no family history of NF2 and are considered founder cases. The presentation and phenotype of NF2 tend to be similar within families. The likelihood of NF2 occurring in related individuals who do not exhibit clinical symptoms similar to those in an affected family member is small. Consideration must still be given to screening these individuals for risks, despite the lack of clinical symptoms. Individuals at risk for developing NF2, including children of NF2-affected patients and their siblings, must be screened to provide an early diagnosis. Fifty percent of all children of patients with NF2 are found to have the disease. Siblings of a patient diagnosed with NF2 are at risk, especially if the parent also has NF2. The type of screening and timing of screening depend on the NF2 center's preference. Early screening is advocated so that tumors may be diagnosed presymptomatically. MRI or genetic blood testing may be used for screening.

Screening for NF2

MRI

MRI screening of potentially affected individuals uses a postcontrast T1-weighted sequence of the full head with thin cuts through the IAC. A dedicated IAC MRI scan identifies most patients with NF2 by showing vestibular schwannomas. Screening of the spine and ophthalmologic examination should be considered if the cranial MRI scan result is positive. An audiogram (pure tone thresholds) or a current clinical standard auditory brainstem response (ABR) testing is likely to miss small vestibular schwannomas. MRI can diagnose presymptomatic lesions.

MRI is recommended for at-risk children when this test can be performed without sedation; this usually can be done when the child is 7 to 9 years old. A recommended first step for children younger than 7 years is an audiogram. Any child with an NF2-associated symptom, such as hearing loss or facial weakness, should be screened irrespective of the need for sedation or age; MRI should be performed as soon as possible after the symptoms become apparent.

Molecular testing

Identification of the NF2 gene and chromosome 22 has made genetic testing possible. Patients with NF2 should see a genetic counselor to discuss the hereditary consequences of the disease. Blood testing for the mutation identifies the defect of the NF2 gene in approximately 70% to 75% of patients with a known diagnosis of NF2. Blood screening of family members is done depending on whether the defect is identified in the affected individual or not. The use of blood screening for patients without a diagnosis of NF2 or with a suspected diagnosis of NF2 is not recommended. New mutations in patients with mild presentation are most likely to be missense mutations and are difficult to identify with genetic testing of patients with NF2. The best molecular testing is performed on fresh vestibular schwannoma tissue. Any patient with a planned vestibular schwannoma removal should be offered the opportunity to have their tumor tissue tested for the genetic mutation. This is the most sensitive test and allows the identification of the genetic mutation in most patients. The results of this test can then be used to screen relatives for NF2. There are currently 2 clinical laboratories that perform this test (the Massachusetts General Hospital, Boston, MA, and the University of Alabama, Tuscaloosa, AL) and many research laboratories associated with NF centers that may perform the test on recently resected tissue. The tissue must be kept frozen, and testing should be coordinated with the laboratories before surgical resection.

SCHWANNOMA TUMOR TYPES

Bilateral vestibular schwannomas (acoustic neuromas) are benign neoplasms of the acoustic or eighth cranial nerve (**Fig. 1**).[21] The tumors are thought to arise from the glioma: Schwann cell junction within the internal auditory meatus. The tumors most commonly arise from the superior vestibular nerve, although with NF2, tumors may be found on the cochlear and facial nerves within the internal auditory meatus. The consequences of a vestibular schwannoma are numerous, including hearing loss progressing to deafness, dizziness and balance problems, tinnitus, facial nerve paralysis, brainstem compression, and, if left untreated, death.

Despite the strong genetic effect in patients with NF2, there is enormous variability in the number of tumor types, rate of progression, and disabilities experienced. This enormous variability is also found in patient presentation (**Table 1**). Some patients may be asymptomatic. Patients who have no symptoms when diagnosed have generally been identified based on either a genetic analysis conducted because a blood relative has NF2 or a presymptomatic MRI screening.

Although the NIH criteria for NF2 require the presence of bilateral vestibular schwannomas for diagnosis, patients may first develop unilateral schwannomas as a young child with no other tumors, or adult patients may present with multiple meningiomas

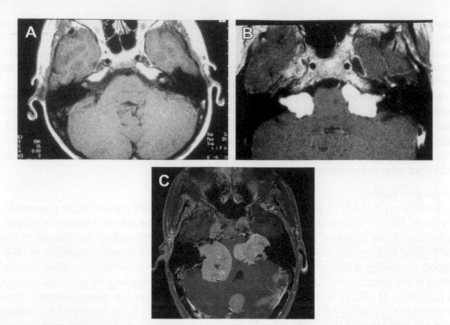

Fig. 1. Bilateral vestibular schwannomas are characteristic of NF2. (*A*) Small bilateral vestibular schwannomas. (*B*) Medium vestibular schwannomas that are compressing the brainstem. (*C*) Giant bilateral vestibular schwannomas that are compressing the brainstem and causing hydrocephalus.

(cranial and spinal) and no vestibular schwannomas.[8,22] Although the NIH criteria for NF2 imply that all patients with NF2 develop bilateral vestibular schwannomas, some researchers are not convinced of this condition.[23] Evans and colleagues[23] based their conclusion on the observation of a possible variant form of NF2 manifesting with skin and spinal tumors in the absence of vestibular schwannomas. Nonetheless, the phenotype generally is reflective of the underlying disorder.

The natural history study of vestibular schwannomas in an NF2 study conducted at the House Ear Institute showed that of the 80 subjects enrolled, 10 (12.5%) had no symptoms at diagnosis and 23 (28.8%) had cranial and spinal meningiomas in addition

Table 1 First symptoms of NF2	
Symptoms	Patients (%)
Neurologic	17.5
Skin tumor	11.7
Vision loss	10.7
Asymptomatic	10.7
Tinnitus	7.8
Weakness	2.9
Vertigo	1.0
Other/unspecified	4.9

Adapted from Slattery WH. Neurofibromatosis 2. In: Brackmann DE, Shelton C, Arriaga MA, editors. Otologic surgery. Philadelphia: Elsevier; 2010. p. 691–701; with permission.

to bilateral vestibular schwannomas. Nearly half (47.5%) of the subjects had 1 vestibular schwannoma removed before enrollment. Generally, the tumor resected before enrollment was removed 1.5 years after discovery and was an average of 2.1 cm at removal. Few patients in the natural history study had spinal tumors or meningiomas removed before enrollment. The preliminary data would indicate that, for this sample of subjects with NF2, the most salient medical issue is the growth of the vestibular schwannomas.

Intracranial Schwannomas

Vestibular schwannomas are the most common intracranial schwannoma associated with NF2. The most frequently identified nonvestibular schwannomas are those of cranial nerves III and V. Bilateral cranial nerve III or V schwannomas are the most common additional schwannomas seen. Lower cranial nerve schwannomas may also be identified but are much less frequently seen. A vestibular schwannoma rarely turns malignant, and sometimes the unilateral vestibular schwannoma may regress in size altogether. Growth of the tumors does not seem to be related either to the loss of heterozygosity (genetic level of analysis) or to the auditory functioning (phenotype level of analysis). For this reason, patients are recommended to have at least yearly MRI scans to track changes in size.[24-29] All newly diagnosed patients should have a full head and spine study to stage their disease. After the disease is staged, a 6-month study is performed to determine if the tumor is fast growing or slow growing.[30]

Cranial nerve V, or trigeminal nerve, schwannomas are the most common type seen after vestibular schwannomas. Oculomotor schwannomas are the third most common schwannomas seen intracranially. Occasionally, it is difficult to distinguish whether these schwannomas have arisen from the oculomotor, trochlear, or abducent nerve, especially when the tumor rises within the cavernous sinus. Trochlear and abducent schwannomas are extremely rare with only a handful of cases reported in the literature.

Facial nerve schwannomas may also be seen, although these are difficult to distinguish radiographically from vestibular schwannomas. Some patients may present with small facial schwannomas that are encountered with large tumors in the eighth nerve whereby the distinction between the facial nerve and cochlear vestibular nerves cannot be found. Cranial nerve III and V schwannomas are usually slow growing and require treatment only when either significant growth has occurred or other intracranial complications are imminent.

Lower cranial nerve schwannomas can be significant in NF2 because these can lead to speech and swallowing disorders. When bilateral lower cranial nerve schwannomas or jugular foramen meningiomas are associated with these tumors, the patient may develop aspiration problems, which can cause significant morbidity. Glossopharyngeal, vagal, and hypoglossal neuropathies resulting from schwannomas on the cranial nerves IX, X, and XII may lead to speech and swallowing disorders. Glossopharyngeal schwannomas are the most common schwannoma of the jugular foramen and may manifest with swallowing difficulty, which may lead to the requirement of gastrostomy feeding tubes for nutritional status.

Vagal nerve defects may contribute to swallowing difficulties related to esophageal dysmotility. Vagal nerve deficits may manifest with voice hoarseness owing to vocal cord paralysis, but the most important issue is aspiration, which occurs because of the loss of sensory innervation to the larynx and other reflexive airway protective mechanisms. Aspiration is often silent in such cases and leads to life-threatening pulmonary complications, including pneumonia. Tracheotomy may be required, leading to other potential life-threatening complications, including pulmonary infection. Lower cranial nerve neuropathies may contribute to NF2-associated mortality.

Hearing Changes in Patients with Vestibular Schwannomas

Hearing loss

Hearing loss is well documented as the most common presenting symptom in patients who have vestibular schwannomas.[31–40] Auditory changes over time in patients with NF2 are less well known. Rosenberg[41] studied the natural history of 80 patients with non-NF2 unilateral vestibular schwannomas for an average of 4.4 years. Rosenberg[41] found a positive correlation between tumor growth and worsening pure tone average. However, there was no statistically significant correlation between positive tumor growth and speech discrimination, change in ABR, and bithermal caloric electronystagmography test result over time.

Pure tone, speech discrimination, and word recognition

Lalwani and colleagues[42] reported that pure tone pattern, speech receptive thresholds and word recognition scores were significantly worse in patients with a mild form of NF2 and large tumors compared with those with mild NF2 and small tumors. Loss of acoustic reflexes and prolonged waves III and V were also associated with larger tumors. In contrast, patients with severe NF2 showed no relationship between tumor size and pure tone levels, speech discrimination thresholds, or word recognition scores. The lack of association may have been because of complete loss of hearing in patients with severe NF2 at the time of the assessment. The larger tumors were also associated with prolonged ABR wave III and V latencies. No data across time were reported. Generally, hearing is progressively impaired with increasing growth of vestibular schwannomas, necessitating the need for surgical intervention or medical treatments for patients with NF2.

Stable hearing

The natural history study evaluated hearing changes prospectively in 63 newly diagnosed patients with NF and found that hearing was stable after diagnosis. During the first 2 years after diagnosis, 27% of patients had a significant change in their hearing and 73% had stable hearing. Patients with a family history of NF2 had more stable hearing after an initial diagnosis compared with those without a family history. Patients with a family history are usually diagnosed at a younger age; the stability of hearing in this group may represent the younger age group. The better the hearing in the newly diagnosed patients, the more stable the hearing. Hearing changes did not vary between ears, with each side acting independently.[43]

OTHER TUMOR TYPES IN NF2
Meningiomas

NF2 has been associated with multiple central nervous system tumors, the most common of which are intracranial meningiomas (**Fig. 2**).[2] Nearly all patients with NF2 develop these tumors in time. Fifty percent of patients with NF2 present with schwannomas and meningiomas; 90% present with spinal tumors in addition to schwannomas. The presence of more than 1 type of tumor in a patient usually indicates a more aggressive disease course. The co-occurrence of vestibular schwannomas and meningiomas has been linked to an increase in the growth rate of schwannomas and meningiomas beyond that expected of sporadic tumors.[44,45] Despite the high number of patients with multiple tumors initially, most meningiomas and spinal tumors are asymptomatic and are first seen on an MRI. In addition, multiple tumors in the skin may be found in patients with NF2 (**Table 2**).

In patients with NF2, meningiomas, unless very large, are generally monitored with imaging. Growing meningiomas may be removed surgically, and they may result in

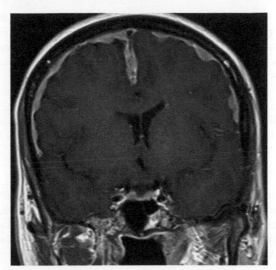

Fig. 2. Multiple meningiomas are seen in severe forms of NF2. Meningiomas may occur throughout the cranium and skull base.

increased intracranial pressure, intractable headaches, hydrocephalus, and seizure disorders.

Spinal Tumors

Various spinal tumors may occur in patients with NF2 and can be found in the cervical, thoracic, and lumbar regions. These tumors are categorized further as either extramedullary or intramedullary tumors depending on their presentation relative to the spinal cord. Extramedullary tumors are commonly schwannomas or meningiomas, whereas intramedullary tumors are often ependymomas but can be astrocytomas or schwannomas.[2] Spinal tumors may often be numerous in the cauda equina. Tumors located in the cervical or thoracic region are usually solitary tumors and may grow to cause spinal cord compression. These tumors may have a solid or cystic component similar to schwannomas and meningiomas seen intracranially. These tumors may extend out the spinal foramen into the soft tissue, causing spinal root compression.[2]

As each NF2-related tumor grows and exerts pressure on the surrounding structures, treatment encompasses surgical resection, radiation therapy, or both. Another treatment choice early in the course of the disease is surgical decompression, in which

Table 2	
Tumor type	
Tumor Type	**Patients (%)**
Bilateral VS	99
Skin	50
Meningioma	46
Spinal	60

Abbreviation: VS, vestibular schwannoma.

Adapted from Slattery WH. Neurofibromatosis 2. In: Brackmann DE, Shelton C, Arriaga MA, editors. Otologic surgery. Philadelphia: Elsevier; 2010. p. 691–701; with permission.

space is created for the growing tumor, relieving the pressure of the tumor on the nerve. Continued growth of spinal tumors causes loss of motion, numbness, tingling, and, eventually, paralysis; 2% to 3% of patients present with numbness or tingling in their arms or legs.[2] Up to 30% of patients with NF2 may undergo surgery to remove the spinal tumors.

Eye Findings

In patients with NF2, cortical and posterior subcapsular cataracts can lead to blindness (see **Table 1**).[2] Retinal hamartomas have been observed in a few patients but are not as frequent.[2,4]

Skin Tumors

Skin tumors can be found in many patients with NF2. These are usually small schwannomas of peripheral nerve origin, asymptomatic, and commonly missed on physical examination unless the patient brings it to the clinician's attention. These are removed only if they present a cosmetic or functional impairment, for example, masses on the hand or foot.

TREATMENT OPTIONS FOR VESTIBULAR SCHWANNOMAS IN PATIENTS WITH NF2

The treatment options for a patient with bilateral vestibular schwannomas vary considerably because of the wide variety of tumor sizes and clinical presentations. Associated symptoms (brainstem compression or hydrocephalus), loss of useful hearing, and the status of other intracranial tumors must be considered when discussing the therapeutic intervention.

Hearing Preservation in NF2

Patients who present with bilateral small tumors (less than 2 cm in greatest diameter) and good hearing may be candidates for hearing preservation procedures. In these patients, total tumor removal is attempted on the side of the larger tumor or on the side with worse hearing. If hearing is successfully preserved on the first side, contralateral tumor removal may be attempted after 6 months. Hearing preservation rates for small unilateral tumors have approached 70%.[40] However, the results in patients with NF2 seem to be worse than those reported in patients with unilateral vestibular schwannomas.[46] Doyle and Shelton[47] found that 67% of patients with NF2 underwent hearing preservation surgery using the middle fossa approach and that 38% of those had serviceable hearing postoperatively. Improvements in the middle fossa surgical approach were introduced in 1992, which led to a significant improvement in the outcomes of tumor removal in patients with NF2. A more recent review of 18 patients with NF2 who had middle fossa removal of their tumors reported that approximately 50% of patients had hearing preserved at the preoperative level compared with 25% in the previous study. The overall ability to preserve any hearing was still close to 68%.[48] The results of this series have led to a more aggressive attempt to preserve hearing in patients with NF2. Patients who present with small tumors and good hearing are now routinely offered an attempt at hearing preservation. Long-term follow-up is still needed in patients with NF2 because additional tumors may arise in the facial or cochlear nerves.

A retrospective chart review reported on 35 children with NF2 and good hearing who had undergone middle fossa resections (47 surgeries) between 1992 and 2004. In 55% of surgeries, hearing of 70 dB or less pure tone average was maintained postoperatively. It is now our practice to perform middle fossa resection in children with NF2.

Results indicate that hearing and facial nerve function can be successfully preserved using this approach. Factors to consider include:

- Patient age
- Severity of additional NF2-related symptoms
- Obtaining high-quality, thin-slice magnetic resonance images before surgery.

Bilateral middle fossa resection after hearing preservation on the first side is also successful and potentially preserves hearing in both ears.[49]

Observation Without Surgical Intervention for NF2

Observation without surgical intervention is the most common treatment option used in patients with NF2 and is used when a small tumor is present in a patient with only 1 hearing ear or when bilateral tumors are too large for hearing preservation procedures. The patient is assessed routinely to ensure that brainstem compression or hydrocephalus does not result. Initially, MRI is performed 6 months after diagnosis, and then, annual MRI scans are performed to document tumor size and determine if intervention is required. Surgical intervention is considered if life-threatening complications occur, the tumors become excessively large (increasing the perioperative morbidity), or the hearing becomes unserviceable.

Middle Fossa Craniotomy and IAC Decompression Without Tumor Removal

Middle fossa craniotomy and IAC decompression without tumor removal allows the tumor to grow without causing compression of cranial nerves VII and VIII. This procedure is recommended when progression of hearing loss occurs in a patient who is being observed. The bone surrounding the IAC is removed extensively, allowing the entire tumor and cranial nerve VII and VIII complex to be decompressed. The tumor itself is not removed because this may increase the risk of hearing loss. Stabilization and improvement of hearing may occur after this procedure. In a review of 49 patients who underwent middle fossa craniotomy with decompression of the IAC, preoperative American Academy of Otolaryngology-Head and Neck Surgery hearing class was preserved in 90% of patients in the immediate postoperative period and in approximately two-thirds of patients for 1 year from surgery.[50] The average duration of hearing preservation was just more than 2 years, with some patients exhibiting hearing preservation for periods up to 10 years.

Retrosigmoid Craniotomy with Partial Removal

Retrosigmoid craniotomy with partial removal in patients with NF2 carries a significant risk because the cochlear fibers are dispersed throughout the tumor, in contrast to unilateral vestibular schwannomas (**Fig. 3**). The risk of hearing loss with partial removal is significant.

Non-Hearing Preservation for NF2

The most common surgical procedures performed in patients with NF2 are the translabyrinthine and retrosigmoid approaches for total tumor removal. Many patients present when the tumor is too large for hearing preservation or when the hearing loss has progressed to a level in which hearing preservation is not considered. These approaches are used for patients with large tumors causing brainstem compression even if serviceable hearing exists. The translabyrinthine or retrosigmoid craniotomy approach may be used in these situations. The risk of a recurrent tumor may be slightly higher with the retrosigmoid approach if the IAC is not fully dissected and the tumor is left in the lateral aspect of the IAC.

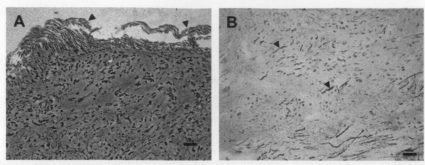

Fig. 3. Histology of vestibular schwannoma. (*A*) Unilateral non-NF2 vestibular schwannoma. Typical schwannoma stain with (*arrowheads*) Bodian silver stain. It stains only the nerve fiber; so the schwannoma cells are not evident. The fibers on the surface of the tumor are visible, however. (*B*) Another (*arrowheads*) Bodian silver stain with black strands embedded within the tumor, representing the nerve fibers invaded by the tumor. This invasion is different from that seen in non-NF2 solitary vestibular schwannomas. Non-NF2 solitary tumors invade the aggregates of cells and push the fibers aside, rather than invading between the fibers. NF2 vestibular schwannomas are histologically different from non-NF2 sporadic, unilateral tumors (Bodian silver stain, original magnification ×200). (*Courtesy of* Linthicum FH Jr, MD, Temporal Bone Histopathology Laboratory, House Research Institute.)

Auditory Brainstem Implant for NF2

The auditory brainstem implant (ABI) was developed to allow electric stimulation of the cochlear nucleus after bilateral vestibular schwannoma removal (**Fig. 4**A). The device is placed in the lateral recess of the brainstem against the dorsal cochlear nucleus (see **Fig. 4**B) during translabyrinthine vestibular schwannoma removal. This device is indicated in individuals with NF2 who have no serviceable hearing and are undergoing vestibular schwannoma removal. Most patients obtain enhanced communication skills with the device. The ABI can be placed with the first tumor removal even when useful hearing may still be present on the contralateral ear. This procedure is recommended when the patient has bilateral large tumors and the probability of hearing loss in the nonsurgical ear is significant. Another advantage of first-side surgery is that the patient has the opportunity to have bilateral ABIs.

Cochlear Implants for NF2

The variability of ABI results has led to a reexamination of the utility of cochlear implantation for auditory rehabilitation in patients with NF2. In the presence of an intact

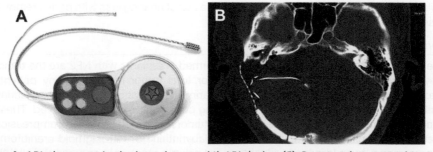

Fig. 4. ABI placement in the lateral recess. (*A*) ABI device. (*B*) Computed tomographic scan showing placement of ABI within the lateral recess of the fourth ventricle on the right. (*Courtesy of* Cochlear Corporation [*A*].)

cochlear nerve, cochlear implantation offers a viable approach for hearing rehabilitation.[51] The use of electrical promontory stimulation to determine the presence of intact and functional cochlear nerve fibers aids in determining the cochlear implant candidacy and selection of the appropriate ear. At least 10 patients have been reported as receiving cochlear implants after they lost hearing following stereotactic radiotherapy.[52] All patients had tumor growth controlled with radiotherapy. Hearing outcome in this select group of patients with their cochlear implant was considered successful in most patients.

Stereotactic Irradiation for NF2

Stereotactic irradiation has been recommended for some patients with NF2, but its use must be carefully considered because irradiation may induce or accelerate tumors in a patient with an inactivated tumor suppressor gene. At least 5 of 106 patients with NF2 who underwent radiotherapy developed radiation-induced malignancies, and although patients with NF2 represent approximately 7% of irradiated patients, nearly 50% of reports of malignant degeneration occur in the context of NF2.[53,54]

Many algorithms have been proposed as treatment plans, but none are widely accepted among NF2 specialists. The range of treatment options is large, larger than for any other nervous system tumor. The potential benefits of treatment are stabilization of tumor growth and hearing preservation. However, it must be noted that the risk of hearing loss is not unsubstantial with radiotherapy. Mathieu and colleagues[55] reported 1-, 2-, and 5-year actuarial serviceable hearing preservation rates of 73%, 59%, and 48%, respectively, in patients with NF2 who underwent stereotactic radiosurgery for vestibular schwannomas. Patients, families, and care providers should be aware of the natural history of these tumors when making recommendations and decisions regarding treatment options. Tumor growth rates and genetic testing may help to guide treatment.

Drug Therapy for NF2

Current investigations into drug therapies for NF2 seek to target multiple intracellular signaling pathways that interact with the NF2 protein, including[4]

- PI3 kinase/Akt
- Raf/MEK/ERK
- Mammalian target of rapamycin
- Integrin/focal adhesion
- Kinase/Src/Ras signaling cascades
- Platelet-derived growth factor receptor beta
- Vascular endothelial growth factor (VEGF).

Current investigations of drugs such as erlotinib, lapatinib, and bevacizumab continue to evaluate their efficacy in the treatment of neurofibromatosis-related tumors. Much attention has been focused recently on anti-VEGF therapies including bevacizumab. Although preclinical studies have demonstrated much interest, current clinical investigations of bevacizumab in patients with NF2 remain ongoing.[56,57] Other clinical trials are investigating lapatinib and rapamycin to stop the growth of NF2 vestibular schwannomas.

Early results of drug therapies have been promising, but long-term studies are needed to demonstrate benefit. As an example, erlotinib was reported to be effective in a case report, but a larger study demonstrated that it was not effective in controlling tumors and many patients suffered side effects.[58,59] Some patients with NF2 have participated in experimental drug therapies only to drop out because of side effects.

MANAGEMENT OF NF2

Initial evaluation of a patient with NF2 can be very complex because this is a multi-system disease. Patients with NF2 may typically see many different physicians, each with experience in a different field of expertise. Patients with NF2 may benefit from 1 physician, leading the treatment team to ensure comprehensive care. A neuro-tologist, geneticist, neurosurgeon, or neurologist may function as the lead physician depending on the NF2 center.

Cranial Tumor Detection and Staging

A comprehensive battery of tests are necessary for tumor detection and adequate staging. The initial MRI study showing the presence of bilateral vestibular schwanno-mas may be inadequate for tumor follow-up. A cranial MRI scan may not have included the IACs, or a spine series may have focused on only 1 segment of the spine. MRI with gadolinium and thin cuts through the IAC is necessary for the study of the head. Particular attention is focused on the IACs, cavernous sinus, and jugular foramen. Any cranial nerve may have tumor formation and hence should be complete imaged. Auditory assessment is necessary to determine the extent of hearing impair-ment. At a minimum, this assessment consists of a standard audiogram, with air and bone pure tone thresholds, and speech testing. Some centers prefer additional testing with ABR to assess cochlear nerve function. ABR testing is particularly helpful when considering a hearing preservation procedure. Electronystagmography testing has benefit in determining tumor location; however, its utility for clinical assessment is unclear.

Neurologic Examination

A complete neurologic examination is required for individuals with suspected NF2. The standard neurologic assessment of dermatomes and muscle strength is required for the assessment of potential spinal cord impairment. Cranial nerve testing may find subtle abnormalities for which the patient has slowly compensated. In addition, the patient may not even be aware of his or her own impairment. This is particularly true of the lower cranial nerves.

Spinal Tumor Detection

A complete spinal cord MRI survey is required to identify tumors within the spine. The use of spine screening is still under investigation for all patients with NF2. Patients with a significant tumor burden, a family history of spinal tumors, or spinal tumor symptoms should have a spine series. A spine series is required for all symptomatic patients.

Neuro-Ophthalmologic Examination

A neuro-ophthalmologic examination is required for all patients with NF2. The potential for deafness in these individuals requires that everything be done to preserve vision for lipreading. A slit-lamp examination is required. It is preferable that a patient be evalu-ated by an ophthalmologist familiar with NF2.

Timing of Testing

The timing of follow-up studies is currently inconsistent among NF2 specialty centers. The authors recommend repeat testing at 6 months and then yearly testing consisting of an MRI of the head and spine, neurology examination, and audiometric testing. When the growth rate of the tumors has been determined, some of these tests may be spread out over time, although individual tumor growth rates can vary over time.

Spinal tumors tend to be very slow growing and after diagnosis may be imaged every several years. The potential for new tumor formation exists especially in patients with severe disease, and this information must be conveyed to the patient with NF2 so that comprehensive follow-up may occur.

Genetic Testing for NF2

Identification of the NF2 gene on chromosome 22 has made genetic testing possible. Patients with NF2 are recommended to see a genetic counselor to discuss the hereditary consequences of this disease. All patients with NF2 should be given the opportunity to have genetic testing performed. The preferred method is testing of the fresh tumor tissue, which is usually accomplished when the first tumor is removed, and the tumor can be frozen and sent to the clinical laboratories that are certified to perform the genetic test. Genetic blood screening identifies the defect on the NF2 gene in approximately 70% to 75% of patients with a known diagnosis of NF2. If the defect is identified, family members may be screened. However, mutation screening may not reveal the causative mutation. Tumor analysis can play a role in genetic testing for the offspring of sporadic patients. Analysis of the tumor can be used to take a targeted approach to the analysis of the blood sample. Once the genetic mutation is identified, screening of at-risk relatives can be performed with a blood test. If the gene is not identified, blood screening of family members cannot be performed. The use of blood screening for patients without a diagnosis or with a suspected diagnosis of NF2 is not recommended. New mutations in patients with mild presentation are most likely missense mutations, which are difficult to identify by genetic testing. If both mutational events are identified in the NF2 gene within the tumor tissue, and neither is present in the blood, then the patient is likely a mosaic for 1 of these mutations.[4] As 25% to 30% of patients with NF2 are thought to be mosaic, tumor specimen should be taken at the time of operation (with patient consent) for genetic testing.

SUMMARY

Care of patients with NF2 requires knowledge of all tumors and symptoms involved with the disorder. Patients are recommended to receive care from a center with expertise in the treatment of NF2 using a multidisciplinary approach.

REFERENCES

1. Guttmann DH, Aylswort A, Carey JC, et al. The diagnostic evaluation and multidisciplinary management of NF1 and NF2. JAMA 1997;278:51–7.
2. Asthagiri AR, Parry DM, Butman JA, et al. Neurofibromatosis type 2. Lancet 2009; 373(9679):1974–86.
3. Evans DG, Howard E, Giblin C, et al. Birth incidence and prevalence of tumor-prone syndromes: estimates from a UK family genetic register service. Am J Med Genet A 2010;152A:327–32.
4. Evans DG. Neurofibromatosis type 2 (NF2): a clinical and molecular review. Orphanet J Rare Dis 2009;4:16.
5. Ruggieri M, Huson SM. The clinical and diagnostic implications of mosaicism in the neurofibromatoses. Neurology 2001;56:1433–43.
6. Baser ME, Mautner VF, Ragge NK, et al. Presymptomatic diagnosis of neurofibromatosis 2 using linked genetic markers, neuroimaging, and ocular examinations. Neurology 1996;47:1269–77.

7. Bijlsma EK, Merel P, Fleury P, et al. Family with neurofibromatosis type 2 and auto-somal dominant hearing loss: identification of carriers of the mutated NF2 gene. Hum Genet 1995;96:1–5.

8. Mautner VF, Baser ME, Kluwe L. Phenotype variability in two families with novel splice-site and frameshift NF2 mutations. Hum Genet 1996;98:203–6.

9. Sainio M, Strachan T, Blomstedt G, et al. Presymptomatic DNA and MRI diag-nosis of neurofibromatosis 2 with mild clinical course in an extended pedigree. Neurology 1995;45:1314–22.

10. Welling DB. Clinical manifestations of mutations in the neurofibromatosis type 2 gene in vestibular schwannomas (acoustic neuromas). Laryngoscope 1998;108:178–89.

11. Shelton C, Brackmann DE, House WF. Middle fossa approach. In: Brackmann DE, Shelton C, Arriaga MA, editors. Otologic surgery. 3rd edition. Philadelphia: Elsevier; 2010. p. 581–9.

12. Antinheimo J, Sankila R, Carpen O, et al. Population-based analysis of sporadic and type 2 neurofibromatosis-associated meningiomas and schwannomas. Neurology 2000;54:71–6.

13. Rouleau GA, Wertelecki W, Haines JL, et al. Genetic linkage of bilateral acoustic neurofibromatosis to a DNA marker on chromosome 22. Nature 1987;329:246–8.

14. Rouleau GA, Merel P, Lutchman M, et al. Alteration in a new gene encoding a putative membrane-organizing protein causes neurofibromatosis type 2. Nature 1993;363:515–21.

15. Trofatter JA, MacCollin MM, Rutter JL, et al. A novel moesin-, ezrin-, radixin-like gene is a candidate for the neurofibromatosis type 2 tumor suppressor. Cell 1993;72:791–800.

16. Merel P, Haong-Xuan K, Sanson M, et al. Predominant occurrence of somatic mutations of the NF2 gene in meningiomas and schwannomas. Genes Chromo-somes Cancer 1995;13:211–6.

17. Merel P, Hoang-Xuan K, Sanson M, et al. Screening for germ-line mutations in the NF2 gene. Genes Chromosomes Cancer 1995;12:117–27.

18. Welling DB, Guida M, Goll F, et al. Mutational spectrum in the neurofibromatosis type 2 gene in sporadic and familial schwannomas. Hum Genet 1996;98:189–93.

19. Wu CL, Thakker N, Neary W, et al. Differential diagnosis of type 2 neurofibroma-tosis: molecular discrimination of NF2 and sporadic vestibular schwannomas. J Med Genet 1998;35:973–7.

20. Irving RM, Harada T, Moffat DA, et al. Somatic neurofibromatosis type 2 gene mutations and growth characteristics in vestibular schwannoma. Am J Otol 1997;18:754–60.

21. Cushing H. Bilateral acoustic tumors, generalized neurofibromatosis and the meningeal endotheliomata. Tumors of the nervous acoustics and the syndrome of the cerebellopontine angle. Philadelphia: Saunders; 1963 (1917 original edition).

22. Mautner VF, Lindenau M, Koppen J, et al. Type 2 neurofibromatosis without acoustic neuroma. Zentralbl Neurochir 1995;56:83–7.

23. Evans DG, Lye R, Neary W, et al. Probability of bilateral disease in people pre-senting with a unilateral vestibular schwannoma. J Neurol Neurosurg Psychiatry 1999;66:764–7.

24. Mathies C, Samii M, Krebs S. Management of vestibular schwannomas (acoustic neuromas): radiological features in 202 cases—their value for diagnosis and their predictive importance. Neurosurgery 1997;40:469–81.

25. Burkey JM, Rizer FM, Schuring AG, et al. Acoustic reflexes, auditory brainstem response, and MRI in the evaluation of acoustic neuromas. Laryngoscope 1996;106:839–41.

26. Levine SC, Antonelli PJ, Le CT, et al. Relative value of diagnostic tests for small acoustic neuromas. Am J Otol 1991;12:341–6.
27. Lhullier FM, Doyon DL, Halimi PM, et al. Magnetic resonance imaging of acoustic neuromas: pitfalls and differential diagnosis. Neuroradiology 1992;34:144–9.
28. Long SA, Arriaga M, Nelson RA. Acoustic neuroma volume: MRI-based calculations and clinical implications. Laryngoscope 1993;103:1093–6.
29. Modugno GC, Pirodda A, Ferri GG, et al. Small acoustic neuromas: monitoring the growth rate by MRI. Acta Neurochir 1999;141:1063–7.
30. Irving RM, Moffat DA, Hardy DG, et al. A molecular, clinical, and immunohistochemical study of vestibular schwannoma. Otolaryngol Head Neck Surg 1997; 116:426–30.
31. Strasnick B, Glasscock ME III, Haynes D, et al. The natural history of untreated acoustic neuromas. Laryngoscope 1994;104:1115–9.
32. Fucci MJ, Buchman CA, Brackmann DE, et al. Acoustic tumor growth: implications for treatment choices. Am J Otol 1999;20:495–9.
33. Brackmann DE, Owens RM, Friedman RA, et al. Prognostic factors for hearing preservation in vestibular schwannoma surgery. Am J Otol 1999;20:495–9.
34. Briggs RJ, Brackmann DE, Baser ME, et al. Comprehensive management of bilateral acoustic neuromas: current perspectives. Arch Otolaryngol Head Neck Surg 1994;120:1307–14.
35. Doyle KJ, Nelson RA. Bilateral acoustic neuromas (NF2). In: House WF, Luetje CM, Doyle KJ, editors. Acoustic tumors: diagnosis and management. San Diego (CA): Singular Publishing Group; 1997. p. 301–8.
36. Evans DG, Huson SM, Donnai D, et al. A genetic study of type 2 neurofibromatosis in the United Kingdom, I: prevalence, mutation rate, fitness, and confirmation of maternal transmission effect on severity. J Med Genet 1992;29:841–6.
37. Gadre AK, Kwartler JA, Brackmann DE, et al. Middle fossa decompression of the internal auditory canal in acoustic neuroma surgery: a therapeutic alternative. Laryngoscope 1990;100:948–52.
38. Kesterson L, Shelton C, Dressler L, et al. Clinical behavior of acoustic tumors: a flow cytometric analysis. Arch Otolaryngol Head Neck Surg 1993;119:269–71.
39. Saunders JE, Luxford WM, Devgan KK, et al. Sudden hearing loss in acoustic neuroma patients. Otolaryngol Head Neck Surg 1995;113:23–31.
40. Slattery WH III, Brackmann DE, Hitselberger W. Middle fossa approach for hearing preservation with acoustic neuromas. Am J Otol 1997;18:596–601.
41. Rosenberg SI. Natural history of acoustic neuromas. Laryngoscope 2000;110: 497–508.
42. Lalwani AK, Abaza MM, Makariou EV, et al. Audiologic presentation of vestibular schwannoma in neurofibromatosis type 2. Am J Otol 1998;19:352–7.
43. Masuda A, Fischer LM, Oppenheimer ML, et al. Hearing changes after diagnosis in neurofibromatosis type 2. Otol Neurotol 2004;25(2):150–4.
44. Pallini R, Tancredi A, Cassalbore P, et al. Neurofibromatosis type 2: growth stimulation of mixed acoustic schwannoma by concurrent adjacent meningioma: possible role of growth factors. Case report. J Neurosurg 1998;89:149–54.
45. Antinheimo J, Haappasalo H, Haltla M, et al. Proliferation potential and histological features in neurofibromatosis 2-associated and sporadic meningiomas. J Neurosurg 1997;87:610–4.
46. Slattery WH III, Brackmann DE. Hearing preservation and restoration in CPA tumor surgery. Neurosurgery 1997;Q7:169–82.
47. Doyle KJ, Shelton C. Hearing preservation in bilateral acoustic neuroma surgery. Am J Otol 1993;14:562–5.

48. Slattery WH, Brackmann DE, Hitzelburger W. Hearing preservation in NF-2. Am J Otol 1998;19:638–43.
49. Slattery WH, Fischer LM, Hitzelburger W, et al. Hearing preservation surgery for NF-2 related vestibular schwannomas in pediatric patients. J Neurosurg 2007; 106:255–60.
50. Slattery WH, Hoa M, Bonne N, et al. Middle fossa decompression for hearing preservation: a review of institutional results and indications. Otol Neurotol 2011;32(6):1017–24.
51. Ahsan S, Telischi F, Hodges A, et al. Cochlear implantation concurrent with trans-labyrinthine acoustic neuroma resection. Laryngoscope 2003;113(3):472–4.
52. Trotter MI, Briggs RJ. Cochlear implantation in neurofibromatosis type 2 after radiation therapy. Otol Neurotol 2010;31:216–9.
53. Baser ME, Evans DG, Jackler RK, et al. Neurofibromatosis 2, radiosurgery and malignant nervous system tumours. Br J Cancer 2000;82(4):998.
54. Evans DG, Birch JM, Ramsden RT, et al. Malignant transformation and new primary tumours after therapeutic radiation for benign disease: substantial risks in certain tumour prone syndromes. J Med Genet 2006;43:289–94.
55. Mathieu D, Kondziolka D, Flickinger JC, et al. Stereotactic radiosurgery for vestibular schwannomas in patients with neurofibromatosis type 2: an analysis of tumor control, complications, and hearing preservation rates. Neurosurgery 2007;60: 460–70.
56. Wong HK, Lahdenranta J, Kamoun WS, et al. Anti-vascular endothelial growth factor therapies as a novel therapeutic approach to treating neurofibromatosis-related tumors. Cancer Res 2010;70(9):3483–93.
57. Plotkin SR, Stemmer-Rachamimov AO, Barker FG 2nd, et al. Hearing improvement after bevacizumab in patients with neurofibromatosis type 2. N Engl J Med 2009;361(4):358–67.
58. Plotkin SR, Singh MA, O'Donnell CC, et al. Audiologic and radiographic response of NF2-related vestibular schwannoma to erlotinib therapy. Nat Clin Pract Oncol 2008;5(8):487–91.
59. Plotkin SR, Halpin C, McKenna MJ, et al. Erlotinib for progressive vestibular schwannoma in neurofibromatosis 2 patients. Otol Neurotol 2010;31(7):1135–43.

The Art of Management Decision Making:
From Intuition to Evidence-based Medicine

Sameer A. Sheth, MD, PhD[a], Churl-Su Kwon, MBBS, MPH[a],
Fred G. Barker II, MD[a,b],*

KEYWORDS

- Vestibular schwannoma • Acoustic neuroma • Evidence-based medicine
- Conservative management • Microsurgery • Radiosurgery • Radiation therapy

Key Abbreviations: VESTIBULAR SCHWANNOMA DECISION-MAKING	
CPA	Cerebellopontine angle
GBI	Glasgow Benefit Inventory
QOL	Quality of life
RCTs	Randomized controlled trials
SRS	Stereotactic radiosurgery
SRT	Stereotactic fractionated radiation therapy
VS	Vestibular schwannoma

Decision-making strategies for management of vestibular schwannomas (VS) reflect this tumor's benign, slow-growing natural history (see the article by Stangerup elsewhere in this issue). Treatment strategies typically emphasize maintenance of quality of life (QOL) and preservation of neurologic function. Radical tumor resection at the expense of neighboring neural tissue is only undertaken when the benefits of surgery, on some realistic time scale, outweigh the anticipated cost in QOL. These tenets have become increasingly important as smaller tumors are discovered earlier and with fewer preoperative neurologic deficits.

There are three main management strategies for VS: (1) observation, (2) radiation treatment, and (3) surgery. Given the natural history of VS, observation with periodic examination and imaging is an acceptable option for many patients and in developed countries has become the dominant initial management strategy for most smaller

The authors have nothing to disclose.
[a] Department of Neurosurgery, Massachusetts General Hospital, 55 Fruit Street, Boston, MA 02114, USA
[b] Department of Surgery, Harvard Medical School, 25 Shattuck Street, Boston, MA 02115, USA
* Corresponding author. Brain Tumor Center, Massachusetts General Hospital, 55 Fruit Street, Yawkey 9E, Boston, MA 02114.
E-mail address: barker@helix.mgh.harvard.edu

Otolaryngol Clin N Am 45 (2012) 333–351
doi:10.1016/j.otc.2012.01.001
0030-6665/12/$ – see front matter © 2012 Elsevier Inc. All rights reserved.

oto.theclinics.com

tumors. When active intervention is indicated, alternatives are microsurgery, which includes retrosigmoid (see the article by Morcos and Telischi elsewhere in this issue), translabyrinthine (see the article by Arriaga and Lin elsewhere in this issue), and middle fossa (see the article by Angeli elsewhere in this issue) approaches, and targeted radiation therapy (see the article by Link and colleagues elsewhere in this issue), including stereotactic radiosurgery (SRS) and stereotactic fractionated radiation therapy (SRT).

Arguments favoring one management strategy over the others hinge on a variety of outcome measures, related to the aforementioned goal of lesion management with preservation of neurologic function and QOL. One important end point or measure of "success" is tumor control or stability, although the precise definition of this end point differs among the three strategies. In the case of observation, it suggests absence of measureable growth or growth slow enough to warrant continued withholding of active intervention; for microsurgery, it implies completeness of resection without recurrence, or failure of residual, unresected tumor to grow after surgery; and for targeted radiation therapy, it denotes freedom from future growth of irradiated tumor. The most common neurologic outcome measures are preservation of hearing and facial function, given the tumor's origin from cranial nerve (CN) VIII and its proximity to CN VII. Balance and tinnitus (CN VIII) and facial sensation (CN V) are other occasionally tested functions. Recent studies have also focused on QOL per se, as measured by various subjective questionnaire instruments, and financial cost to society.

In this article, the reader finds the following:

- Available evidence on the various management options as they relate to the decision-making strategies used to select between them
- Consideration of individual management options
- Literature review directly comparing two or more management options, noting the level of evidence supporting their claims
- Discussion of the strategies developed to guide decision making
- Summary of the evidence-based findings and suggestions for further research.

The focus is on management of sporadic, unilateral VS, because patients with neurofibromatosis type 2 pose different management problems best discussed separately.

OBSERVATION

One strategy that has been widely adopted especially in the management of small VS in older patients is surveillance with regular clinical review and diagnostic imaging to evaluate for tumor growth.[1–3] Traditionally, among the reasons for a trial of conservative management is advanced age (usually >65 years), where the extent of tumor growth in the patient's lifetime is unlikely to mandate intervention. In patients whose medical history poses an increased risk of postoperative complications, a trial of conservative management may also be warranted. Small tumor size and those causing few, if any symptoms, especially when entirely intracanalicular, are often managed with observation. Further indications for observation are risk of deterioration of good hearing, or if the tumor is involving the better or only hearing ear. Some patients choose observation for smaller tumors with good hearing and switch preference to active management only if hearing is lost during observation. Patient preference is another reason that a patient may undergo a "wait and scan" option even for medium-size tumors.

Since 1985 there have been several studies using conservative management of VS. A summary of some of the larger recent studies is provided in **Table 1**. In these, tumor

Table 1
Selected studies on observation management of VS

Study	N	Follow-Up[a] (mo)	Growth Rate (mm/yr) Overall	Growth Rate (mm/yr) Treated[b]	Failure Rate (%)
Suryanarayanan et al,[3] 2010	327	43 (12–168)	1.1	4.8	24.5
Bakkouri et al,[51] 2009	386	NA (12–108)	1.15	NA	23.7
Godefroy et al,[52] 2009	70	40 (11–73)	0.45	NA	39
Malhotra et al,[53] 2009	202	30 (1–192)	NA	NA	9.4
Ferri et al,[54] 2008	123	58 (6–182)	0.3	NA	36.3
Hajioff et al,[1] 2008	72	121 (80–271)	1	NA	35
Stangerup et al,[55] 2008	636	47 (4–137)	NA	NA	20.8
Raut et al,[56] 2004	72	80 (52–234)	1	3.1	32
Hoistad et al,[57] 2001	102	29 (6–120)	NA	NA	33.3
Walsh et al,[58] 2000	72	40 (12–194)	1.42	4.2	15.3

Abbreviation: NA, not available.
[a] Mean or median follow-up period, with range indicated in parentheses.
[b] Growth rate of tumors requiring intervention (either microsurgery or targeted radiation therapy).

growth ranged between 30% and 40% and regression between 2% and 19.4%. The mean annual growth rates of all tumors varied from 0.3 to 1.42 mm/yr. In studies that specifically mentioned growth rates of tumors needing treatment because of failure of conservative management, rates ranged from 3 to 4.8 mm/yr (see **Table 1**).

Failure of conservative management was seen in 9.4% to 40% of patients in the various recently published studies with the mean follow-up ranging from 2.5 to 4.8 years. One study from Canada with the longest follow-up to date (median, 10 years) has shown a failure rate of 35%, of which 75% failed within the first 5 years of follow-up.[1] Reasons for failure of conservative management include tumor growth rate greater than or equal to 3 mm/yr; increasing cochleovestibular symptoms (disabling vertigo, hearing deterioration); and patient choice.

As seen from the studies, almost two-thirds of patients show favorable results with the conservative "wait and scan" management option. For many patients the conservative approach is a reasonable initial management of VS, and in the authors' clinic it is the most frequent initial choice for patients with smaller tumors.

MICROSURGERY FOR VS

The aim of microsurgery of VS is to accomplish complete tumor removal while preserving CN function and brainstem and cerebellar integrity. Since the introduction of microsurgical VS resection in the early 1960s, studies have demonstrated tumor control rates of approximately 95%, irrespective of approach.[4] A summary of several of the larger surgical series is provided in **Table 2**.

Recurrence rate after microsurgery is highly dependent on the extent of removal. In the largest series to date, Samii and Matthies[5] have shown that 979 of 1000 tumors were completely resected, with a recurrence rate of 0.8%. Total resection rates of 97% to 99% are associated with recurrence rates of 0% to 3%.[4,6–8]

Recent microsurgical studies have shown that in more than 90% of patients there is complete tumor removal, with anatomic and functional preservation of the facial

Table 2
Selected studies on microsurgical management of VS

Study	N	Large[a] (%)	Follow-Up[b] (mo)	Approach	GTR (%)	RR (%)	CN VII[c] (%)		CN VIII[d] (%)
							Anat.	Func.	
Lanman et al,[59] 1999	190	100	12	TL	96.3	NA	93.7	52.6	0
Samii & Matthies,[5] 1997	1000	80	NA	RS	97.9	0.8	93	NA	39.5
Gormley et al,[4] 1997	179	59	65 (3–171)	RS	99	1	98	NA	38
Sampath et al,[8] 1997	611	NA	NA	TL/RS	99.5	0.82	97.5	89.7	NA
Buchman et al,[9] 1996	96	NA	≥12	RS	77	6	95	75	48
Glasscock et al,[60] 1993	161	46	78 (12–144)	RS/MF	100	1	99	NA	36
Ebersold et al,[6] 1992	255	62	NA	RS	97	3	92.6	64	19

Abbreviations: Anat., anatomic preservation; Func., functional preservation; RR, recurrence rate; RS, retrosigmoid approach; TL, translabyrinthine approach; GTR, gross total resection; MF, middle fossa approach; NA, not available; RR, recurrence rate with House-Brackmann 1–2.
[a] Fraction of patients with tumors >3 cm.
[b] Mean or median follow-up period, with range indicated in parentheses.
[c] Rate of facial nerve preservation.
[d] Rate of hearing preservation with Gardner-Robertson I–II.

nerve.[8,9] The risk of developing facial nerve damage from microsurgery depends on the tumor size. Gormley and colleagues[4] found that the likelihood of a favorable outcome (House Brackmann grade I–II) was 96% for tumors smaller than 2 cm^3, 74% for tumors 2 to 4 cm^3, and 38% for tumors larger than 4 cm^3. Other studies have also supported this relationship of greater preservation rates with smaller tumor size.[10]

Hearing preservation after microsurgery has presented a greater challenge compared with preserving the facial nerve. Preservation of hearing is critically dependent on the size of the tumor. Functional hearing preservation (Gardner-Robertson Class I–II) was seen in 48% of tumors smaller than 2 cm^3, 25% in tumors 2 to 4 cm^3, and none in those larger than 4 cm^3.[4] Other surgical series have reported a 14% to 50% rate of preservation of serviceable hearing (pure tone average <50 dB, speech discrimination score >50%).[5,6,8,11,12] Recurrence of tumor after complete resection is rare in most series.

STEREOTACTIC RADIOSURGERY

Since its introduction in 1969 as a treatment for VS, SRS has been applied increasingly more often, because of favorable demonstrated outcomes and because it offers an outpatient alternative to an inpatient procedure requiring general anesthesia. SRS offers single fraction dose administration and thus short treatment times, which is convenient for patients. LINAC radiation therapy (using a linear accelerator adapted for SRS) is an alternative to gamma knife radiosurgery and similar outcomes have been seen for both in terms of tumor control and side effects.[13] A summary of several recent series is presented in **Table 3**.

Indications for SRS have included advanced age, failure of prior microsurgery, patient preference, and medical comorbidities precluding general anesthesia. SRS has also been preferred for smaller tumors because of the increased risk of trigeminal and facial nerve neuropathies after radiation treatment of larger tumors,[14] and increased risk of tumor swelling causing posterior fossa crowding and obstructive or communicating hydrocephalus. Studies have tended to use size criteria of less than 3 cm in mean diameter or less than 15 cm^3 in volume.[15,16]

As opposed to microsurgery, in which the goal is tumor resection, the goal of SRS is tumor control, or freedom from progression of tumor growth. In the early Swedish experience, of 14 tumors ranging in size from 7 to 30 mm, eight (57%) decreased in size, two (14%) remained stable, and three (21%) increased.[17] In a large series of 829 patients treated by the Pittsburgh group, long-term tumor control (absence of the need for further intervention) was 98% in the 252 patients with 10-year follow-up or longer.[18] Of these, 73% experienced a decrease in tumor volume, and 25% had no change. Notably, however, these results reflect changing radiation doses during the first 5 years of their experience. From initial tumor margin doses of 18 to 20 Gy, adapted from the early Swedish experience,[17] the dose gradually decreased to 14 to 16 Gy by 1992. Their results during this early period, in which the mean dose was 16.6 Gy, showed a high overall growth control rate of 98%, with a decrease in size in 62%, no change in 53%, and increase in 6%.[19] Since 1992 they used a margin dose of 12 to 13 Gy, and reported actuarial 6-year control rates of 98.6% in 313 patients with median 24 months of follow-up.[20]

Another study with comparable follow-up duration (over 10 years) to that by Kondziolka and colleagues,[19] but using a lower mean margin dose of 14.6 Gy, showed a lower control rate of 87% overall, and 93% in tumors smaller than 10 cm^3.[16] A later study by the same group in 346 patients with median follow-up of 7.8 years and lower mean margin dose of 13.2 Gy showed actuarial 10-year control rates of 92% overall, and 97% in tumors smaller than 15 cm^3.[15] Treatment failures observed in these

Table 3
Selected studies on radiosurgical management of VS

Study	N	Marginal Dose (Gy)		Follow-Up[a] (mo)	Control[b] (%)	CN V[c] (%)	CN VII[d] (%)	CN VIII[e] (%)	Failure (%)
		Median	Range						
Lobato-Polo et al,[26] 2009	55	13	11–20	64 (48–240)	96	96.4	98.2	87	5.5
Chopra et al,[23] 2007	216	13	12–13	68	98.3	94.9	100	NA	1.4
Hasegawa et al,[15] 2005	317	13.2	10–18	94	92	NA	98	68	6.9
Hasegawa et al,[16] 2005	73	14.6	10–18	135	87	NA	89	68	12.3
Flickinger et al,[20] 2004	313	13	12–13	24	98.6	95.6	100	78.6	0.6
Iwai et al,[25] 2003	51	11.7	8–12	60 (18–96)	92	100	100	56	4
Spiegelmann et al,[21] 2001	44	14.6	11–20	32 (12–60)	98	82	76	71	2.3
Petit et al,[27] 2001	47	12	7.5–14	43 (12–84)	96	100	96	88	4.2
Foote et al,[13] 2001	149	14	10–22.5	34 (6–94)	93	71/98[f]	71/95[f]	NA	4
Flickinger et al,[24] 2001	190	13	11–18	30	91	97.4	98.9	74	5
Prasad et al,[28] 2000	153	13	11–18	52 (12–120)	92	97	98	65	NA

Abbreviation: NA, not available.
[a] Mean or median follow-up period, with range indicated in parentheses.
[b] Rate of tumor growth control, often representing actuarial results.
[c] Rate of trigeminal nerve preservation.
[d] Rate of facial nerve preservation.
[e] Rate of hearing preservation.
[f] Different values refer to different time periods in the study (before/after 1994).

studies tended to occur within the first 3 years.[15,19] A summary of recent SRS studies is shown in **Table 3**, with reported failure rates (defined by tumor progression) ranging from 0.6% to 12%. Thus, whereas the early studies using higher marginal doses showed a high rate of tumor control, longer follow-up is needed to confirm whether such rates are durable using lower doses.

The risk of CN neuropathy is similarly margin dose-dependent. Foote and colleagues[13] stratified 149 patients by marginal dose level and showed that those receiving 20 or 22.5 Gy experienced a 100% rate of CN (V or VII) neuropathy, whereas those receiving 10 or 12.5 Gy experienced a rate of 0% and 2.9%, respectively. Dichotomizing results with a cutoff of 12.5 Gy, those receiving less had a 2-year incidence of CN V or VII neuropathy of 2%, whereas those receiving more had an incidence of 24%.

Consistently, studies using higher doses have reported lower rates of facial nerve preservation. In one study of 162 patients receiving 16.6 Gy, facial nerve preservation was 79%.[19] Other studies using mean margin doses of 14.6 and 19.4 Gy reported rates of 76%[21] and 79%,[22] respectively. In contrast, studies using lower doses (mean, 12–13) have reported facial preservation rates ranging from 96% to 100% (see **Table 3**).[15,20,23–28]

Similarly, rates of trigeminal nerve preservation show that higher doses (mean, 14.6–19.4 Gy) are associated with lower preservation rates of 73% to 86%,[19,21,22] whereas lower doses (mean, 12–13 Gy) are associated with higher preservation rates of 95% to 100%.[20,23–28] Hearing preservation rates show more variability, but follow the same trend. Rates using 14.6 to 19.4 Gy have ranged from 50% to 71%,[19,21,22] whereas rates using 12 to 13 Gy have ranged from 56% to 88%.[15,20,23–28]

As experience has accumulated during the past few decades, marginal tumor dose prescriptions have been lowered to reduce CN neuropathies. With magnetic resonance imaging replacing computed tomography and improved treatment-planning software, a large number of isocenters can be used to attain more precise conformality and sharper dose fall-off.[19,24,29] The more recent studies have thus demonstrated less neurologic morbidity, but the question is whether this is achieved at a cost to tumor growth control. A comparison between two contemporary studies at different centers with similar long-term follow-up (≥10 years) suggests lower control rates (87% vs 98%) with lower margin dose (14.6 vs 16.6 Gy).[16,19] Consistently, Pollock and colleagues[30] reviewed their experience in 293 patients with minimum 24-month follow-up, and found that those treated before 1997 with an average marginal dose of 16 Gy had a 7-year actuarial tumor control rate of 98%, but those treated after 1997 with an average marginal dose of 12 Gy had a 90% control rate. Further studies and longer follow-up are needed to address this important issue.

STEREOTACTIC FRACTIONATED RADIATION THERAPY

SRT has been used in the treatment of acoustic neuromas since 1987. SRT combines the precision of target and dose localization of the stereotactic system with the biologic benefits of delivering multiple doses of radiation over time. A conceived advantage of SRT over SRS is that with fractionation, VS greater than 3 cm or those that involve adjacent CNs or abut the brainstem can be treated while minimizing radiation-attributed side effects. SRS, however, is delivered in a single fraction, which carries with it dosing limitations.

Indications for SRT include patient preference, failure of previous surgical removal, adjuvant treatment after surgical debulking of large tumors, poor general health or advanced age, hearing preservation in bilateral VS after contalateral tumor removal, partial excision or high risk of recurrence after subsequent surgery for relapse, and nonsurgical tumor recurrence.

There are only a few long-term studies that have examined SRT and its effects on tumor control and resultant complications. SRT can be separated into two categories: conventionally fractionated and hypofractionated.

Conventional Fractionation

Conventional fractionation generally involves 5 to 6 weeks of treatment with total radiation doses ranging from 45 to 57.6 Gy. A summary of the main studies of conventionally fractionated SRT in the treatment of acoustic neuromas is provided in **Table 4**. The longest follow-up study to date was performed by Maire and colleagues[31] with median follow-up of 80 months. This study showed that the 15-year actuarial local tumor control rate (freedom from surgery) was 86%. Interestingly, local tumor control rates in the other studies using conventional SRT have been consistently higher than 90%, but median follow-up time has been shorter (19–49 months). In these series, tumor recurrence rates after SRT have ranged from 1.4% to 5.9%.[31–34]

New facial nerve weakness after conventional fractionated therapy is a rarity. The major studies to date have shown strong maintenance of the same House-Brackmann grade, with 94% to 100% preservation of good function (see **Table 4**). Trigeminal nerve complications are more common than those of the facial nerve, with preservation rates of the former ranging from 90% to 100%. Current treatment goals in SRT are targeted toward better hearing preservation. Actual hearing preservation in patients presenting with useful hearing ranges from 63% to 100%, although there may be a trend for declining preservation rates with longer follow-up.

Hypofractionation

Hypofractionated SRT involves shorter lengths of treatment but with larger and fewer doses. A summary of series examining hypofractionated SRT is shown in **Table 5**. Studies have mostly described 100% local tumor control with minimal complications of CN V and VII. Hearing preservation rates varied from 61% to 74%. As yet there is no general consensus regarding the optimal dosing or fraction size for treating VS.

STUDIES DIRECTLY COMPARING TREATMENT OPTIONS FOR VS

In the last two decades, an increasing number of studies have directly compared outcomes from two or more management strategies for VS. Although most have been retrospective comparisons,[35–43] a few recent studies have used prospective designs.[44–46] Notably, however, randomized controlled trials (RCTs) do not exist comparing treatment strategies for VS patients. The results of the existing studies by outcome measure, indicating the level of available evidence, are discussed next and summarized in **Table 6**.

Tumor Control Rate Studies

Although tumor control rate is potentially a very important distinguishing characteristic between microsurgery and targeted radiation, currently available studies do not provide meaningful comparative measures, because of the relatively short follow-up intervals for these slow-growing tumors. The best information regarding failures caused by recurrence (in the case of surgery) or progression (in the case of radiation therapy) therefore remains in the single-therapy series described previously. These studies report rates of 0.8% to 7% for surgery,[4–8] compared with rates of 0.6% to

Table 4
Selected studies on conventionally fractionated radiotherapy management of VS

Study	N	Dose (Gy)[a] Total	Dose (Gy)[a] Fraction	Follow-Up[b] (mo)	Control[c] (%)	CN V[d] (%)	CN VII[e] (%)	CN VIII[f] (%)	Failure (%)
Thomas et al,[34] 2007	34	45	1.8	37 (12–85)	97	100	94	63	5.9
Horan et al,[61] 2007	52	50	1.66	19 (4–78)	97	100	96.8	100	NA
Koh et al,[62] 2007	60	50	2	32 (6–107)	96	100	100	77.3	NA
Maire et al,[31] 2006	45	51	1.8	80 (4–227)	86	100	100	77.7	4.3
Combs et al,[63] 2005	106	57.6	1.8	49 (3–172)	93	96.6	97.7	94.5	NA
Chan et al,[32] 2005	70	54	1.8	45	94	96	99	82	1.4
Sawamura et al,[33] 2003	101	48	2	45 (6–128)	97	86	96	78	3
Szumacher et al,[64] 2002	39	50	2	22 (4–50)	95	95	95	68	NA
Andrews et al,[35] 2001	56	50	2	29	NA	93	98	81	4.3

Abbreviation: NA, nct available.
[a] Total dose and dose of each fraction.
[b] Mean or median follow-up period, with range indicated in parentheses.
[c] Rate of tumor growth control, often representing actuarial results.
[d] Rate of trigeminal nerve preservation.
[e] Rate of facial nerve preservation.
[f] Rate of hearing p'eservation.

Table 5									
Selected studies on hypofractionated radiotherapy management of VS									
Study	N	Dose (Gy)[a] Total	Dose (Gy)[a] Fraction	Follow-Up[b] (mo)	Control[c] (%)	CN V[d] (%)	CN VII[e] (%)	CN VIII[f] (%)	Failure (%)
Chang et al,[65] 2005	61	21/18	7/6	48 (36–62)	98	100	100	74	2
Meijer et al,[66] 2003	80	20/25	4/5	33 (12–107)	100	92	93	75	NA
Williams[67] 2002	125	25/30	5/3	22 (12–68)	100	100	100	61	0
Kalapurakal et al,[68] 1999	19	30	5/6	54 (34–65)	100	100	100	NA	0

Abbreviation: NA, not available.
[a] Total dose and dose of each fraction; multiple values refer to varying dose schedules, either by time period of study or tumor size.
[b] Mean or median follow-up period, with range indicated in parentheses.
[c] Rate of tumor growth control, often representing actuarial results.
[d] Rate of trigeminal nerve preservation.
[e] Rate of facial nerve preservation.
[f] Rate of hearing preservation.

12% for SRS,[13,15,16,20,21,23–27] although the latter rates are notably dependent on tumor margin dose.[18]

Hearing Preservation Studies

Hearing preservation has been studied in two prospective studies comparing microsurgery with SRS. Pollock and colleagues[45] prospectively observed patients with unilateral, unoperated VS less than 3 cm. Therapy selection was determined by patient preference without randomization. Of the 82 patients, 36 received microsurgery, and 46 received gamma knife SRS with mean tumor margin dose of 12.2 Gy. The SRS cohort was slightly older, but other demographic and clinical variables were similar. Mean tumor size was 12 to 14 mm in the cerebellopontine angle (CPA). Hearing preservation was statistically better in the SRS cohort at 3 months (77% vs 5%) and at last follow-up (63% vs 5%), which ranged from 12 to 62 months (mean, 42 months).

The other prospective trial including hearing preservation was conducted by Myrseth and colleagues.[46] This trial similarly included patients with unilateral unoperated VS less than 25 mm, and therapy was determined largely by patient selection. Of the 91 patients, 28 received microsurgery and 63 received gamma knife SRS with margin dose of 12 Gy. Notably, microsurgery procedures did not include the middle fossa approach or use CN VIII monitoring. Demographic and clinical variables were similar, and mean tumor size in the CPA was 16 to 18 mm. Hearing preservation at 2 years was 68% for the SRS cohort compared with 0% for the microsurgery cohort.

These two studies provide Level IIa evidence that SRS is superior to microsurgery for hearing preservation in small-to-medium sized tumors (CPA diameter, 10–18 mm). Several retrospective case-control studies (Level IIb) have arrived at similar conclusions favoring SRS for hearing preservation.[38,39,41] This finding should be tempered, however, with two important points regarding the prospective studies. In both, hearing preservation rates after microsurgery (5% and 0%) are lower than other series of microsurgery for VS from high-volume centers, which report rates ranging from 40% to 50%.[4,5,9,12] Secondly, the study by Myrseth and colleagues[46] did not use the middle fossa approach or CN VIII monitoring, both of which might have improved hearing preservation rates.

Table 6
Selected studies comparing treatments for VS

Study	Outcomes	Limitations
Hearing preservation		
Pollock et al,[45] 2006	Tumor size <3 cm • Microsurgery (N = 36) vs SRS (N = 46, 12.2 Gy) • At 3 months: 5% vs 77% • At 42 months: 5% vs 63%	Hearing preservation rates for microsurgery notably lower than high-volume centers (40%–50%)
Myrseth et al,[46] 2009	Tumor size <2.5 cm • Microsurgery (N = 28) vs SRS (N = 63, 12 Gy) • At 24 months: 0% vs 68%	• Did not use middle fossa approach or CN VIII monitoring • Hearing preservation rates for microsurgery notably lower than high-volume centers (40%–50%)
Facial nerve preservation		
Pollock et al,[45] 2006	Tumor size <3 cm • Microsurgery (N = 36) vs SRS (N = 46, 12.2 Gy) • At 3 months: 61% vs 100% • At 12 months: 69% vs 100%	See above regarding microsurgical expertise
Myrseth et al,[46] 2009	Tumor size <2.5 cm • Microsurgery (N = 28) vs SRS (N = 63, 12 Gy) • At 12 months: 57% vs 100% • At 24 months: 54% vs 98%	See above regarding microsurgical expertise
Balance preservation		
Coelho et al,[37] 2008	Tumor size <15 mm, no serviceable hearing • Microsurgery (N = 10) vs SRS (N = 12) • Balance significantly better with microsurgery	Translabyrinthine resection only
Pollock et al,[45] 2006	Tumor size <3 cm • Microsurgery (N = 36) vs SRS (N = 46, 12.2 Gy) • Balance significantly better with SRS	All three common surgical approaches used
QOL		
Sandooram et al,[42] 2004	All tumor sizes included • GBI as outcome measure • Observation (N = 42) vs microsurgery (N = 102) vs SRS (N = 10) • Observation similar to SRS, trend toward better than microsurgery Subset of tumor with size <2 cm • Observation better than microsurgery	• Retrospective design with patients required to recall their QOL before treatment • Small sample size of radiosurgery group • Short length of follow-up of radiosurgical patients

(continued on next page)

Study	Outcomes	Limitations
Table 6 (*continued*)		
Di Maio & Akagami,[44] 2009	All tumor sizes included • Short Form 36 as outcome measure • Observation (N = 47) vs microsurgery (N = 134) vs • SRS (n = 48) • Observation and SRS: no change in QOL • Microsurgery: improvement in QOL	• Nonrandomization of patients and effect of selection bias • Fewer patients in observation and SRS groups
Brooker et al,[36] 2010	All tumor sizes included • Short Form 12 and GBI • Observation (N = 36) vs microsurgery (N = 102) vs SRS (N = 42) • No difference in QOL among three groups	Cross-sectional design • Generic measure of Short Form 12 not specific to concern of VS patients

Facial Nerve Function Studies

In terms of facial nerve function, the same two prospective studies mentioned previously found improved rates of CN VII preservation for SRS over microsurgery. Pollock and colleagues[45] found significant differences in the number of patients with normal facial function (House-Brackmann I) at 3 months (100% vs 61%), 1 year (100% vs 69%), and last follow-up (96% vs 75%). Myrseth and colleagues[46] found similar rates of House-Brackmann I outcomes favoring SRS at 1 year (100% vs 57%) and at 2 years (98% vs 54%). In both studies, the SRS patients who developed facial weakness did so after microsurgery for tumor progression after SRS. Retrospective comparative studies are split on this outcome measure, with some showing an advantage for SRS (77%–100%) over microsurgery (48%–80%),[38–41] and one showing no difference (100% vs 100%).[37] The results therefore provide Level IIa evidence that SRS for small-to-medium VS permits better facial nerve preservation than microsurgery. However, a similar caveat regarding microsurgical CN VII preservation rates applies here. Rates of good facial function at last follow-up in the two prospective studies (75% and 54%) were somewhat lower than are found in other modern microsurgical literature.[47]

Balance and Dizziness Studies

Results regarding balance and dizziness are equivocal. One retrospective study found an advantage for microsurgery over SRS.[37] Of 22 patients with small (<15 mm) tumors and nonserviceable hearing, 10 patients underwent translabyrinthine resection, and the remaining 12 underwent SRS. Although CN V and VII function were similar between the groups, balance was significantly worse in the SRS cohort. A prospective study mentioned previously[45] with 82 patients found the opposite effect: a significant difference in favor of SRS over microsurgery. This difference may be caused by heterogeneities in lesion size (<15 vs <30 mm, although mean diameter was 12–14 mm in the latter); approach (only translabyrinthine vs all three common approaches); or other factors. Other studies have not found any significant difference in balance.[38,46] Thus, there are insufficient data for any evidence-based conclusion to be drawn regarding balance or dizziness outcomes in VS treatment.

QOL Studies

QOL, although a somewhat elusive quantity to measure, is ultimately extremely important to the patient, and can help inform decision making between alternatives. Three studies have investigated QOL as the primary outcome measure across all three management strategies. Sandooram and colleagues[42] included 165 patients with tumors of all sizes, treated with observation (N = 42 successfully + N = 11 failed, requiring surgery or SRS); microsurgery (N = 102); and SRS (N = 10). Tumors treated by the two interventional options were approximately twice the size of those treated conservatively (mean, 18–20 vs 10 mm). Total Glasgow Benefit Inventory (GBI) scores for observation were not significantly different than those for SRS, and showed a trend over microsurgery. When considering only tumors less than 20 mm, the trend of observation over microsurgery attained significance. Thus, for small tumors this study suggested an advantage for a conservative approach.

A prospective study of the three management strategies was performed by Di Maio and Akagami[44] in 205 patients. According to their treatment strategy, most patients with tumors less than 10 to 15 mm were recommended a conservative management trial. Criteria for intervention included larger size at diagnosis, documented enlargement, and sufficient symptoms. Tumors greater than 30 mm were generally referred for surgery, and smaller tumors were treated with either intervention. In the observation and SRS-SRT group, there was no change in QOL (as measured by the Short Form 36 questionnaire) between baseline and either 2 years or last follow-up (mean, 32 months). The surgery group was divided into tumors 3 cm or less and greater than 3 cm, both of which experienced improvements in QOL. In the smaller tumor group, mental health and total QOL scores showed significant improvement at 2 years, but not at last follow-up. In the larger tumor group, total scores were significantly increased at 2 years and last follow-up. Patients with any tumor size undergoing surgery were significantly more likely to be "very satisfied" with their treatment, and those with smaller tumors were significantly less likely to report that the "VS affected their QOL" at the time of last follow-up. The authors suggested that this last finding might be caused by the decreased psychological burden of knowing that the tumor was completely removed, as opposed to the observation and radiation therapy groups.

Brooker and colleagues[36] compared the three strategies in 180 VS patients using a retrospective questionnaire administered at a mean follow-up interval of 30 to 33 months. They found no difference in overall QOL scores (Short Form 12 and GBI) among the three groups. In comparison, two prospective studies comparing microsurgery with SRS found an advantage for SRS in some QOL scores.[45,46]

The heterogeneity of these results is likely a consequence of several factors, including differences in treatment selection algorithms, surgical and radiation therapy technique, patient interpretation of questionnaire meaning, and the metrics themselves. This lack of consistency precludes a firm evidence-based recommendation regarding QOL in the management of VS.

Treatment Cost Studies

Regarding differences in cost between SRS and microsurgery, an early retrospective study from the Netherlands showed lower costs associated with SRS.[43] A more recent study from the Mayo Clinic provided more nuanced results by analyzing initial and follow-up costs. Although total costs of microsurgery were higher, follow-up costs of SRS were higher, leading the authors to suggest that SRS may be less expensive overall if follow-up costs remain low because of preserved low recurrence rates.

A retrospective Canadian study comparing all three management paradigms noted a cost advantage for conservative management, provided that complications requiring active treatment because of tumor growth were minimal.[48] Thus, although there is a lack of prospective studies specifically powered to address cost, Level III evidence suggests that observation is least expensive provided that conservative management does not produce increased complication-associated treatments, and that between the two interventions, radiosurgery may be a less expensive treatment modality if tumor growth after treatment is infrequent.

DECISION-MAKING ALGORITHMS

Implicitly or explicitly, the aforementioned studies frequently use similar strategies for choosing management modalities, based on a variety of patient- and tumor-related characteristics. Small tumors (<10–15 mm), especially when entirely intracanalicular or with minimal symptoms, are often observed with serial imaging and neurologic examination. A recent study using Markov decision analysis supports this practice, with the authors advocating an initial observation period for all tumors smaller than 15 mm, regardless of patient age, as the "best" strategy.[49] Large tumors (>30 mm or >15 cm^3) or those causing brainstem compression or hydrocephalus are almost always referred for microsurgery in modern practice.

The most complex decisions arise in the management of medium-sized tumors. In elderly patients or those with significant medical comorbidities, a trial of observation may be recommended. In patients potentially eligible for either active intervention, there is no clear consensus. Arguments favoring microsurgery include its ability to provide complete resection, with the attendant psychological relief, and low recurrence rates if resection is complete. Morbidity of resection for medium tumors is quite low in modern practice, especially in high-volume centers with experienced surgeons. Detractors cite its up-front discomfort and nonnegligible complication rate, including such factors as headache and balance difficulty that are ill-reported in most surgical series. Arguments favoring targeted radiation therapy include its lack of anesthesia risk, reduced discomfort, high tumor control rate, and low cranial neuropathy rate. Opponents emphasize the yet-unknown rate of tumor control with the lower radiation doses currently used, with poor surgical success on radiated tumors that have grown progressively. Additional factors include the still not fully characterized rate of secondary malignancy,[50] and the probable necessity for more intensive postprocedural imaging surveillance than after complete removal. As more data become available regarding the safety and efficacy of SRS and SRT, more evidence-based recommendations will be possible. Until then, these decisions continue to depend on patient and surgeon preferences.

SUMMARY

Although all three management strategies for VS have been available for decades, there remain many open questions regarding patient choice and outcome. Regarding the two active interventions, it is unlikely that an RCT comparing microsurgery and targeted radiation therapy will occur soon, given the anticipated resistance of patients and surgeons to randomization.[35,46] Such a trial may be feasible between SRS and SRT, however, and would certainly help elucidate the effect of fractionation on tumor control and neurologic morbidity. In addition, existing literature assumes that patients will weigh information on measureable qualities, such as facial weakness, hearing loss, and QOL, in a linear rational manner. Studies in other fields of decision making, such as economics, show that few human decisions are actually made in this manner.

Instead, factors that are not strictly rational are important in many observed decisions. An example is "loss aversion," which is the tendency to go to extreme lengths to preserve an existing good, compared with the smaller value subjects place on the same good when they do not presently possess it. Loss aversion could explain the preference for surgery with small, asymptomatic VS when patients believe this offers the best chance of preserving hearing, even at the risk of incurring other problems, such as postoperative headache or imbalance that might outweigh the benefits of surgery for some individuals. The influence of nonrational decision-making processes probably explains much observed patient behavior and awaits further study for elucidation.

Lessons learned from the existing literature suggest that future comparative studies should have certain characteristics. Microsurgery should be performed by experienced surgeons, in a high-volume center, using standard techniques, such as CN monitoring and all possible surgical approaches. Follow-up of patients receiving radiation therapy should be prospectively collected for at least 5 years (ideally ≥10 years) to capture the actual rates of tumor progression, the effects of subsequent treatments, and the incidence of secondary malignancy. Outcome measures should include QOL, using scales or metrics specifically developed for this pathology. Analysis should use multivariate techniques to control for treatment-unrelated effects, such as age, number of pretreatment symptoms, and comorbidities.

Many present-day VS patients will have to make their treatment decisions in the absence of perfect information, and in some cases with hardly any relevant information at all. For new patients in their practice, the authors try to provide at least a summary of information on all three management options, even when one seems strongly preferable. For example, in recommending surgery to a young patient with a large tumor, the authors take care to also briefly discuss observation and radiation therapy, even if only to explain why these options are not appropriate for the specific clinical situation at hand. This explanation avoids patients' later discovery that others have been managed using means they were never informed about, which can easily foster distrust.

In the present medical environment many patients are actually good candidates for all three management options. For the foreseeable future, such factors as patients' personal tendency toward risk-aversion, the relative weight of present discomfort versus future possible loss of function, and comfort with uncertain long-term prognoses during observation or after radiation will weigh heavily in many treatment decisions. In addition to better objective data on treatment comparisons in VS management, further study is needed on the obscure processes that sometimes drive strong patient preferences without rational bases before clinicians can truly understand many treatment decisions made by patients with VS.

REFERENCES

1. Hajioff D, Raut VV, Walsh RM, et al. Conservative management of vestibular schwannomas: third review of a 10-year prospective study. Clin Otolaryngol 2008;33(3):255–9.
2. Stangerup SE, Tos M, Thomsen J, et al. Hearing outcomes of vestibular schwannoma patients managed with "wait and scan": predictive value of hearing level at diagnosis. J Laryngol Otol 2010;124(5):490–4.
3. Suryanarayanan R, Ramsden RT, Saeed SR, et al. Vestibular schwannoma: role of conservative management. J Laryngol Otol 2010;124(3):251–7.
4. Gormley WB, Sekhar LN, Wright DC, et al. Acoustic neuromas: results of current surgical management. Neurosurgery 1997;41(1):50–8 [discussion: 58–60].

5. Samii M, Matthies C. Management of 1000 vestibular schwannomas (acoustic neuromas): hearing function in 1000 tumor resections. Neurosurgery 1997; 40(2):248–60 [discussion: 260–2].

6. Ebersold MJ, Harner SG, Beatty CW, et al. Current results of the retrosigmoid approach to acoustic neurinoma. J Neurosurg 1992;76(6):901–9.

7. Fischer G, Fischer C, Remond J. Hearing preservation in acoustic neurinoma surgery. J Neurosurg 1992;76(6):910–7.

8. Sampath P, Holliday MJ, Brem H, et al. Facial nerve injury in acoustic neuroma (vestibular schwannoma) surgery: etiology and prevention. J Neurosurg 1997; 87(1):60–6.

9. Buchman CA, Chen DA, Flannagan P, et al. The learning curve for acoustic tumor surgery. Laryngoscope 1996;106(11):1406–11.

10. Lalwani AK, Butt FY, Jackler RK, et al. Facial nerve outcome after acoustic neuroma surgery: a study from the era of cranial nerve monitoring. Otolaryngol Head Neck Surg 1994;111(5):561–70.

11. Nadol JB, Chiong CM, Ojemann RG, et al. Preservation of hearing and facial nerve function in resection of acoustic neuroma. Laryngoscope 1992;102(10): 1153–8.

12. Brackmann DE, Owens RM, Friedman RA, et al. Prognostic factors for hearing preservation in vestibular schwannoma surgery. Am J Otol 2000;21(3):417–24.

13. Foote KD, Friedman WA, Buatti JM, et al. Analysis of risk factors associated with radiosurgery for vestibular schwannoma. J Neurosurg 2001;95(3):440–9.

14. Linskey ME, Martinez AJ, Kondziolka D, et al. The radiobiology of human acoustic schwannoma xenografts after stereotactic radiosurgery evaluated in the subrenal capsule of athymic mice. J Neurosurg 1993;78(4):645–53.

15. Hasegawa T, Fujitani S, Katsumata S, et al. Stereotactic radiosurgery for vestibular schwannomas: analysis of 317 patients followed more than 5 years. Neurosurgery 2005;57(2):257–65 [discussion: 257–65].

16. Hasegawa T, Kida Y, Kobayashi T, et al. Long-term outcomes in patients with vestibular schwannomas treated using gamma knife surgery: 10-year follow up. J Neurosurg 2005;102(1):10–6.

17. Norén G, Arndt J, Hindmarsh T. Stereotactic radiosurgery in cases of acoustic neurinoma: further experiences. Neurosurgery 1983;13(1):12–22.

18. Lunsford LD, Niranjan A, Flickinger JC, et al. Radiosurgery of vestibular schwannomas: summary of experience in 829 cases. J Neurosurg 2005;102(Suppl): 195–9.

19. Kondziolka D, Lunsford LD, McLaughlin MR, et al. Long-term outcomes after radiosurgery for acoustic neuromas. N Engl J Med 1998;339(20):1426–33.

20. Flickinger JC, Kondziolka D, Niranjan A, et al. Acoustic neuroma radiosurgery with marginal tumor doses of 12 to 13 Gy. Int J Radiat Oncol Biol Phys 2004; 60(1):225–30.

21. Spiegelmann R, Lidar Z, Gofman J, et al. Linear accelerator radiosurgery for vestibular schwannoma. J Neurosurg 2001;94(1):7–13.

22. Martens F, Verbeke L, Piessens M, et al. Stereotactic radiosurgery of vestibular schwannomas with a linear accelerator. Acta Neurochir Suppl 1994;62:88–92.

23. Chopra R, Kondziolka D, Niranjan A, et al. Long-term follow-up of acoustic schwannoma radiosurgery with marginal tumor doses of 12 to 13 Gy. Int J Radiat Oncol Biol Phys 2007;68(3):845–51.

24. Flickinger JC, Kondziolka D, Niranjan A, et al. Results of acoustic neuroma radiosurgery: an analysis of 5 years' experience using current methods. J Neurosurg 2001;94(1):1–6.

25. Iwai Y, Yamanaka K, Shiotani M, et al. Radiosurgery for acoustic neuromas: results of low-dose treatment. Neurosurgery 2003;53(2):282–7 [discussion: 287–8].
26. Lobato-Polo J, Kondziolka D, Zorro O, et al. Gamma knife radiosurgery in younger patients with vestibular schwannomas. Neurosurgery 2009;65(2):294–300 [discussion: 300–1].
27. Petit JH, Hudes RS, Chen TT, et al. Reduced-dose radiosurgery for vestibular schwannomas. Neurosurgery 2001;49(6):1299–306 [discussion: 1306–7].
28. Prasad D, Steiner M, Steiner L. Gamma surgery for vestibular schwannoma. J Neurosurg 2000;92(5):745–59.
29. Flickinger JC, Kondziolka D, Lunsford LD. Dose and diameter relationships for facial, trigeminal, and acoustic neuropathies following acoustic neuroma radiosurgery. Radiother Oncol 1996;41(3):215–9.
30. Pollock BE, Link MJ, Foote RL. Failure rate of contemporary low-dose radiosurgical technique for vestibular schwannoma. J Neurosurg 2009;111(4):840–4.
31. Maire JP, Huchet A, Milbeo Y, et al. Twenty years' experience in the treatment of acoustic neuromas with fractionated radiotherapy: a review of 45 cases. Int J Radiat Oncol Biol Phys 2006;66(1):170–8.
32. Chan AW, Black P, Ojemann RG, et al. Stereotactic radiotherapy for vestibular schwannomas: favorable outcome with minimal toxicity. Neurosurgery 2005; 57(1):60–70 [discussion: 60–70].
33. Sawamura Y, Shirato H, Sakamoto T, et al. Management of vestibular schwannoma by fractionated stereotactic radiotherapy and associated cerebrospinal fluid malabsorption. J Neurosurg 2003;99(4):685–92.
34. Thomas C, Di Maio S, Ma R, et al. Hearing preservation following fractionated stereotactic radiotherapy for vestibular schwannomas: prognostic implications of cochlear dose. J Neurosurg 2007;107(5):917–26.
35. Andrews DW, Suarez O, Goldman HW, et al. Stereotactic radiosurgery and fractionated stereotactic radiotherapy for the treatment of acoustic schwannomas: comparative observations of 125 patients treated at one institution. Int J Radiat Oncol Biol Phys 2001;50(5):1265–78.
36. Brooker JE, Fletcher JM, Dally MJ, et al. Quality of life among acoustic neuroma patients managed by microsurgery, radiation, or observation. Otol Neurotol 2010; 31(6):977–84.
37. Coelho DH, Roland JT, Rush SA, et al. Small vestibular schwannomas with no hearing: comparison of functional outcomes in stereotactic radiosurgery and microsurgery. Laryngoscope 2008;118(11):1909–16.
38. Karpinos M, Teh BS, Zeck O, et al. Treatment of acoustic neuroma: stereotactic radiosurgery vs. microsurgery. Int J Radiat Oncol Biol Phys 2002;54(5): 1410–21.
39. Myrseth E, Moller P, Pedersen PH, et al. Vestibular schwannomas: clinical results and quality of life after microsurgery or gamma knife radiosurgery. Neurosurgery 2005;56(5):927–35 [discussion: 927–35].
40. Pollock BE, Lunsford LD, Kondziolka D, et al. Outcome analysis of acoustic neuroma management: a comparison of microsurgery and stereotactic radiosurgery. Neurosurgery 1995;36(1):215–24 [discussion: 224–9].
41. Régis J, Pellet W, Delsanti C, et al. Functional outcome after gamma knife surgery or microsurgery for vestibular schwannomas. J Neurosurg 2002;97(5): 1091–100.
42. Sandooram D, Grunfeld EA, McKinney C, et al. Quality of life following microsurgery, radiosurgery and conservative management for unilateral vestibular schwannoma. Clin Otolaryngol Allied Sci 2004;29(6):621–7.

43. van Roijen L, Nijs HG, Avezaat CJ, et al. Costs and effects of microsurgery versus radiosurgery in treating acoustic neuroma. Acta Neurochir (Wien) 1997;139(10): 942–8.
44. Di Maio S, Akagami R. Prospective comparison of quality of life before and after observation, radiation, or surgery for vestibular schwannomas. J Neurosurg 2009;111(4):855–62.
45. Pollock BE, Driscoll CL, Foote RL, et al. Patient outcomes after vestibular schwannoma management: a prospective comparison of microsurgical resection and stereotactic radiosurgery. Neurosurgery 2006;59(1):77–85 [discussion: 77–85].
46. Myrseth E, Moller P, Pedersen PH, et al. Vestibular schwannoma: surgery or gamma knife radiosurgery? A prospective, nonrandomized study. Neurosurgery 2009;64(4):654–61 [discussion: 661–3].
47. Ojemann RG. Management of acoustic neuromas (vestibular schwannomas) (honored guest presentation). Clin Neurosurg 1993;40:498–535.
48. Verma S, Anthony R, Tsai V, et al. Evaluation of cost effectiveness for conservative and active management strategies for acoustic neuroma. Clin Otolaryngol 2009; 34(5):438–46.
49. Morrison D. Management of patients with acoustic neuromas: a Markov decision analysis. Laryngoscope 2010;120(4):783–90.
50. Loeffler JS, Niemierko A, Chapman PH. Second tumors after radiosurgery: tip of the iceberg or a bump in the road? Neurosurgery 2003;52(6):1436–40 [discussion: 1440–2].
51. Bakkouri WE, Kania RE, Guichard JP, et al. Conservative management of 386 cases of unilateral vestibular schwannoma: tumor growth and consequences for treatment. J Neurosurg 2009;110(4):662–9.
52. Godefroy WP, Kaptein AA, Vogel JJ, et al. Conservative treatment of vestibular schwannoma: a follow-up study on clinical and quality-of-life outcome. Otol Neurotol 2009;30(7):968–74.
53. Malhotra PS, Sharma P, Fishman MA, et al. Clinical, radiographic, and audiometric predictors in conservative management of vestibular schwannoma. Otol Neurotol 2009;30(4):507–14.
54. Ferri GG, Modugno GC, Pirodda A, et al. Conservative management of vestibular schwannoma. The Laryngoscope 2008;118:951–7.
55. Stangerup SE, Caye-Thomasen P, Tos M, et al. Change in hearing during 'wait and scan' management of patients with vestibular schwannoma. J Laryngol Otol 2008;122(7):673–81.
56. Raut VV, Walsh RM, Bath AP, et al. Conservative management of vestibular schwannomas - second review of a prospective longitudinal study. Clin Otolaryngol Allied Sci 2004;29(5):505–14.
57. Hoistad DL, Melnik G, Mamikoglu B, et al. Update on conservative management of acoustic neuroma. Otol Neurotol 2001;22(5):682–5.
58. Walsh RM, Bath AP, Bance ML, et al. The role of conservative management of vestibular schwannomas. Clin Otolaryngol Allied Sci 2000;25(1):28–39.
59. Lanman TH, Brackmann DE, Hitselberger WE, et al. Report of 190 consecutive cases of large acoustic tumors (vestibular schwannoma) removed via the translabyrinthine approach. J Neurosurg 1999;90(4):617–23.
60. Glasscock ME 3rd, Hays JW, Minor LB, et al. Preservation of hearing in surgery for acoustic neuromas. J Neurosurg 1993;78(6):864–70.
61. Horan G, Whitfield GA, Burton KE, et al. Fractionated conformal radiotherapy in vestibular schwannoma: early results from a single centre. Clin Oncol (R Coll Radiol) 2007;19(7):517–22.

62. Koh ES, Millar BA, Menard C, et al. Fractionated stereotactic radiotherapy for acoustic neuroma: single-institution experience at The Princess Margaret Hospital. Cancer 2007;109(6):1203–10.
63. Combs SE, Volk S, Schulz-Ertner D, et al. Management of acoustic neuromas with fractionated stereotactic radiotherapy (FSRT): long-term results in 106 patients treated in a single institution. Int J Radiat Oncol Biol Phys 2005;63(1):75–81.
64. Szumacher E, Schwartz ML, Tsao M, et al. Fractionated stereotactic radiotherapy for the treatment of vestibular schwannomas: combined experience of the Toronto-Sunnybrook Regional Cancer Centre and the Princess Margaret Hospital. Int J Radiat Oncol Biol Phys 2002;53(4):987–91.
65. Chang SD, Gibbs IC, Sakamoto GT, et al. Staged stereotactic irradiation for acoustic neuroma. Neurosurgery 2005;56(6):1254–61 [discussion: 1261–53].
66. Meijer OW, Vandertop WP, Baayen JC, et al. Single-fraction vs. fractionated linac-based stereotactic radiosurgery for vestibular schwannoma: a single-institution study. Int J Radiat Oncol Biol Phys 2003;56(5):1390–6.
67. Williams JA. Fractionated stereotactic radiotherapy for acoustic neuromas. Int J Radiat Oncol Biol Phys 2002;54(2):500–4.
68. Kalapurakal JA, Silverman CL, Akhtar N, et al. Improved trigeminal and facial nerve tolerance following fractionated stereotactic radiotherapy for large acoustic neuromas. Br J Radiol 1999;72(864):1202–7.

Radiation Therapy and Radiosurgery for Vestibular Schwannomas:

Indications, Techniques, and Results

Michael J. Link, MD[a],*, Colin L.W. Driscoll, MD[b],
Robert L. Foote, MD[c], Bruce E. Pollock, MD[d]

KEYWORDS

• Acoustic neuroma • Radiosurgery • Radiotherapy • Vestibular schwannoma

Stereotactic radiosurgery (SRS) and stereotactic radiotherapy (SRT) are similar but distinctly different techniques to treat vestibular schwannomas (VSs). These techniques have evolved over the past 50 years as alternatives to microsurgery (MS) of VS, with the common goal of providing long-term tumor control with minimal treatment-related morbidity. The Swedish neurosurgeon Lars Leksell[1] is deservedly credited as the father of SRS. He tested a variety of radiation delivery techniques in the 1950s before putting his primary efforts into a fixed cobalt 60 (Co 60) source unit. SRS combines stereotactic localization with radiation physics to distribute energy (photons, protons) to an imaging-defined target in 1 to 5 sessions. SRT uses similar principles but delivers the radiation dose in more than 5 sessions, depending on the technique and indication. Effective SRS relies on conformal radiation dose plans with steep radiation falloff to minimize injury to adjacent normal tissues, whereas SRT typically does not use the same dose conformality as SRS, but a similar degree of safety is achieved by dose fractionation.

The authors have nothing to disclose.

[a] Department of Neurologic Surgery, Mayo Clinic and Mayo Foundation; Department of Otolaryngology, Mayo Clinic and Mayo Foundation, 200 First Street Southwest, Rochester, MN 55902, USA
[b] Department of Otolaryngology, Mayo Clinic and Mayo Foundation; Department of Neurologic Surgery, Mayo Clinic and Mayo Foundation; 200 First Street Southwest, Rochester, MN 55902, USA
[c] Department of Radiation Oncology, Mayo Clinic and Mayo Foundation, 200 First Street Southwest, Rochester, MN 55902, USA
[d] Department of Neurologic Surgery, Mayo Clinic and Mayo Foundation; Department of Radiation Oncology, Mayo Clinic and Mayo Foundation, 200 First Street Southwest, Rochester, MN 55902, USA
* Corresponding author.
E-mail address: link.michael@mayo.edu

Otolaryngol Clin N Am 45 (2012) 353–366
doi:10.1016/j.otc.2011.12.006
0030-6665/12/$ – see front matter © 2012 Elsevier Inc. All rights reserved.

oto.theclinics.com

Key Abbreviations: RADIATION THERAPY AND RADIOSURGERY FOR VESTIBULAR SCHWANNOMAS: INDICATIONS, TECHNIQUES, AND RESULTS	
MS	Microsurgery
NF2	Neurofibromatosis 2
PTA	Pure tone audiometry
QOL	Quality of life
SDS	Speech discrimination score
SRS	Stereotactic radiosurgery
SRT	Stereotactic radiotherapy
VS	Vestibular schwannoma

SRS

SRS can be performed using a variety of devices that have been continually improved over the past several decades.

Leksell Gamma Knife

- The Leksell Gamma Knife (Elekta Instruments, Norcross, GA, USA) uses either 201 (models U, B, C, 4-C) or 192 (model Perfexion) fixed Co 60 radiation sources that can be collimated to radiation beams of 4 to 18 mm (16 mm with Perfexion).
- Dose plans generally consist of several weighted isocenters to create a conformal 3-dimensional volume to cover the desired target.
- A stereotactic headframe is used to provide reference fiducials for stereotactic accuracy and fixation in the device.

Linear Accelerator

- Multiple linear accelerator (LINAC) systems have also been developed during the second half of the last century. These include X-knife (Radionics Inc, Burlington, MA, USA), Novalis (BrainLAB, Heimstetten, Germany), and Cyberknife (Accuray Inc, Sunnyvale, CA, USA), which are commercially available.
- Rather than relying on multiple fixed radiation sources collimated to a set point, the radiation source moves around the patient usually as multiple arcs with the radiation entering the skull through many different points.
- Various techniques have been developed to improve dose conformality, including dynamic techniques, in which both the patient couch and arc radiation delivery system move to shape target volume, and the addition of minileaf or microleaf collimators.
- These systems are also used in conjunction with a stereotactic headframe.

Cyberknife

- The Cyberknife uses a LINAC mounted on a 6-axis robot. The robot positions the LINAC at different beam positions, always aiming the center of the radiation beam at the target.[2]
- This technology does not require a stereotactic headframe but relies on orthogonal radiographs and an optical tracking system that scans the patient multiple times throughout the treatment, and any patient movement is detected and dose delivery corrected by the robot in real time.

Proton beam

- Charged particles, mainly in the form of protons, have the advantage of delivering most of their energy at a fixed point, the Bragg peak, with minimal entry and exit radiation compared with photon-based radiation delivery systems.

- This technology is theoretically appealing when treating intracranial targets surrounded by sensitive critical structures such as the brainstem or cochlea. However, the cost of charged particle centers is much greater than that of other technologies, and its application to VS is fairly limited.[3–5]

This article reviews the technique, indications, and results of SRS and SRT for the treatment of VS.

TECHNIQUE
SRS

The precise technique of SRS varies based on the device used as detailed earlier. The general principles, however, are very similar. Our experience at the Mayo Clinic, Rochester, MN, USA, has been with the Leksell Gamma Knife and the associated software (GammaPlan) that allows the rapid creation of conformal 3-dimensional dose planning.

SRS is typically performed as an outpatient procedure.

- After administration of low-dose oral benzodiazepine, the patient's head is cleaned with alcohol.
- The Leksell Model G stereotactic headframe is applied using 4-point fixation after the infiltration of local anesthesia. This is generally well tolerated in patients older than 14 years. For younger patients, the procedure is done under general anesthesia. We have encountered very few superficial pin site infections in more than 5000 headframe applications using this technique, and the pins do not leave any permanent marks on the skin once removed.
- Detailed stereotactic imaging of the VS and adjacent critical temporal bone structures is then performed using magnetic resonance imaging (MRI) and computed tomography (CT). A postgadolinium axial spoiled gradient recalled acquisition in the steady state, MRI with 1 mm thick, volumetrically acquired slices (28–60 images) is performed to encompass the tumor and surrounding pertinent anatomy. The patient is then taken to the CT scanner where a noncontrast axial CT scan of the temporal bones is obtained with 1-mm thick slices. This imaging is directly transferred to the computer workstation. MRI and CT can also be fused using the Gamma Plan software (Elekta Instruments, Norcross, GA, USA).
- A conformal radiation dose plan is then developed by using a combination of isocenters using various-sized collimators and differential weighting. The Perfexion model divides 192 Co 60 radiation sources into 8 sectors of 24 sources each. Each sector can be completely blocked from contributing to the isocenter or collimated to sizes of 4, 8, or 16 mm. Previous models only resulted in ovoid isocenters of radiation using collimator helmets of 4, 8, 14, or 18 mm. The Perfexion allows for more complex-shaped isocenters by varying the sizes or blocking different combinations of the 8 sectors.[6] See **Box 1** for evolution of dose planning and treatment at Mayo Clinic
- Patients typically tolerate the noiseless painless delivery of the radiation well and are discharged from the outpatient observation ward of the hospital within several hours of completing treatment. They can resume all daily activities after treatment with no restrictions.
- Patients are requested to take follow-up audiograms and MRI scans at 6-month intervals for the first year, then yearly for the next several years, eventually moving to MRI imaging every 3 to 4 years if no evidence of tumor growth is detected.

Box 1
Dose planning and treatment of SRS

- Dose planning and treatment evolved significantly during the first decade of experience at Mayo Clinic. Between 1990 and 1993, 44 VSs were treated with a mean tumor margin dose of 18 Gy (range, 16–20 Gy). The mean number of isocenters used was 5 (range, 1–12). The tumor control rate was excellent, and most tumors showed a dramatic decrease in size on follow-up imaging. However, there was a rate of new facial weakness of 21% and a chance of trigeminal paresthesias or sensory loss of 36%, and 75% of patients with serviceable hearing before SRS had hearing loss.

- To reduce the cranial nerve morbidity associated with VS SRS, the prescribed tumor margin dose was reduced in 1994 and then again in 1996.

- Between 1997 and 2000, 84 patients were treated with a mean tumor margin dose of 13 Gy (range, 12–16 Gy). In addition, the mean number of isocenters used increased to 8 (range, 2–20), reflecting the overall improved dose conformality. Over this interval, there were no cases of new facial weakness, trigeminal symptoms occurred in less than 4% of patients, and hearing loss was reduced to 23%.

- At present at Mayo Clinic, we typically prescribe 12 to 13 Gy for patients with serviceable hearing and 13 to 14 Gy for patients with poor hearing. Most cases are treated using the 50% to 60% isodose line, which maintains a high intratumoral dose with a steep radiation falloff. Single-fraction SRS using LINAC-based units is very similar, except that the tumor margin dose of 12 to 14 Gy is usually prescribed to the 80% or 90% isodose line.[7] This results in a more homogeneous radiation distribution, but the maximum dose is less than typically used in Gamma Knife procedures. Hypofractionated (multisession) SRS procedures for patients with VS generally use 18 to 21 Gy in 3 daily fractions up to 20 to 25 Gy in 5 daily fractions.[8,9]

SRT

Several fractionation schemes have been used and reported in the literature to treat VS.[10–15]

- Typical fractionation schemes in radiation oncology involve delivering 1.8 to 2.0 Gy per fraction with a maximum dose of 45.0 to 57.6 Gy. This dose has historically been proven to be safe for adjacent normal tissues and allows for total doses in excess of 50 Gy to be delivered over a course of approximately 6 weeks.

- To allow repeatable radiation delivery over several weeks, a molded mask and bite block is created for each patient. Similar fractionation schemes have been developed for proton beam SRT with the radiation dose being expressed as cobalt Gray equivalents (CGE). These doses have ranged from 1.8 to 2.0 CGE per fraction delivered in 30 to 33 fractions with a maximum dose of 54 to 60 CGE for patients with useful hearing before treatment.[3–5]

- Follow-up after treatment is similar to SRS, with MRIs and audiograms being performed at roughly 6-month intervals initially and less frequent examinations after several years.

INDICATIONS AND RESULTS FOR SRS AND SRT FOR VS

The debate regarding the role of SRS and SRT in the management of patients with VS with small to medium-sized tumors has been fairly contentious. Advocates for or against using radiation to treat VS have even reached opposite conclusions after reviewing the same body of literature.[16,17] However, increasing evidence regarding the safety and efficacy of SRS has been established, initially from retrospective case series (level 4 evidence) and case-control series (level 3 evidence)[18-26] up to more recent prospective cohort studies (level 2 evidence).[27-29]

The best evidence (levels 2 and 3) shows improved cranial nerve outcomes in short-term follow-up (<5 years) for patients with VS using SRS compared with MS. Two prospective studies have shown that MS is associated with a decline in quality-of-life (QOL) measures, whereas SRS did not affect patients' day-to-day living in a significant manner.[28,29] Conversely, one prospective study found no difference in QOL measures for patients with VS undergoing observation, MS, or radiation treatment (included were patients who underwent either SRS or SRT).[27]

Sporadic VS

In the 1980s and early 1990s, the primary indications for VS SRS were recurrent tumors after prior MS resection, patients with neurofibromatosis type 2 (NF2), and patients considered poor candidates for general anesthesia.[19] As our and other academic centers gained more experience, SRS became a popular treatment option for all patients with small to medium-sized VSs (**Table 1**).

At our institution between 2000 and 2002, patients being evaluated for newly diagnosed sporadic VS smaller than 3 cm in posterior fossa diameter were offered to participate in a prospective observational outcome analysis comparing MS and SRS.[29] Data were collected preoperatively and at 3 months, 1 year, and last follow-up. Mean follow-up was 3.5 years. Facial nerve outcome was assessed by an independent observer in a blinded review of photographs of the patients (at rest, eye closure, eyebrow raising, smiling, frowning) taken at each time interval. Hearing was assessed by an independent blinded audiologist reviewing pure tone audiometry (PTA) and speech discrimination scores (SDS) on preoperative and follow-up audiograms. Patients completed questionnaires evaluating dizziness, tinnitus, headache, and general QOL. Forty-six patients were in the SRS cohort, and no patient withdrew from the study.

- The only facial weakness seen in this group occurred in 2 patients who required salvage MS for continued tumor growth after SRS, for a treatment failure and new facial nerve weakness rate of 4%.
- Sixty-three percent of patients maintained serviceable hearing (PTA<50 dB, SDS>50%) at last follow-up.
- One patient (2%) developed new trigeminal neuralgia after SRS, requiring medication.
- The SRS group had no decline at 3 months, 1 year, or last follow-up on any component of the health status questionnaire compared to prior to treatment.
- There was no difference in tinnitus or headache at any time comparing SRS and MS.
- At last follow-up, patients who underwent SRS had a lower dizziness handicap inventory score.

Table 1 VS SRS at the Mayo Clinic from 1990 to 2011	
Indication	**Number of Patients (Percentage of Series [%])**
Sporadic VS	526 (94)
NF2 (bilateral)[a]	28 (5)
NF2 (unilateral)	6 (1)

[a] Patients who have undergone SRS on both sides, but procedures performed at different times.

Table 2 reviews some of the prospective and retrospective data available in the literature regarding the use of SRS to treat patients with VS. The results of LINAC-based SRS on tumor control and facial nerve weakness are comparable to published Gamma Knife reports, but less information is available to compare hearing preservation.[7] Advocates of dose fractionation have posited that SRT may provide better hearing outcomes than single-fraction SRS (Table 3). However, multiple reports on VS SRT have relied on patients' subjective hearing perception and not objective comparison of audiometry performed before and after treatment.[11,14] In addition, both single-center experiences using both SRT and SRS[12] and a recent review of the SRT literature found that hearing preservation rates for conventional and hypofractionated schemes are no better than what has been reported for single-session SRS.[30] Proton beam radiotherapy seems to have similar tumor control and facial nerve outcomes, with hearing preservation rates reported from 31% to 42%.[3–5]

Dose to cochlea factor in hearing preservation

There is growing evidence that dose to the cochlea may be one of the most important factors for hearing preservation after SRS or SRT.[15,31–33] For single-session SRS, a maximum cochlear dose less than 4.0 to 4.2 Gy has been shown to correlate with better hearing preservation. In a study by Kano and colleagues,[31] all patients (n = 12) younger than 60 years who received a radiation dose of less than 4.2 Gy to the central cochlea retained serviceable hearing at 2 years after SRS. Thomas and colleagues[15] used a variety of SRT techniques and demonstrated better

Table 2
Selected published results of SRS for the treatment of VS

Institution	N	Mean or Median F/U (y)	New VII Weakness (%)	Hearing Preservation (%)	Failure Rate (%)
Retrospective					
University of Pittsburgh[18]	216	5.7	0.0	71[a]	1.4[b]
Komaki City[20]	317	7.8	1.6	58[c]	7.0[d]
Baylor, Houston[24]	96	4.0	6.1[e]	51[f]	9.0[g]
Marseille, France[26]	104	4.0[h]	2.0[i]	50[c]	3.0[b]
Bergen, Norway[25]	103	5.9	5.2[j]	43[c]	10.8[g]
Stanford University[8]	61	4.0	0.0	74[c]	2.0[g]
University of Florida[7]	295	3.3	4.4	NR	10.0[g]
Prospective					
Mayo Clinic[31]	46	3.5	4.0[k]	63[c]	4.0[b]
Bergen, Norway[30]	60	2.0	1.7	68[c]	1.7[b]

Abbreviations: F/U, follow-up; NR, not reported; VII, facial nerve.
[a] Defined as unchanged Gardner-Robertson hearing level.
[b] Defined as need for salvage surgery.
[c] Defined as maintained Gardner-Robertson grade 1 to 2 hearing.
[d] Defined as any tumor growth or development of peritumoral edema.
[e] Defined as any change in preoperative function.
[f] Defined as any change in preoperative function.
[g] Defined as any tumor enlargement.
[h] Minimum F/U, mean or median not given.
[i] Temporary deficit only.
[j] Facial nerve function House-Brackmann grade 3 to 6.
[k] Facial weakness after salvage surgery for failed SRS.

Table 3
Selected published results of SRT for the treatment of VS

Institution	N	Mean or Median F/U (y)	New VII Weakness (%)	Hearing Preservation (%)	Failure Rate (%)
University of Toronto[14]	60	2.7	0	77[a]	4[b]
University of British Columbia[15]	34	3.0	0	56[c]	4[d]
Harvard University[11]	70	3.5	1	84[e]	2[b]
University of Heidelberg[12]	172	6.3	2	69[f]	4[g]

Abbreviations: F/U, follow-up; NR, not reported; VII, facial nerve.
[a] Based on 22 pts with serviceable hearing at baseline as defined as any hearing allowing both use of the telephone on the affected side and any intelligible words to be heard.
[b] 5 year actuarial tumor control defined as no growth on serial MRI scans.
[c] 5 year actuarial rates of <15 dB loss of speech reception threshold.
[d] 4 year actuarial tumor control rates.
[e] 5 year actuarial self assessed hearing preservation with hearing loss defined as inability to use a telephone in the affected ear or need to use visual aids for communication.
[f] 10 year actuarial rates of maintaining pre treatment Gardner Robertson class.
[g] 10 year actuarial tumor control rates.

hearing outcomes by reducing the dose to the cochlea as much as possible. Although every effort is made to minimize radiation dose to the cochlea during dose planning for VS, if the tumor extends out into the fundus of the internal auditory canal, it is often not possible to completely cover the tumor with the prescribed radiation dose and maintain the cochlear dose below 4 Gy (**Fig. 1**).[33]

Imaging Assessment After Radiation

Although facial nerve and hearing outcomes can be objectively assessed in follow-up after SRS or SRT using standardized grading scales, tumor control or treatment failure

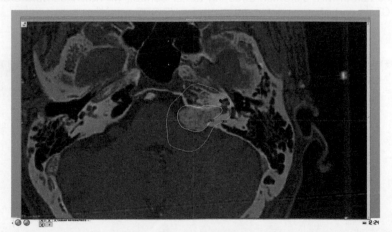

Fig. 1. Axial fused gadolinium-enhanced SPGR MRI and stereotactic CT showing the dose plan for a 2.1-cm³ left-sided VS. The tumor margin dose was 12 Gy. Note that the entire cochlea (*blue outline*) is covered by at least 4 Gy of radiation (*green isodose line*) when the entire tumor is treated with the prescribed 12 Gy at the 50% isodose line (*yellow line*). Maximum calculated cochlea dose, 9.8 Gy.

is a more controversial metric. Over the years, treatment failure after SRS or SRT has been variously defined as any tumor enlargement, symptomatic tumor growth, or the need for any additional treatment after SRS. Although most patients do achieve tumor control (absence of tumor growth) or a reduction in tumor volume after SRS or SRT (**Fig. 2**), the imaging changes observed after radiation are variable and must be interpreted correctly to ensure that the procedures are not prematurely deemed a failure (**Fig. 3**). Tumor expansion after VS radiosurgery is common but rarely denotes a failed procedure, and most patients only require further imaging.[34,35] Approximately 5% of tumors enlarge and remain increased in size when compared with the time of radiosurgery but do not show sequential growth (**Fig. 4**). We define treatment failure as serial growth seen on more than 1 follow-up imaging study before considering additional intervention. Additional tumor treatment should be reserved only for patients who demonstrate progressive tumor enlargement on serial imaging. Based on our own experience and that in the literature, we counsel patients with sporadic VS that single-fraction SRS with a tumor margin dose of 12 to 13 Gy has a chance of 92% to 95% of long-term tumor control.

It is important to recognize that the decline in cranial nerve morbidity after VS SRS correlates with dose reduction and other technical changes to this procedure. We recently reviewed 293 patients with VS who underwent radiosurgery from 1990 to 2004 with a minimum of 24 months of imaging follow-up to determine the effect that dose reduction and increased dose conformality has had on tumor control rates.[36] Failure was defined as progressive tumor enlargement noted on 2 or more MRI scans. The mean follow-up was 61 months. Tumor control was 96% at 3 years and 94% at 7 years. Although univariate analysis found 2 factors that correlated with failed VS radiosurgery: increasing number of isocenters and tumor margin doses of 13 Gy or less, multivariate analysis only found increasing number of isocenters correlated with failed VS radiosurgery.

We concluded that image distortion of stereotactic MRI coupled with increased radiosurgical conformality and progressive dose reduction likely caused some VSs to receive less than the prescribed radiation dose to the entire tumor volume. To minimize the risk of MRI distortion affecting tumor control, we now incorporate stereotactic CT as part of our imaging database for VS SRS.

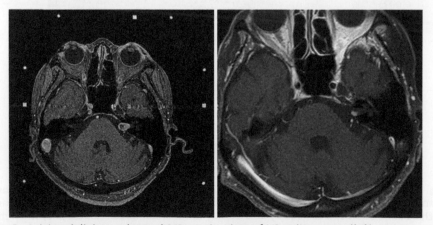

Fig. 2. Axial gadolinium-enhanced MRI at the time of VS radiosurgery (*left*) and 12 years after SRS (*right*). The tumor margin dose was 12 Gy.

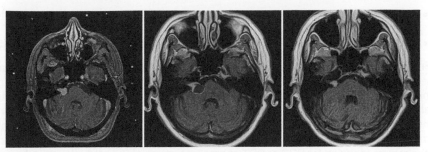

Fig. 3. Axial gadolinium-enhanced MRI at the time of VS radiosurgery (*left*), 8 years after SRS (*middle*), and 10 years after SRS (*right*). The patient had developed a cystic enlargement 8 years after SRS but remained neurologically stable, and further imaging was recommended. Two years later, the cyst resolved and the tumor remains smaller than at the time of SRS.

Large Tumors

Tumor size has been a significant limiting factor in deciding the appropriate application of SRS and SRT for VS. Typically, only tumors smaller than 3 cm are considered acceptable. Between 1997 and 2006, 305 VSs were treated at our institution with SRS.

- Thirty-four patients (11%) had tumors with a volume more than 1 SD above the mean during that period.
- The median tumor volume for these 34 tumors was 7.3 cm^3 (range, 5.3–19.1 cm^3).
- The corresponding median maximum posterior fossa diameter, usually measured parallel to the petrous temporal bone, was 2.6 cm (range, 2.2–3.9 cm).
- Fourteen patients had serviceable hearing before SRS.
- Failure after SRS was defined as either tumor growth on serial MRI or surgical resection for symptoms related to progressive mass effect. At a median follow-up of 55.2 months, 6 patients (18%) met the criteria for SRS failure. This included one patient who developed an undifferentiated high-grade pleomorphic sarcoma 7 years after SRS.[37]
- The 5-year actuarial rates of tumor control, normal facial nerve function, and hearing preservation were 83%, 86%, and 35%, respectively.
- Corticosteroid therapy for symptomatic radiation-induced changes in the brainstem and/or cerebellum was required in 5 patients (15%) for a mean of 12 weeks (range, 2–37 weeks).

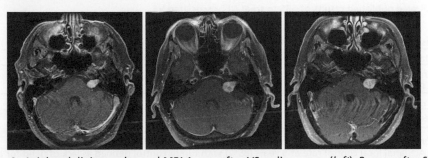

Fig. 4. Axial gadolinium-enhanced MRI 1 year after VS radiosurgery (*left*), 2 years after SRS (*middle*), and 6.5 years after SRS (*right*). The patient's tumor initially enlarged after SRS but has not shown progressive enlargement, and the patient has remained neurologically stable.

- Three patients required ventriculoperitoneal shunting for hydrocephalus after SRS.
- At last follow-up, 85% of tumors were smaller than the size at the time of SRS.

Fractionation has been used as an alternative to SRS to reduce morbidity for treating patients with larger VS. Mandl and colleagues[38] reported a cohort with large tumors treated with 5 Gy per fraction for 5 fractions to the 80% isodose line. The actuarial 5-year maintenance of pretreatment hearing level, facial nerve function, and tumor control was 30%, 80%, and 82%, respectively. Although these results are comparable to what is reported for MS for large VSs, they are clearly not as good as the results reported for SRS or SRT of smaller tumors. Unless the patient is thought to be at high risk for general anesthesia, we prefer MS for tumors larger than approximately 2.7 cm in posterior fossa greatest diameter.

NF2-Associated VS

The role of SRS or SRT in treating patients with NF2 with VS is perhaps even more controversial than the radiation treatment of sporadic VSs. **Table 4** outlines several reports on the treatment of NF2-associated VS with SRS.[39-42] Rowe and colleagues[42] reported the outcomes on 92 tumors using current techniques (MRI localization) and dose (mean tumor margin dose, 13.4 Gy). If failure was defined as the need for an additional procedure, 79% of tumors were successfully controlled at 8 years. However, if a more strict definition of failure is defined as any progressive growth with increasing symptoms, the control rate decreases to 52% at 8 years. In this series, tumor volume at the time of treatment was the most significant determinant of failure, with tumors larger than 10 cm^3 having a higher chance of failure. Overall, 23 of 61 (38%) patients who had serviceable hearing before SRS maintained their hearing grade, whereas 42% had some deterioration of their hearing and 20% became deaf. Permanent facial weakness occurred in 5% of patients, and 2% developed permanent trigeminal dysfunction related to the SRS.

Our results at the Mayo Clinic are similar. We have treated 29 VSs in 24 patients with NF2 between 1999 and 2007 with imaging follow-up available for 24 tumors. At a median follow-up of just more than 3 years, 20 tumors (83%) have remained stable or decreased in volume and 4 tumors (17%) have shown progressive enlargement. Before SRS, 15 "ears" had measurable hearing before SRS and 14 were deaf. Thirteen

Table 4
Selected published results of SRS to treat NF2-associated VS

Institution	N	Mean or Median F/U (y)	New VII Weakness (%)	Hearing Preservation (%)	Failure Rate (%)
Marseille[44]	35	2.7	3	57	26
University of Pittsburgh[42]	74	4.4	8	42	15[a]
Sheffield[45]	92	NR	5	38	21[b]
Seoul[43]	36	3.0	3	33[c]	34[c]

Abbreviations: F/U, follow-up; NR, not reported; VII, facial nerve.
  [a] Actuarial local control rate at 5 years (85%) with tumor control defined as lack of need for an additional intervention.
  [b] Actuarial control rate at 8 years depending on if control is defined as lack of need for additional intervention (79%).
  [c] Actuarial 5-year hearing preservation and tumor control rates.

sides were evaluable after SRS, with 6 maintaining their pretreatment hearing and 7 progressing to nonservicable hearing, for a hearing preservation rate of 46%.

In addition to the concern that NF2-associated VS may not respond as well as sporadic VS to SRS or SRT, there has been a great concern of malignant tumor formation after radiation in these patients who are already missing a tumor suppressor gene.[43] There are only 14 potential cases of histologically verified intracranial malignancy arising in a stereotactically irradiated field, and, in 4 of these cases, the patient had NF2.[44] Although the concern of secondary malignancy should always be discussed, there has not been any definitive evidence that there is an increased risk of malignancy in patients with NF2 after SRS.

One of the potential advantages of SRS compared with MS is that SRS guarantees an anatomically intact cochlear nerve.[45] We have placed ipsilateral cochlear implants (CIs) in 3 patients with NF2 after SRS for VS. The mean age of these patients was 68 years, and they had been deaf in the implanted ear for 1 to 10 years before CI. Mean tumor volume was 1 cm^3. All patients experienced significant restoration of hearing after CI, achieving consistently greater than 85% correction on hearing in noise sentence testing. For patients with large tumors (>2.5 cm), we prefer MS followed by auditory brainstem implant placement.

Cystic Tumors

Cystic VS may represent a unique subtype of tumor. One difficulty in evaluating this morphologic factor is deciding what percentage of the tumor needs to be cystic to be included in this subgroup. Pendl and colleagues[46] noted that 3 of 6 cystic VSs had fairly rapid and significant expansion of the cysts and required surgery for progressive neurologic decline after SRS. The Marseille group reported 54 cystic VSs treated with SRS with a median follow-up of 26 months.[47] The failure rate, defined as need for a second procedure, was 6.4%, approximately 3 times what they report for noncystic tumors. There was no increased cranial nerve morbidity in this study. Although a cystic tumor morphology is not an absolute contraindication in our view for VS SRS, we do take into account the tumor volume, including the cyst, when deciding on the appropriateness of SRS for these tumors.

Repeated SRS

A percentage of patients with VS who underwent SRS or SRT will fail treatment and have progressive tumor enlargement, requiring further tumor-directed therapy. It has been our experience, and that of other surgeons, that MS resection of VS after failed SRS is more difficult than untreated tumors.[48] Acknowledging the high morbidity of MS in this situation, several centers have repeated SRS for failed VSs.[49,50] To date, the experience with repeating VS SRS is limited, with each center only reporting a small number of cases and short follow-up after repeated SRS. Using tumor margin doses similar to the initial treatment (11–13 Gy), control rates have ranged from 90% to 100%. The morbidity of repeating SRS has been low, with most patients already deaf before a second SRS and new facial weakness occurring in less than 10%.

SUMMARY

SRS and SRT have been shown to be safe and effective for the treatment of patients with small to medium-sized VS. Contemporary single-session SRS using tumor margin doses of 12 to 13 Gy and limiting the cochlear dose whenever possible is associated with hearing preservation rates of 60% to 80%, and the risk of facial weakness is approximately 1%. It remains to be proved whether hearing preservation rates will be higher with multisession SRS or SRT. Proper patient selection is critical when considering larger tumors, tumors associated with NF2, and cystic VS. Further evaluation is needed to determine the usefulness of repeat SRS or SRT for VSs that fail prior radiation treatment.

REFERENCES

1. Leksell L. The stereotaxic method and radiosurgery of the brain. Acta Chir Scand 1951;102:316–9.
2. Adler JR Jr, Chang SD, Murphy MJ, et al. The Cyberknife: a frameless robotic system for radiosurgery. Stereotact Funct Neurosurg 1997;69:124–8.
3. Bush DA, McAllister CJ, Loredo LN, et al. Fractionated proton beam radiotherapy for acoustic neuroma. Neurosurgery 2002;50:270–5.
4. Vernimmen FJ, Mohamed Z, Slabbert JP, et al. Long-term results of stereotactic proton beam radiotherapy for acoustic neuromas. Radiother Oncol 2009;90: 208–12.
5. Weber DC, Chan AW, Bussiere MR, et al. Proton beam radiosurgery for vestibular schwannoma: tumor control and cranial nerve toxicity. Neurosurgery 2003;53: 577–88.
6. Yomo S, Tamura M, Carron R, et al. A quantitative comparison of radiosurgical treatment parameters in vestibular schwannomas: the Leksell Gamma Knife Perfexion versus Model 4C. Acta Neurochir (Wien) 2010;152:47–55.
7. Friedman WA, Bradshaw P, Myers A, et al. Linear accelerator radiosurgery for vestibular schwannomas. J Neurosurg 2006;105:657–61.
8. Chang SD, Gibbs I, Sakamoto G, et al. Staged stereotactic irradiation for acoustic neuromas. Neurosurgery 2005;56:1254–63.
9. Lederman G, Lowry J, Werthiem S, et al. Acoustic neuroma: potential benefits of fractionated stereotactic radiosurgery. Stereotact Funct Neurosurg 1997;69: 175–82.
10. Andrews DW, Werner-Wasik M, Den RB, et al. Toward dose optimization for fractionated stereotactic radiotherapy for acoustic neuromas: comparison of two dose cohorts. Int J Radiat Oncol Biol Phys 2009;74:419–26.
11. Chan AW, Black PM, Ojemann RG, et al. Stereotactic radiotherapy for vestibular schwannomas: favorable outcome with minimal toxicity. Neurosurgery 2005;57: 60–70.
12. Combs SE, Welzel T, Shculz-Ertner D, et al. Differences in clinical results after LINAC-based single-dose radiosurgery versus fractionated stereotactic radiotherapy for patients with vestibular schwannomas. Int J Radiat Oncol Biol Phys 2010;76:193–200.
13. Fuss M, DeBus J, Lohr F, et al. Conventionally fractionated stereotactic radiotherapy (FSRT) for acoustic neuromas. Int J Radiat Oncol Biol Phys 2000;48:1381–7.
14. Koh E, Millar B, Menard C, et al. Fractionated stereotactic radiotherapy for acoustic neuroma: single-institution experience at the Princess Margaret Hospital. Cancer 2007;109:1203–10.
15. Thomas C, Di Maio S, Ma R, et al. Hearing preservation following fractionated stereotactic radiotherapy for vestibular schwannomas: prognostic implications of cochlear dose. J Neurosurg 2007;107:917–26.
16. Pollock BE, Lunsford LD, Noren G. Vestibular schwannoma management in the next century: a radiosurgical perspective. Neurosurgery 1998;43:475–83.
17. Sekhar LN, Gormley WB, Wright DC. The best treatment for vestibular schwannoma (acoustic neuroma): microsurgery or radiosurgery? Am J Otol 1996;17:676–82.

18. Chopra R, Kondziolka D, Niranjan A, et al. Long-term follow-up of acoustic schwannoma radiosurgery with marginal tumor doses of 12 to 13 Gy. Int J Radiat Oncol Biol Phys 2007;68:845–51.
19. Foote RL, Coffey RC, Swanson JW, et al. Stereotactic radiosurgery using the gamma knife for acoustic neuromas. Int J Radiat Oncol Biol Phys 1995;32: 1153–60.
20. Hasegawa T, Fujitani S, Katsumata S, et al. Stereotactic radiosurgery for vestibular schwannomas: analysis of 317 patients followed more than 5 years. Neurosurgery 2005;57:257–64.
21. Brooker JE, Fletcher JM, Dally MJ, et al. Quality of life among acoustic neuroma patients managed by microsurgery, radiation, or observation. Otol Neurotol 2010; 31:977–84.
22. Karpinos M, The BS, Zeck O, et al. Treatment of acoustic neuroma: stereotactic radiosurgery vs. microsurgery. Int J Radiat Oncol Biol Phys 2002;54:1410–21.
23. Myrseth E, Moller P, Pedersen P, et al. Vestibular schwannomas: clinical results and quality of life after microsurgery or gamma knife radiosurgery. Neurosurgery 2005;56:927–35.
24. Pollock BE, Lunsford LD, Kondziolka D, et al. Outcome analysis of acoustic neuroma management: a comparison of microsurgery and stereotactic radiosurgery. Neurosurgery 1995;36:215–23.
25. Regis J, Pellet W, Delsanti C, et al. Functional outcome after gamma knife surgery or microsurgery for vestibular schwannomas. J Neurosurg 2002;97:1091–100.
26. Van Roijen L, Nijs HG, Avezaat CJ, et al. Costs and effects of microsurgery versus radiosurgery in treating acoustic neuromas. Acta Neurochir (Wien) 1997;139: 942–8.
27. Di Maio S, Akagami R. Prospective comparison of quality of life before and after observation, radiation, or surgery for vestibular schwannomas. J Neurosurg 2009;111:855–62.
28. Myrseth E, Moller P, Pedersen PH, et al. Vestibular schwannoma: surgery or gamma knife radiosurgery? A prospective, nonrandomized study. Neurosurgery 2009;64:654–63.
29. Pollock BE, Driscoll CL, Foote RL, et al. Patient outcomes after vestibular schwannoma management: a prospective comparison of microsurgical resection and stereotactic radiosurgery. Neurosurgery 2006;59:77–85.
30. Yang I, Aranda D, Han SJ, et al. Hearing preservation after stereotactic radiosurgery for vestibular schwannoma: a systematic review. J Clin Neurosci 2009;16:742–7.
31. Kano H, Kondziolka D, Khan A, et al. Predictors of hearing preservation after radiosurgery for acoustic neuroma. J Neurosurg 2009;111:863–73.
32. Massager N, Nissim O, Delbrouk C, et al. Irradiation of cochlear structures during vestibular schwannoma radiosurgery and associated hearing outcome. J Neurosurg 2007;107:733–9.
33. Timmer FC, Hanssens PE, van Haren AE, et al. Gamma Knife radiosurgery for vestibular schwannomas: results of hearing preservation in relation to the cochlear radiation dose. Laryngoscope 2009;119:1076–81.
34. Nagano O, Higuchi Y, Serizawa T, et al. Transient expansion of vestibular schwannoma following stereotactic radiosurgery. J Neurosurg 2008;109:811–6.
35. Pollock BE. Management of vestibular schwannomas that enlarge after stereotactic radiosurgery: treatment recommendations based on a 15 year experience. Neurosurgery 2006;58:241–8.
36. Pollock BE, Link MJ, Foote RL. Failure rate of contemporary low-dose radiosurgical technique for vestibular schwannoma. J Neurosurg 2009;111:840–4.

37. Schmitt WR, Carlson ML, Giannini C, et al. Radiation-induced sarcoma in a large vestibular schwannoma following stereotactic radiosurgery: case report. Neurosurgery 2011;68:E840–6.
38. Mandl ES, Meijer OW, Slotman BJ, et al. Stereotactic radiation therapy for large vestibular schwannomas. Radiother Oncol 2010;95:94–8.
39. Mathieu D, Kondziolka D, Flickinger JC, et al. Stereotactic radiosurgery for vestibular schwannomas in patients with neurofibromatosis type 2: an analysis of tumor control, complications, and hearing preservation rates. Neurosurgery 2007;60: 460–70.
40. Phi JH, Kim DG, Chung HT, et al. Radiosurgical treatment of vestibular schwannomas in patients with neurofibromatosis type 2. Cancer 2009;115:390–8.
41. Roche PH, Regis J, Pellet W, et al. Neurofibromatosis type 2. Preliminary results of gamma knife radiosurgery of vestibular schwannomas. Neurochirurgie 2000;46: 339–53 [in French].
42. Rowe JG, Radatz M, Kemeny A. Radiosurgery for type II neurofibromatosis. Prog Neurol Surg 2008;21:176–82.
43. Baser ME, Evans DGR, Jackler RK, et al. Neurofibromatosis 2, radiosurgery and malignant nervous system tumours [letter]. Br J Cancer 2000;82:998.
44. Carlson ML, Babovic-Vuksanovic D, Messiaen L, et al. Radiation-induced rhabdomyosarcoma of the brainstem in a patient with neurofibromatosis type 2. J Neurosurg 2010;112:81–7.
45. Lustig LR, Yeagle J, Driscoll CL, et al. Cochlear implantation in patients with neurofibromatosis type 2 and bilateral vestibular schwannoma. Otol Neurotol 2006;27:512–8.
46. Pendl G, Ganz JC, Kitz K, et al. Acoustic neurinomas with macrocysts treated with Gamma Knife radiosurgery. Stereotact Funct Neurosurg 1996;66(Suppl 1): 103–11.
47. Delsanti C, Regis J. Cystic vestibular schwannomas. Neurochirurgie 2004;50: 401–6 [in French].
48. Slattery WH 3rd. Microsurgery after radiosurgery or radiotherapy for vestibular schwannomas. Otolaryngol Clin North Am 2009;42:707–15.
49. Dewan S, Noren G. Retreatment of vestibular schwannomas with gamma knife surgery. J Neurosurg 2008;109(Suppl):144–8.
50. Yomo S, Arkha Y, Delsanti C, et al. Repeat gamma knife surgery for regrowth of vestibular schwannomas. Neurosurgery 2009;64:45–52.

Management of Radiation/ Radiosurgical Complications and Failures

Pierre-Hugues Roche, MD[a],*, Rémy Noudel, MD[a],
Jean Régis, MD, PhD[b]

KEYWORDS

- Acoustic neuroma • Morbidity • Complications • Gamma knife surgery
- Radiosurgery • Vestibular schwannoma

Key Abbreviations: MANAGEMENT OF RADIATION/RADIOSURGICAL COMPLICATIONS AND FAILURES	
AICA	Anteroinferior cerebellar artery
CNN	Cranial nerve neuropathies
GKRS	Gamma knife radiosurgery
RS	Radiosurgery
SAH	Subarachnoid hemorrhage
VS	Vestibular schwannoma

After several decades of technical refinements, radiosurgery (RS) is now considered an efficient treatment of vestibular schwannomas (VS), despite the fact that the goal of RS is not the removal of the tumor mass but the avoidance of tumor growth. Today, thousands of patients harboring VS have been treated with this technique all over the world with an excellent tumor control rate in the long-term setting and a reduced number of complications when the treatment is delivered in centers of excellence. However, there are several concerns about possible complications linked to this option that deserve special comments. Based upon the authors' personal experience and an extensive review of the literature, we report the whole spectrum of the adverse effects of radiosurgery will be highlighted.

Before starting with specific complications, it must be stressed that, basically, complications due to the cranial and dural opening cannot occur. Likewise, complications that are more or less linked to the general anesthesia are not reported, since the procedure is carried on under local anesthesia.

[a] Service de neurochirurgie, CHU Nord, Chemin des Bourrely, 13915, Marseille Cedex 20, France
[b] Service de neurochirurgie fonctionnelle et stéréotaxique, CHU la Timone, 13005 Marseille, France
* Corresponding author.
E-mail address: proche@ap-hm.fr

Otolaryngol Clin N Am 45 (2012) 367–374
doi:10.1016/j.otc.2011.12.007
0030-6665/12/$ – see front matter © 2012 Elsevier Inc. All rights reserved.

oto.theclinics.com

FAILURE OF RADIOSURGERY IN VESTIBULAR SCHWANNOMA

In modern series of radiosurgery, failure is considered as a very unusual event and published in less than 5% of cases (**Table 1**). Considering that this complication deserves a proactive treatment, there is a need to identify the patterns of tumor growth after RS. These patterns justify a sequential clinical and radiological follow-up after RS, and it is recommended to perform a magnetic resonance imaging (MRI) scan at 6 months, 1 year, and 2, 3, 5, 7, and 9 years after the treatment.

A transient growth in the year that follows RS is a frequent situation encountered in 15% to 30% of cases. Another situation is an initial growth followed by stabilization at a higher volume in the long term. This scenario is found in 5% to 10% of patients.[9,10] The knowledge of these 2 patterns has to be known by the patients and referring physician when considering a misleading anticipated decision of treatment. Therefore, a reasonable definition of failure is a continuous growth for more than 3 years after RS. The factors that are linked with failure are ill-known, but large tumor volume at the time of treatment, inadequate dose coverage, and cystic texture of the VS are predictive of poor tumor control. In **Fig. 1** we show a flowchart of our own contemporary management of these patterns of growth.

When a true failure is confirmed, it can be decided to operate or to retreat the tumor with RS, depending on the tumor size and clinical tolerance. When surgery is chosen, the surgeon may expect to observe some degree of arachnoid thickening. Modification of the vascularity and tumor texture is usually noted, and there is probably more adhesion with the brainstem and acousticofacial bundle.[11] However, there is no scientific evidence that this surgery is systematically more difficult than in previously nonirradiated patients.[3,9,12] To minimize the risk of facial nerve injury, it may be preferable to leave a small piece of tumor capsule along the facial nerve in case of excessive adherence. To avoid microsurgery (MS), the other option (see **Fig. 1**) is to propose a second procedure of RS if tumor size is still compatible with such treatment. In a recent series, such strategy was published by the Marseille team,[13] whereby the results of additional Gamma knife RS (GKRS) in a series of 8 patients followed more than 2 years were reported. No failure was observed, and significant decrease of tumor size was shown in 6 patients, without any additional morbidity.

RADIO-INDUCED CRANIAL NERVE NEUROPATHIES

Due to various mechanisms, the cranial nerves that run in the close vicinity of the tumor may malfunction after radiosurgery (see **Table 1**). High doses delivered at the tumor margin and inadequate dose planning are clearly identified as risk factors. Considering the technical refinements of the machines and the accumulated expertise of the radiosurgeons/radiation oncologists, rates of cranial nerve neuropathies (CNNs) have dramatically decreased. However, there is still a risk of new deficit or worsening of a pre-existing deficit in the 2 years that follow RS. Their management is a matter of controversy. A short course of steroid therapy can be proposed if the hypothesis of edema is suggested. Above all, it is recommended to check the MRI to make sure that there is no local complications in the field of irradiation (eg, tumor volume modification, brainstem edema).

Facial Nerve Deficit

Facial palsy is a major concern after the treatment of VS Thankfully, this is a very rare complication in the modern series. In the series from Sheffield,[14] the rate of facial nerve deficit involved 4.5% of patients with less than 1% of permanent deficits. In

Table 1
Main series of vestibular schwannomas treated with gamma knife radiosurgery and reporting complications.

Center/Author/Reference	Number of Patients	Period of Study	Follow-Up (Months)	Tumor Volume (cc)	Peripheral Dose	Tumor Failure	Permanent Facial Palsy	Permanent Trigeminal Dysfunction	Hearing Loss
Charlottesville/Prasad et al[1]	153	89–99	51	2.7	13.2 Gy	6%	1%	1%	60%
Graz/Unger et al[2]	192	92–98	62	—	12–14	2%	1%	1.5%	38%
Sheffield/Rowe et al[19]	238	96–99	35	3.7	14.6	8%	1%	1.5%	25%
Tilburg Timmer et al[4]	97	03–07	21	2.7	11.1	—	8%	16%	22%
Pittsburg Chopra et al[5]	216	92–00	70	1.3	12–13	2%	0%	5% (10 years)	29%
Pittsburg/Ogunrinde et al[6]	31	87–92	20	<2	16.9	6%	5%	6%	50%
Marseille/Regis et al[7]	97	92–98	48	—	12–14	3%	0%	4%	30%
Bergen/Myrseth et al[8]	103	88–99	69	—	10–12	11%	5%	—	—

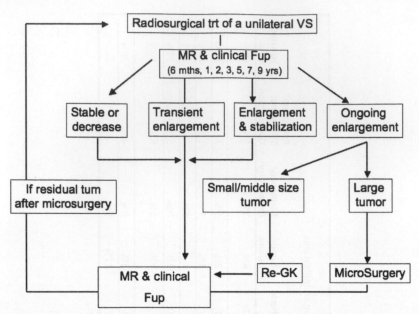

Fig. 1. Flowchart of management of vestibular schwannoma after gamma knife radiosurgery, depending on tumor volume modifications.

Marseille, rates of less than 0.5% of facial palsy and 8% of hemifacial spasm were mentioned.[15] Yang and colleagues[16] provided a metanalysis that studied 2204 patients extracted from 23 series of GKRS for VS The overall facial nerve preservation rate (House & Brackmann grades 1–2) was 96.2%. Higher risk was found in elderly patients (older than age 60 years), high dose (<13 Gys), and tumor volumes superior to 1.5 cc.

Another issue, which is usually not reported in the main series, is the assessment of the intermedius nerve (Wrisberg nerve). As reported by the Marseille team,[17] a careful analysis of lacrimation and taste before and after RS found a deterioration (ocular problems, taste disturbance) after the treatment in 14% of cases despite excellent facial nerve motility.

Hearing Loss

The known influencing parameters are: (1) tumor size, (2) hearing level (Gardner-Robertson class), (3) auditory brainstem response, (4) delivered dose at the tumor margin, and (5) dose delivered to the cochlea. The authors also showed that young age and presentation with tinnitus were predictive of hearing preservation.[7]

Early hearing loss within 1 week may be related to direct neural radiation injury or edema, whereas delayed hearing loss may be related to vascular effects. A slow deterioration of hearing over a period of months, as observed after RS, has been considered to be preferable to the sudden deafness that occurs after microsurgical excision.

The hypothesis is that with lower marginal doses and longer follow-up, hearing loss may continue through a number of mechanisms, including direct radiation effects, vascular effects, and changes in the tumor remnant.[5]

Taken together, the main series of the literature of GKRS indicate a loss of serviceable hearing in 30% to 50% of cases in the 2 years following treatment.[1,15]

This result has to be compared with the risk of spontaneous deafness in the natural course of the disease and with the potential of hearing deterioration after MS.

Vertigo, Tinnitus, Imbalance

Sughrue and colleagues[18] made an extensive metanalysis of 63 articles reporting the results of 5631 patients treated for VS smaller than 25 mm in their largest diameter. They distinguished 2 cohorts of patients according to the marginal dose of radiation delivered:

1. Lower dose cohort: less than 13 Gy for 3248 patients/58%
2. Higher dose cohort: greater than 13 Gy for 2383 patients/42%

They found that 84 out of 5631 patients (1.5%) experienced vertigo or balance disturbance after their treatment. Surprisingly, they found in the lower dose cohort:

- An increased rate of vertigo and imbalance: 1.1% for less than 13 Gy versus 1.8% for greater than 13 Gy, $P = .001$
- An increased rate of tinnitus: 1.7% for less than 13 Gy versus 0.1% for greater than 13 Gy, $P = .001$

To explain this paradoxic phenomenon, the hypothesis is that patients treated with higher doses have more complete dysfunction of this nerve before treatment, while those treated with lower doses have enough function left to detect vertigo and tinnitus. In separate series, occurrence of tinnitus was described in 6% to 25% of patients after RS. It is of paramount importance to inform patients before treatment that RS will not provide better results than MS for these symptoms.

Nonaudiofacial Cranial Nerve Neuropathy

Trigeminal neuropathy (facial numbness) was defined as any temporary or permanent, subjective or objective decrease in facial sensation, or new pain within the ipsilateral trigeminal nerve distribution after radiosurgery.

Sughrue and colleagues[18] reported that:

- Incidence of new trigeminal neuropathy was 2.3% and significantly increased with higher doses (3.15% for patients treated with doses >13 Gy and 1.63% for doses <13 Gy: $P<0.001$)
- Risk of VI nerve palsy was 0.03% (0.08% for doses >13 Gy and 0% for doses <13 Gy).
- Risk of XII nerve neuropathy was 0.08% overall (0.15% for doses <13 Gy, 0% for doses >13 Gy).
- Onset of the deficit occurred at 6 to 24 months after RS.

Ogunrinde and colleagues[6] reported a 6% rate of delayed sensory trigeminal nerve dysfunction. Onset of new trigeminal dysfunction occurred at 11 and 22 months. At last follow-up, no patient in this series developed any deafferentation pain.

Rowe and colleagues[19] published a rate of persistent trigeminal neuropathy of about 1.5%. Chopra and colleagues[5] indicated that at 10 years, 95% of patients were free of trigeminal nerve problems.

HYDROCEPHALUS

In separate series, the incidence of hydrocephalus diagnosed on computed tomography (CT) or MRI is reported in around 4% of cases,[8,20] and usually appears at 4 to 18 months after RS.

In the aforementioned metanalysis[18]:

- 0.85% of patients displayed hydrocephalus, and 75% of them required a shunt.
- The reported incidence of hydrocephalus was not affected by marginal doses of radiation (0.6% for both cohorts), but patients with hydrocephalus who were receiving greater than 13 Gy had a higher rate of symptomatic hydrocephalus requiring shunt treatment than those receiving lower doses ($P<0.001$).

Communicating hydrocephalus accompanying a VS is supposed to be caused by tumor necrosis with subsequent elevation of cerebrospinal fluid (CSF) protein concentration and secondary obstruction of CSF resorption at the level of the arachnoid granulation. Radiosurgery may play a role in exacerbating the mechanism of tumor necrosis. More rarely, the hydrocephalus is due to the mass effect. It has been particularly shown in several cases of RS failure after simultaneous treatment of bilateral tumors involving neurofibromatosis type 2 patients.

VASCULAR COMPLICATIONS

Vessel occlusion and hemorrhage are complications that are seldom described. Hemorrhage due to potentially de novo ruptured aneurysm have been reported in 3 cases[21-23] with an uncertainty, because no angiography was performed before RS.

Park and colleagues[22] reported a case of subarachnoid hemorrhage (SAH) secondary to an anteroinferior cerebellar artery aneurysm occurring 5 years after GKRS done for an ipsilateral VS. In this case

- Before GKRS, the MR angiogram was normal.
- Anatomically, the aneurysm suggested a pseudoaneurysm.
- Endovascular treatment failed.
- At 1 month, angiography demonstrated spontaneous occlusion of the aneurysm.
- The lesion originated directly from the arterial wall rather than from a branching site.

The mechanism underlying aneurysm formation associated with low-dose radiosurgery has not been elucidated, but a focal vasculopathy may be induced by the radiation on the vessel wall considering that the aneurysm developed in the irradiated field.

Karampelas and colleagues[24] described the unique case of spontaneaous intratumoral hemorrhage in a VS occurring more than 2 years after GKRS (the patient was treated with microsurgical resection 13 years earlier). Intratumoral infarction following GKRS led to an increase in intratumoral pressure, which could have changed the local hemodynamics and weakened the vessel wall. Another hypothesis for hemorrhage is the increase in vascular outflow resistance due to radiation-induced venous obliteration after RS.

MALIGNANT TRANSFORMATION & RADIO-INDUCED TUMORS

This is probably the most polemic issue, because little data are available and because it appears unacceptable to bear the potential risk of malignancy after irradiation of a benign lesion. This potential risk is an argument still used by some colleagues not to recommend RS in the treatment of VS.

Currently, it is known that the incidence of malignant transformation is very low. In an extensive recent review of the literature, Demetriades and colleagues[25] reported 14 cases of malignant VS. Only 6 of them were irradiated, and 3 had a histologic confirmation of a benign lesion before radiotherapy.

To be recognized as a radiation-induced tumor, the lesion should fulfill the following criteria as defined by Cahan:

1. The tumor must occur at the irradiated site.
2. Time latency is longer than 5 years.
3. Tumor is of different pathologic type from the initial irradiated tissue.

This complication is well described in the case of fractionated radiation therapy but cannot be extrapolated to RS considering that radiobiology of both techniques and responses of tissues to these techniques are very different. Whole brain volume is exposed to low doses of radiation (1 Gy) by the radiosurgical procedure.

An estimate of the incidence of radiosurgery-induced tumor ranges from 0 to 3 per 200,000 patients.[26] The influencing factors are[27] age at exposure and individual susceptibility.

In a retrospective study conducted by a single center in the United Kingdom on a patient database of about 5000 patients and 30,000 patient-years of follow-up, a single case of astrocytoma was diagnosed. Rowe and colleagues[19] did not find any excess incidence of cerebral malignancy in a large group of patients radiosurgically treated in a single center, and compared with cancer registries.

SUMMARY

As a rule, RS is an efficient and safe treatment of small to middle-sized VS. CNNs are the most frequent complications, and they are usually transient. To be confirmed and before taking any unjustified decision of surgery, diagnosis of failure needs a sequential survey of the images after RS. Potential complications should be explained to the patients and referring physician at the time of the decision-making process.

REFERENCES

1. Prasad D, Steiner M, Steiner L. Gamma surgery for vestibular schwannoma. J Neurosurg 2000;92:745–59.
2. Unger F, Walch C, Haselberger K, et al. Radiosurgery of vestibular schwannomas: a minimally invasive alternative to microsurgery. Acta Neurochir (Wien) 1999;141: 1281–5.
3. Roche PH, Khalil M, Soumare O, et al. Hydrocephalus and vestibular schwannomas: considerations about the impact of gamma knife radiosurgery. Prog Neurol Surg 2008;21:200–6.
4. Timmer FC, Van Haren AE, Mulder JJ, et al. Quality of life after gamma knife radiosurgery treatment in patients with a vestibular schwannoma: the patient's perspective. Eur Arch Otorhinolaryngol 2010;267:867–73.
5. Chopra R, Kondziolka D, Niranjan A, et al. Long-term follow-up of acoustic schwannoma radiosurgery with marginal tumor doses of 12 to 13 Gy. Int J Radiat Oncol Biol Phys 2007;68:845–51.
6. Ogunrinde OK, Lunsford LD, Flickinger JC, et al. Cranial nerve preservation after stereotactic radiosurgery for small acoustic tumors. Arch Neurol 1995;52:73–9.
7. Régis J, Tamura M, Delsanti C, et al. Hearing preservation in patients with unilateral vestibular schwannoma after gammaknife surgery. Prog Neurol Surg 2008; 21:142–52.
8. Myrseth E, Moller P, Pedersen PH, et al. Vestibular schwannomas: clinical results and quality of life after microsurgery or gamma knife radiosurgery. Neurosurgery 2005;56:927–35.

9. Pollock BE, Lunsford D, Kondziolka D, et al. Vestibular schwannoma management. Part II. Failed radiosurgery and the role of delayed microsurgery. J Neurosurg 1998;89:949–55.
10. Pollock BE. Management of vestibular schwannomas that enlarge after stereotactic radiosurgery: treatment recommendations based on 15-year experience. Neurosurgery 2006;58:241–7.
11. Friedman RA, Brackmann DE, Hitselberger WE, et al. Surgical salvage after failed irradiation for vestibular schwannoma. Laryngoscope 2005;115:1827–32.
12. Limb CJ, Long DM, Niparko JK. Acoustic neuroma after failed radiation therapy: challenges of surgical salvage. Laryngoscope 2005;115:93–8.
13. Yomo S, Arkha Y, Delsanti C, et al. Repeat gamma knife surgery for regrowth of vestibular schwannomas. Neurosurgery 2009;64:48–55.
14. Rowe JG, Radatz MW, Walton L, et al. Gamma knife radiosurgery for unilateral acoustic neuromas. J Neurol Neurosurg Psychiatry 2003;74:1536–42.
15. Régis J, Pellet W, Delsanti C, et al. Functional outcome after gamma knife surgery or microsurgery for vestibular schwannomas. J Neurosurg 2002;97:1091–100.
16. Yang I, Sughrue ME, Han SJ, et al. Facial nerve preservation after vestibular schwannoma gamma knife radiosurgery. J Neurooncol 2009;93(1):41–8.
17. Tamura M, Murata N, Hayashi M, et al. Facial nerve function insufficiency after radiosurgery versus microsurgery. Prog Neurol Surg 2008;21:108–18.
18. Sughrue ME, Yang I, Han SJ, et al. Nonaudiofacial morbidity after gamma knife surgery for vestibular schwannoma. Neurosurg Focus 2009;27(6):1–8.
19. Rowe J, Grainger A, Walton L, et al. Risk of malignancy after gamma knife stereotactic radiosurgery. Neurosurgery 2007;60:60–7.
20. Roche PH, Régis J, Devèze A, et al. Surgical removal of unimateral vestibular schwannomas after failed gammaknife radiosurgery. Neurochirurgie 2004;50:383–93.
21. Akamtsu Y, Sugawara T, Mikawa S, et al. Ruptured pseudoaneurysm following gamma knife surgery for a vestibular schwannoma. Case report. J Neurosurg 2009;110:543–6.
22. Park KY, Ahn JY, Lee JW, et al. De novo intracranial aneurysm formation after gamma knife radiosurgery for vestibular schwannoma. Case report. J Neurosurg 2009;110:540–2.
23. Takao T, Fukuda M, Kawaguchi T, et al. Ruptured intracranial aneurysm following gamma knife surgery for acoustic neuroma. Acta Neurochir (Wien) 2006;148: 1317–8.
24. Karampelas I, Alberico RA, Plunkett RJ, et al. Intratumoral hemorrhage after remote subtotal microsurgical resection and gamma knife radiosurgery for vestibular schwannoma. Acta Neurochir 2007;149(3):313–6.
25. Demetriades AK, Saunders N, Rose P, et al. Malignant transformation of acoustic neuroma/vestibular schwannoma 10 years after gammaknife streotactic radiosurgery. Skull Base 2010;20(5):381–7.
26. Ganz JC. Gamma knife radiosurgery and its possible relationship to malignancy: a review. J Neurosurg 2002;9:644–52.
27. Muracciole X, Régis J. Radiosurgery and carcinogenesis risk. Prog Neurol Surg 2008;21:207–13.

Retrosigmoid Approach:
Indications, Techniques, and Results

Mohamed Samy Elhammady, MD[a],*, Fred F. Telischi, MEE, MD[b],
Jacques J. Morcos, MD, FRCS (Eng.), FRCS (Ed)[a]

KEYWORDS

- Vestibular schwannoma • Acoustic neuroma • Retrosigmoid • Surgical technique

KEY POINTS

- The retrosigmoid or lateral suboccipital approach is the most commonly used approach for vestibular schwannoma; indicated for tumors of all sizes, particularly when hearing preservation is the goal.
- The excellent exposure of the brainstem and cranial nerves via the retrosigmoid approach permits complete excision of small-to-medium-sized tumors when hearing preservation is the goal and safe resection of larger tumors that compress the brainstem and adjacent neurovascular structures.
- Expertise in retrosigmoid surgery is very much experience dependent, as one incrementally learns new technical pearls in complication avoidance.

As in any other discipline, many of today's accomplishments in the treatment of acoustic neuromas owe their existence to the brilliance (or good fortune) of the many pioneers who came before and paved an ever more refined path. The year 1777 seems to be the accepted time stamp that marks the recognition by Sandifort during an autopsy of the entity of acoustic neuroma.[1] Fast-forward to 1890, the year that von Bergmann earned the distinct honor of attempting to become the first to resect surgically an acoustic neuroma.[1] The patient sadly succumbed before von Bergmann's localizing the tumor.

EARLY SURGICAL APPROACHES

In spite of reports by many authors, most today would recognize Krause as the architect of the suboccipital approach.[2] It is quite amazing to realize that an early version of the "translabyrinthine" approach was suggested by Panse in 1904[3]; the tireless

[a] Department of Neurological Surgery, University of Miami School of Medicine, Lois Pope LIFE Center, 1095 NW 14th Terrace, 2nd Floor, (D4-6), Miami, FL 33136-1060, USA
[b] Department of Otolaryngology, Neurological Surgery and Biomedical Engineering, University of Miami School of Medicine, Clinical Research Building, 1120 NW 14th Street, 5th Floor, Miami, FL 33136, USA
* Corresponding author.
E-mail address: melhammady2@med.miami.edu

Otolaryngol Clin N Am 45 (2012) 375–397
doi:10.1016/j.otc.2012.02.001
0030-6665/12/$ – see front matter © 2012 Published by Elsevier Inc.

debate between proponents of both approaches has been raging ever since. Cushing criticized the translabyrinthine approach for its narrow confines, proximity of vascular structures, risk of CSF leak, and unsuitability for large tumors.[4] Remarkably, a hundred years later, many modern neurosurgeons have similar reservations.

The advent of ventriculography, pneumoencephalography and angiography improved the diagnostic accuracy of acoustic neuromas and Cairns is credited with the first successful total resection of an acoustic neuroma with facial nerve preservation in 1931.[5] While Cushing had advocated a bilateral suboccipital craniotomy in all cases to prevent cerebellar herniation, and intentional subtotal resection, Dandy much favored the small unilateral retrosigmoid flap and gross total resection, which he first reported in 1917.[6] McKenzie, Alexander[7] and Olivecrona[8] modified his technique, and popularized the shift from prone to sitting position, a trend that remained significant for several decades, to be supplanted by the three-quarter prone and supine positions in more recent years.

SURGICAL MICROSCOPE

The distinction of introducing the surgical microscope to the resection of acoustic neuromas, undoubtedly, the most influential technical advance in this 120 year history belongs to an otological surgeon, Bill House, although he used it to re-introduce successfully the transtemporal approaches (translabyrinthine and middle fossa).[9]

EARLY SURGICAL OUTCOMES

Safety of surgery improved steadily through the century. Surgical mortality started in the 80% range in the early days, and dropped to below 10% in House's hands in the 1960s, and is today below 1%. Similarly, anatomic facial nerve preservation rates started at 0% and today are virtually 100%.[2]

INDICATIONS

Treatment options for acoustic neuromas include observation, radiosurgery, and microsurgery. The factors involved in decision-making are discussed in this issue in the article by Sheth et al. Once a decision has been made to operate, the surgeon must choose from among three main surgical approaches:

1. Middle fossa
2. Translabyrinthine
3. Retrosigmoid.

The choice of surgical approach is dependent on several factors including:

- Patient's age
- Paitent's hearing status
- Tumor size
- Surgeon preference.

The middle fossa approach is used for small tumors ($\approx$ 1 cm) that are primarily intracanalicular and when hearing preservation is the goal.

The translabyrinthine approach is generally used for tumors of any size when hearing preservation is not an issue.

The retrosigmoid or lateral suboccipital approach is the most commonly used approach and is also indicated for tumors of all sizes, particularly when hearing preservation is the goal. The retrosigmoid approach offers an excellent exposure of the brainstem and cranial nerves IV through XII. This permits complete excision of small-to-medium-sized tumors when hearing preservation is the goal and safe resection of larger tumors that compress the brainstem and adjacent neurovascular structures.

PREOPERATIVE ASSESSMENT

Preoperative evaluation includes:

- Standard preoperative labs
- Electrocardiogram
- Chest radiograph
- Assessment of the patient's general health.

It is important to obtain a preoperative audiogram with pure tones and speech discrimination to ascertain baseline hearing function.

Magnetic resonance imaging with and without gadolinium administration including IAC views provides vital information regarding the soft tissue anatomy.

The tumor size, including its rostro-caudal and intracanalicular extensions, is determined.

T2-weighted images provide details regarding tumor consistency (hyperintense lesions are suggestive of softer and more suckable tumors), associated edema, and the plane between the tumor and surrounding structures.

The location and size of the sigmoid sinus and jugular bulb should also be assessed, particularly to be aware of a high jugular bulb that may hinder drilling of the caudal posterior lip of the IAC.

Computed tomography of the temporal bone provides information regarding aeration of the mastoid process and the location of the posterior semicircular canal in relation to the IAC.

ANESTHESIA FOR VESTIBULAR SCHWANNOMA

The anesthetic technique is similar to that of other brain tumors:

- After anesthesia is induced an arterial line is obtained and an indwelling Foley catheter inserted.
- All pressure points are padded.
- Sequential compression devices are placed to prevent deep venous thrombosis.
- Preoperative antibiotics are administered one-half hour before skin incision and 10 mg of dexamethasone is given at the beginning of the operation. Antibiotics are re-dosed as necessary based on the length of the procedure.
- At the time of skin incision, a 20% solution of mannitol in a dosage of 0.5 to 1 mg/kg body weight is administered intravenously over a period of 15 to 20 minutes.
- The patient is hyperventilated to obtain an end-tidal CO_2 of 28 mmHg.
- Although a lumbar drain can be inserted, we have found that, in most cases, adequate brain relaxation can be obtained with corticosteroids, hyperventilation, and cisterna magna drainage.
- It is important not to give paralytics to allow monitoring of facial nerve function. However, once the tumor has been removed, inhalation anesthetics may be administered to allow a rapid and smooth awakening from anesthesia.

MONITORING DURING SURGERY

Neurophysiologic monitoring during acoustic neuroma surgery allows continuous assessment of brain stem, facial nerve, and auditory nerve function throughout the procedure. Facial nerve function is monitored by inserting EMG electrodes into the orbicularis oculi and oris muscles and placing a motion sensor on the patient's face. Brainstem auditory evoked potentials and electrocochleography using a trans-tympanic electrode allows monitoring of auditory function in cases where hearing preservation is attempted. We have been very satisfied with near-field direct cochlear nerve recordings as a reliable measure of cochlear nerve functioning during dissection. More details about intraoperative monitoring are discussed in another Chapter.

SURGICAL TECHNIQUE
Position

The patient can be positioned sitting, supine, or in a lateral decubitus.
In the sitting position:

- The patient is placed upright on several cushions and hips and knees are bent approximately 90°.
- The head is turned 30° toward the side of the lesion, flexed slightly in an antero-posterior plane, and fixed in a 3-pin Mayfield head clamp.

The sitting position facilitates drainage of blood and cerebrospinal fluid out of the wound and thus provides a bloodless and clear operative field. However, it carries a higher risk of air embolism and spinal cord ischemia and, in our opinion is more cumbersome and exhausting for the surgeon's arms as compared with the other positions. For these reasons, we prefer either the supine or lateral decubitus position based on the patient's body habitus.

We used the supine position in our earlier experience, but more recently have adopted the lateral decubitus position exclusively.

- In the supine position, the shoulder that is ipsilateral to the tumor is elevated with a gel roll to allow turning of the head without excessive tension on the neck.
- In the lateral position, the patient is placed with the side of the lesion upward while the dependant arm hangs off the bed and is cradled in a padded sling between the table and edge of the Mayfield head holder.
- With the lateral position, it is important to retract the patient's superior shoulder toward the patient's feet using adhesive tape, taking special care not to create a brachial plexus stretch injury.

Regardless of the position used, the head is fixed in a 3-pin Mayfield clamp and positioned with 3 movements:

1. Contralateral rotation so that the temple is parallel to the floor.
2. Contralateral bending so that the vertex is slightly tilted toward the floor.
3. Flexion in the anteroposterior plane until the chin is two finger breadths from the clavicle to open the cervical-suboccipital angle. Over-flexion could compress the jugular veins.

The operating table is placed in slight reverse Trendelenberg so as to position the patient's head above the level of the heart to reduce cerebral venous congestion.

Incision and Exposure

The retroauricular region of the scalp is shaved. Several surface landmarks can be identified and marked to plan the skin incision. We use 3 reference points:

1. External auditory canal (EAC)
2. Inion
3. Tip of the mastoid process.

The course of the sigmoid sinus is represented by the posterior border of the mastoid process. The EAC-inion line is generally parallel to and slightly lower than the lower border of the transverse sinus.

- We mark a point along the EAC-inion line at which we start our drilling to expose the transverse sigmoid junction. This point is placed 4 cm and 4.5 cm from the external auditory canal in females and males, respectively.

Technical pearl
Although the asterion may be used to approximate the transverse-sigmoid junction, it is frequently difficult to accurately identify intraoperatively. We have found that these points are useful safe areas to start the drilling to expose the venous sinuses. They are almost always medio-caudal to the actual TS junction.

- The size of the planned craniotomy is approximately 3.0 to 3.5 cm, immediately posterior to the sigmoid sinus.
- A C-shaped retroauricular incision is then marked extending approximately 2 cm below the tip of the mastoid to a point approximately 2 cm above the pinna. It is crucial that the apex of the C-shaped incision extend beyond the medial edge of the planned craniotomy because it is difficult to retract the skin posteriorly. It is for this reason that we do not use a linear incision, which generally results in the skin edges lifting up with traction and compromising the medial exposure.
- The scalp is prepped and draped in a standard fashion and the planned incision infiltrated with 0.5% lidocaine with epinephrine 1:200,000.
- The scalp incision is elevated sparing the pericranium above the superior nuchal line and the fascia overlying the suboccipital musculature.
- The suboccipital fascia and muscles are then incised in a T-shaped fashion.
- The horizontal limb is made leaving a small muscular cuff attached to the superior nuchal line.
- The vertical limb is carried down caudally until the occipital bone changes orientation from a horizontal to a more vertical plane (floor of the posterior fossa).

Technical pearl
Caution must be exercised during the lower end of the exposure. Overzealous use of the Bovie in the region between the occipital bone and C1 may result in a vertebral artery injury. In this region it is only necessary to incise the superficial muscle fibers. Adequate exposure can then be achieved with several fishhooks retracting in an upward direction, a maneuver that creates significant depth.

- Once the muscular incisions have been made, the muscles are elevated in a subperiosteal fashion to uncover the suboccipital bone and the base of the mastoid process including the digastric groove. The exposure is maintained by retracting the scalp flap and suboccipital muscles with fish hooks.
- The transverse and sigmoid sinuses are then exposed using a combination of 5 mm round cutting and diamond burrs.
- An initial burr hole is placed just medio-caudal to the presumed location of the transverse-sigmoid junction based on the surface landmarks described above.
- Once the dura is identified, the drilling is continued in a superolateral direction until the transverse-sigmoid junction is identified.

- Drilling is then continued in a caudal direction to expose the edge of the sigmoid sinus. It should be noted that the outer wall of the sigmoid sinus is curved and more adherent to the overlying bone than the transverse sinus.

Technical pearl
Bleeding from the mastoid emissary vein is frequently encountered during drilling. This may be controlled with bone wax until its bony canal has been drilled, at which point it may be coagulated and sectioned. The emissary vein may also be used as a landmark and followed to the sinus.

- Once the sigmoid sinus has been exposed, the dura is carefully separated from the overlying bone in the region of the transverse sinus and cerebellum.
- A craniotomy is then performed extending from the transverse sinus to the caudal level of the sigmoid sinus where it curves anteriorly. Frequently, it is necessary to remove additional bone inferiorly beyond the craniotomy flap to expose the floor of the posterior fossa to gain access to the lateral cerebellomedullary cistern. Any mastoid air cells that have been entered during the drilling are occluded now with bone wax.
- At this stage of the procedure the operative microscope is used.
- The dura is opened in a C-shaped fashion based medially.
- Initially only a small horizontal dural opening at the caudal portion of the exposure is made to avoid outward herniation of the cerebellum. It is helpful here for the surgeon to position himself at the patient's vertex, looking caudally with the microscope.
- A 0.25 × 3 in telfa is placed over the cerebellum and the latter is depressed to expose the lateral recess of the cisterna magna.
- The arachnoid membrane is then sharply incised under direct vision and cerebrospinal fluid is allowed to drain for several minutes.

Technical pearl
Occasionally there may be a small vein in this region which may be injured if the cerebellum is excessively retracted or the arachnoid is blindly incised.

- Once the cerebellum is adequately relaxed, the remaining dura is opened approximately 5 mm parallel to the sigmoid and transverse sinuses, and the dural flap placed under tension medially to avoid it shrinking during the surgery. The dural edge along the sigmoid and transverse sinuses is also retracted with 4–0 neurolon sutures.

Tumor Exposure and Removal

- The midportion of the cerebellum is covered with telfa patties and gently mobilized to expose the cerebellopontine angle. A self-retaining retractor is never used, no matter how small or large the tumor is.

Technical pearl
The key to exposure is not forceful cerebellar retraction, but rather thorough arachnoidal lysis in the upper, middle and lower components of the CP angle cistern, as well as the cerebellomedullary cistern. Working from caudally to rostrally is usually the best strategy.

- The next step is to open the arachnoid over the inferior tumor pole and the lower cranial nerves and establish the appropriate plane of dissection.

Technical pearls

Acoustic neuromas are invested in two arachnoidal layers. The first of these layers represents the peripheral arachnoidal layer of the posterior fossa whereas the second layer comprises the arachnoid membrane that envelops the tumor itself and was invaginated by it. Ideally the dissection should be performed between these two layers so that cranial nerves and major arteries can be shielded from the dissection. However, in the event that there is a poor arachnoidal plane, it may be necessary to carry out the dissection between the tumor and the deep arachnoidal layer.

Unless the tumor is very large and occupies all available space, the initial view reveals the lateral portion of the tumor and the anterior inferior cerebellar artery with its subarcuate branch. The lower cranial nerves and posterior inferior cerebellar artery are identified caudally and the trigeminal and petrosal vein rostrally.

Occasionally, with small-to-medium-sized tumors the eighth nerve complex may be identified entering the inferomedial side of the tumor with its fibers splayed over the posterior surface of the capsule. In such cases the vestibular nerve remnant proximal to the tumor is divided, enabling dissection of the tumor from the cochlear and facial nerve.

- The AICA is dissected and mobilized off the capsule; branches to the tumor are coagulated and sectioned.
- The subarcuate artery that arises from the AICA and enters the subarcuate fossa (located superior and posterior to the IAC) is coagulated and divided.

Technical pearl

Rarely, a subarcuate variant of the AICA is identified in which the main vessel forms a loop with the apex embedded in the dura and possibly the petrous bone just posterior to the IAC. To free the AICA, the dura and bone surrounding the artery must be carefully removed.

Technical pearl

At this stage in the procedure, the posterior surface of the tumor capsule is inspected and stimulated to ensure that the facial nerve has not been displaced posteriorly, a rare surgical variant that carries tremendous consequences if unrecognized. In most cases the facial nerve can be found along the anterior or anterosuperior surface of the tumor capsule as it courses laterally. However on rare occasions, particularly in patients with recurrent tumors or those with neurofibromatosis type 2, the facial nerve may be found on the inferior or even the posterior aspect of the tumor. In small-to-medium-sized tumors, where the root entry zone of the eighth cranial nerve may be visualized early in the procedure, the facial nerve is identified or stimulated beneath and deep to the vestibulo-cochlear nerve. The facial nerve can be differentiated from the eight cranial nerve and adjacent brainstem by its characteristic color and of course by direct stimulation.

- After confirming that the facial nerve has not been displaced posteriorly, internal decompression of the tumor is then performed to gain surgical space.
- The posterior surface of the capsule is entered and the intracapsular contents of the lateral portion of the tumor are evacuated using a combination of suctioning, bipolar coagulation, cup forceps, and ultrasonic aspiration. The goal should be to thin the tumor to within a few millimeters from the remaining capsule. This creates a space for delivery and subsequent internal decompression of the more medially situated tumor. Furthermore, it reduces the tension on the VII/VIII nerve complex during the dissection.

Technical pearl
Over-aggressive debulking should be avoided as it may breach the tumor capsule and potentially injure the brainstem and adherent cranial nerves.

- Once adequate internal decompression has been achieved, the tumor capsule is dissected along the double layer of arachnoid away from the surrounding neurovascular structures. The dissection usually begins caudally separating the glossopharyngeal and vagus nerves from the lower pole of the tumor capsule.

Technical pearl
Loops of the posterior and anterior inferior cerebellar arteries may be encountered and need to be dissected from the tumor and protected.

- The dissection is continued medially along the medulla to the foramen of Luschka and flocculus.
- After carefully elevating the inferiomedial capsule laterally and superiorly, the facial and vestibulocochlear nerves are identified at their exit from the pons at the pontomedullary sulcus.
- A useful landmark to identify the root entry zone of the VII/VIII complex is to trace a line superiorly from the root entry zone of the glossopharyngeal and vagus nerves. As previously mentioned the facial nerve is usually located just under the vestibulocochlear nerve. These nerves are often splayed out and appear as a thin membrane over the anterior surface of the tumor.
- The tumor capsule is sharply dissected away from the nerves using a combination of microscissors, a sharp nerve hook, or a Rhoton no. 3 dissector. Because the cochlear nerve exits the IAC at the fundus through a "cribriform" plate, its individual fibers are prone to be avulsed easily if retracted medially. There, Rhoton advocates using only medial-to-lateral traction of the tumor if hearing preservation is the goal.[10]

Technical pearl
Dissection of these nerves beyond the point at which they become splayed, thinned out, or enter through the porus acousticus is not advisable at this stage in the procedure. The internal auditory (labyrinthine) branch of the AICA, which frequently accompanies the eighth cranial nerve should be preserved if hearing is to be saved.

- Next, the upper pole of the tumor capsule is separated from the trigeminal nerve and petrosal vein. In most cases it is unnecessary to sacrifice the petrosal vein;

however it may be coagulated and divided, if absolutely necessary, particularly with larger tumors to facilitate dissection of the upper pole.

- The superior cerebellar artery is encountered and freely dissected.
- As the cranial, caudal, and medial portions of the tumor are dissected from the surrounding neurovascular structures, the cleavage plane is maintained using telfa patties.
- Redundant tumor capsule is excised and repeated internal decompression performed to allow further centripetal mobilization of the tumor.

Technical pearl

Any maneuver that results in deterioration in the brainstem auditory evoked responses or abnormal firing of the facial nerve require immediate cessation to allow recovery. Irrigation with warm saline frequently quiets the facial nerve. Deterioration secondary to surgically induced vasospasm may be managed by local application of papaverine.

- When the porus is reached or when further dissection of the tumor from medial to lateral becomes difficult, the posterior wall of the IAC is drilled and the intracanalicular tumor removed.
- If the porus cannot be easily appreciated, a blunt microhook may be used to probe the canal and delineate its superior and inferior margins.

Technical pearl

The tumor is frequently constricted by the thickened dura at the porus, which may give a false impression as to the true caliber of the meatus and the amount of bone removal required.

- Several landmarks on the posterior surface of the petrous bone provide orientation to the labyrinth and IAC:
  1. The entrance of the subarcuate artery at the subarcuate fossa marks the center of the superior semicircular canal.
  2. The bony operculum which overlies the aperture of the vestibular aqueduct approximates the floor of the internal auditory meatus.
  3. The medial border of the endolymphatic sac can be used as a lateral boundary to avoid the common crus and ampullated end of the superior semicircular canal.
- Gelfoam sponges are placed in the subarachnoid space to prevent dissemination of bone dust during drilling.
- The dura is excised along the axis of the IAC, extending no more that 1 cm lateral to the porus acousticus. Alternatively, the dura may be incised in a C-shaped fashion from the porus, elevated, and reflected over the posterior aspect of the tumor, to be used later to cover the exposed perilabyrinthine air cells following drilling.
- The posterior wall of the IAC is then drilled under constant suction and irrigation until the posterior 180 to 270° of the canal circumference has been removed.
- The dura lining the IAC is gradually exposed along its long axis from medial to lateral using progressively smaller cutting then diamond burrs. The safe drilling zone tapers as one reaches the fundus.

- An extensive bony removal as described is necessary to adequately expose the tumor and facilitate its dissection.

Technical pearl
Caution should be exercised while drilling the superior aspect of the canal to avoid injury to the facial nerve as it runs in the facial canal located in the antero-superior quadrant of the IAC. Similarly, drilling of the inferior aspect of the canal should be performed judiciously to avoid injury to a high jugular bulb.
The drilling should be carried as far laterally as the tumor extends without entering the labyrinth.
A clue to the lateral extent of the tumor is the transition in color of the canal dura from white to blue indicating presence and absence of tumor, respectively. Occasionally the lateral exposure requires blue-lining of the common crus or ampullated end of the superior semicircular canal.
In the event that a semicircular canal is entered, it should be immediately closed with bone wax in hopes of preserving hearing. The endoscope may also be used to visualize residual tumor in the lateral end of the canal.

- Once the drilling has been completed, the dura lining the IAC is opened to expose the intracanalicular portion of the tumor.
- The tumor and/or superior vestibular nerve are displaced inferiorly to expose and stimulate the facial nerve near the origin of the facial canal.
- The vestibular nerve remnant distal to the tumor is sectioned, whereas normal vestibular fascicles are preserved.
- We also attempt to maintain continuity of the cochlear nerve, even if hearing preservation is not a goal, because it provides support and limits movement of the facial nerve. Furthermore it may reduce the risk of facial nerve ischemia.
- The intracanalicular tumor is then removed and the facial nerve identified to the porus. In most cases this part of the tumor has few adhesions to the nerves and can be removed without difficulty. However, in some instances the tumor can expand the porus irregularly and cause significant adhesions and displacement of the nerves making identification of the nerves and tumor resection challenging.

Technical pearl
The most difficult part of the tumor to dissect is the transitional or junctional zone. This is a 1 cm long area along the ventrolateral portion of the tumor just proximal to the porus acousticus. In this region the tumor capsule and nerves are extremely adherent as a result of tumor invasion of the arachnoid. Facial nerve stimulation is vital as it facilitates identification of the facial nerve fibers which may be difficult, despite high magnification, to distinguish from arachnoidal adhesions or filaments of the eighth cranial nerve.

- If the adhesions between the tumor and nerves prove to be extremely difficult to dissect, a small piece of tumor may be left to avoid facial or cochlear nerve injury.

385

Case 1. Illustrates a typical case with hearing preservation. The surgical steps are demonstrated in partial detail

35 year old woman who was diagnosed with a right acoustic neuroma in 2008. She was advised conservative follow-up. The tumor grew from 9mm to 18mm in 3 years, with decline in hearing. We first saw her in 2011 and recommended a retrosigmoid approach.

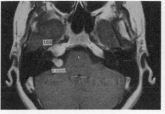
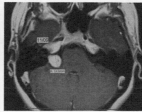
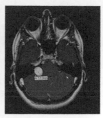

MRI axial T1 Gad in 2008. Tumor size 8mm.

MRI axial T1 Gad in 2009. Tumor size 15mm.

MRI T1 axial Gad.

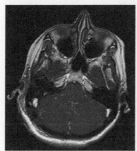
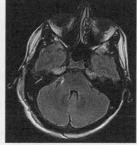
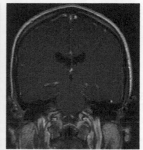

Postoperative MRI on POD2 (axial T1 Gad, axial FLAIR and coronal T1 Gad, respectively). Gross total resection confirmed. Patient retained serviceable hearing.

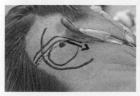
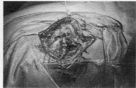
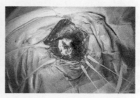

Surface landmarks for the transverse/sigmoid, the mastoid tip, the external auditory meatus-inion line, the proposed bone flap, the curved incision and the mark for the initial drilling site.

Skin incision, T-shaped incision in musculature.

Fishhook retraction of soft tissues.

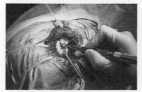
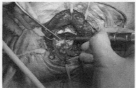
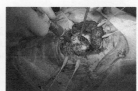

Initial drilling just below transverse-sigmoid junction.

Once dura secured, drill with foot plate used to elevate free bone flap.

Bone flap lifted.

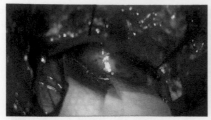

CP angle approached, arachnoid incised, tumor exposed. Self-retaining retractors never used.

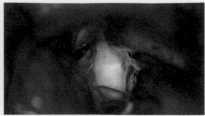

Trigeminal nerve visualized at superior pole.

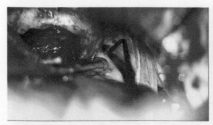

Stimulator (with its tip bent) searching for facial nerve on anterior-caudal surface of tumor.

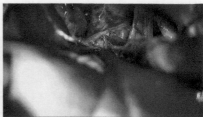

Sharp dissection to separate arterial branches (here AICA branches).

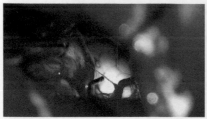

Facial nerve traced along anterior tumor surface.

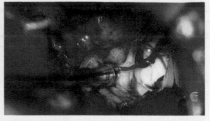

Dissection begins between vestibulo-cochlear bundle and tumor.

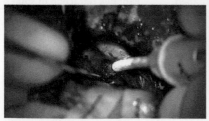

Low profile, curved, shaft-insulated, diamond tipped drill used to drill posterior wall of IAC from medially to laterally.

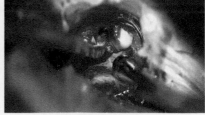

Curved sickle knife used to mobilize intracanalicular tumor from laterally to medially.

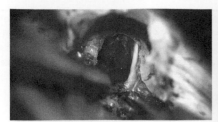

Intracanalicular tumor completely removed. Vestibulo-cochlear bundle well seen.

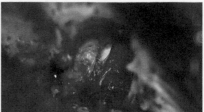

Tumor mobilized from lateral to medial, with careful attention to cochlear nerve signal.

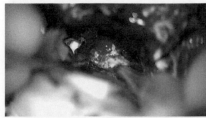

Further intracapsular debulking with CUSA.

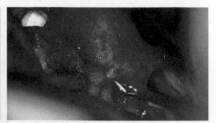

Sharp microhook used to tease out adherent tumor off nerves.

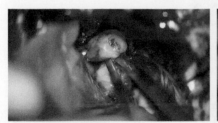

Free tumor removed.

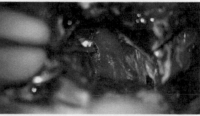

Final microscopic view. No packing needed in IAC, since no air cells encountered.

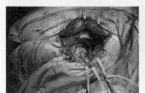

Dural flap closed primarily.

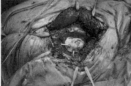

Bone flap replaced with 3 simple titanium plates.

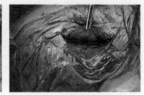

Muscles and fascia re-approximated to cuff, ensuring absence of dead space.

Case 2. Illustrates an unusual case (that must always be timely recognized intraoperatively) where the facial nerve was draped on the posterior surface of the tumor, resulting in subtotal resection

55 year old female with a left acoustic neuroma and Class A hearing, complaining of imbalance and tinnitus.

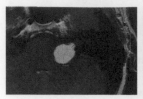 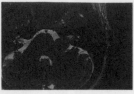 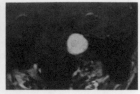

Preop MRI (axial T1 Gad, axial T2 and coronal T1 Gad, respectively). The intracanalicular portion measures 4.5 mm; the extracanalicular portion measures 17 mm.

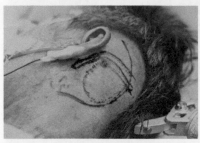 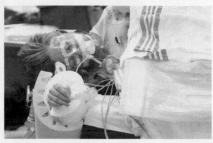

Surface markings of sigmoid/transverse sinus, bone flap, incision and location of initial drilling near TS junction.

Surgical positioning in right lateral decubitus position, with dependent arm carefully "cocooned" in soft foam.

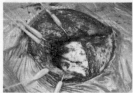 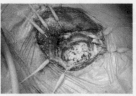 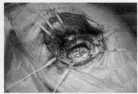

Following skin incision, the muscle layers are incised in a T-shape, leaving a cuff of attachment on the superior nuchal line. Fish hooks are judiciously applied in a fashion that minimizes muscle incisions.

Following a craniectomy that exposes the inner edges of the sigmoid and transverse sinuses, a free bone flap is lifted.

The dura is incised in a line parallel to the sinuses.

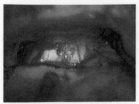 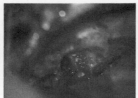 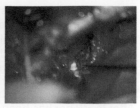

Under the microscope, the dorsal surface of the tumor is interrogated with the stimulator. Facial nerve activity is unfortunately obtained from the posterior superior surface of the tumor, in a diffuse manner. This case illustrates the importance of performing this step prior to debulking the tumor, in order to recognize this unusual configuration and avoid facial nerve injury.

Partial drilling of the posterior wall of the IAC, to uncover the lateral extent of the tumor.

After resecting the caudal portion of the tumor. Note the shiny white brainstem surface.

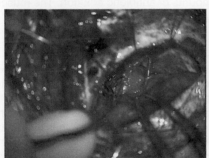 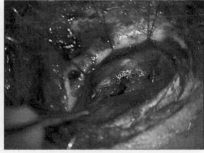

The tumor resection line goes up to the edge of the stimulation zone. The fibers of the facial nerve are diffusely covering the rest of the unresected tumor.

Final view after forced subtotal resection. The facial nerve still stimulates with 0.05 mA of current. The auditory evoked potentials have weakened significantly.

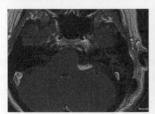 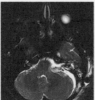 

Postop MRI on postop day 2. Axial T1 Gad, Axial T2 and Coronal T1 Gad, respectively. Note the residual tumor. Hearing was not preserved.

- An efficient method to dissect tumor and identify simultaneously the nature of the tissue being mobilized, is to use special dissecting-stimulating instruments.
- Prior to closure, the facial nerve is stimulated at its exit from the brainstem and, if a current of 0.05 mA achieves stimulation, then long term normal facial nerve function is almost guaranteed.

Closure

- After the tumor has been removed, the surgical bed is irrigated and is inspected for hemostasis. Bleeding along the nerves generally stops spontaneously or with Surgicel (Ethicon, Inc. Somerville, NJ, USA).
- The bony edges of the drilled internal auditory meatus are thoroughly waxed to occlude any air cells.
- A fat graft, harvested from the abdomen, or a local piece of muscle is used to fill loosely the IAC.
- A single layer of Surgicel is laid over the surface of the retracted cerebellum.
- The dura is closed in a watertight fashion either primarily or using a pericranial graft or dural substitute.
- The bone flap is replaced and fixed with titanium plates.
- Bone loss is usually not excessive, because of the initial targeted opening, and therefore cranioplasty is usually not needed.
- The wound is irrigated with copious amounts of antibiotic solution. The muscles and skin are meticulously closed in layers.

POSTOPERATIVE CARE

The patient should be placed in an intensive care unit for hourly neurologic assessments and continuous monitoring of vital signs. The patient's head is elevated approximately 30° to minimize the incidence of a postoperative cerebrospinal fluid leakage through the wound or development of a local pseudomeningocele. Assessment of lower cranial nerve function should be performed before initiation of an oral diet. In patients with House-Brackmann grade 4 to 6 facial paresis, exposure keratopathy is prevented by instillation of saline eye drops every 2 hours during the day and use of an eye patch and lubricant at night. A lateral tarsorrhaphy or placement of an upper eyelid gold weight is performed if delayed or no recovery of facial function is expected. Postoperative brain MRI with and without gadolinium including views of the internal auditory canal and fat suppression sequences is obtained within 2 days of surgery to determine the degree of resection and rule out postoperative hematoma or hydrocephalus.

SURGICAL RESULTS

There have been numerous series reporting surgical outcomes for acoustic neuromas. A popular strategy has been to compare the results of radiosurgery versus open surgery, as well as the results between the 3 different approaches: middle fossa, retrosigmoid and translabyrinthine. The validity of most of these comparisons is generally limited because of the retrospective nature of the studies, enrollment bias, heterogeneity of studied populations, skewed expertise within various institutions, and other factors. Nonetheless, **Table 1** is a snapshot summary of the most recent series (last 5 years) regarding outcomes and complications.

COMPLICATIONS AND THEIR MANAGEMENT

There are several complications unique to the retrosigmoid approach and resection of acoustic neuromas. These include injury to the cerebellum, venous sinuses, posterior fossa vasculature, cranial nerves, and brain stem as well as postoperative cerebrospinal fluid leaks.

Cerebellar Injury

Cerebellar edema, hematoma, or contusion may occur. The causes are varied: Poor positioning of the head and neck, careless elevation of the bone flap, opening the dura in the face of a swollen brain and before obtaining CSF egress, excessive cerebellar retraction, venous sinus injury or compromise. Such complications can be avoided by careful surgical technique and adequate cerebellar relaxation using corticosteroids, mannitol, hyperventilation and early release of cerebrospinal fluid from the posterior fossa cisterns. In the event of a hematoma or contusion, surgical evacuation of the clot or resection of the contused cerebellum is necessary. It should be noted that approximately one third of the cerebellum can be resected without producing a permanent cerebellar deficit. Cerebellar swelling secondary to compromise of venous sinus drainage can be prevented by avoiding excessive head turning or flexion during positioning. Management of venous sinus injury is discussed below. If the cerebellum remains swollen, it may be necessary to decompress the posterior fossa including the foramen magnum.

Venous Sinus Injury

Transverse and sigmoid sinus injuries can occur during the craniotomy. Sharp tears are easily repaired with 6–0 prolene. Other tears may be controlled by carefully layering (NOT packing) with Surgicel. Over-packing should be avoided as it may easily occlude the sinus. If the tear is large, it is best to cover the bleeding with gelfoam and a cottonoid, elevate the head of the bed to decrease venous pressure, and then expose more of the sinus. The tear may then be repaired primarily with a 6–0 suture or using a small dural patch.

Cranial Nerve Deficits

Trigeminal nerve
Injury to the trigeminal nerve is rare and may occur in large acoustic neuromas during dissection of the upper pole of the tumor. Deficits include diminished facial sensation and loss of the corneal reflex. If there is an associated facial paralysis the potential for exposure keratitis is high and thus preventive measures should be started early as described above.

Facial nerve
Injury to the facial nerve may occur during drilling of the internal auditory canal or as a result of transection or excessive traction on the nerve during tumor resection. The facial nerve is particularly vulnerable to injury in large-sized lesions where it may be thinned out over the tumor capsule and may be difficult to visualize or dissect. The most vulnerable site is the junction between the cisternal and meatal segments. Several options exist for facial nerve reconstruction in the event of transection or persistent postoperative facial paralysis.

Primary repair of a transected nerve provides the best opportunity for functional recovery. Prerequisites for primary repair include identification of both proximal and distal stumps of the nerve and sufficient nerve length to allow trimming of the damaged ends and approximation without any tension. This is frequently possible because the nerve is often elongated by the tumor. The technique of primary repair consists of direct end-to-end epineural or perineural anastomosis with a minimal number of tension-free sutures.

Table 1
Summary of surgical results of recent series as published since 2006

Authors	Year	N	Size	Extent of Surgery Resection	FP (Anatomic Preservation)	FP (HB 1-2)	HP	Death	Comments
Li et al[11]	2011	176	>3 cm	RS	96%	82%	41%	1.7%	
Tringali et al[12]	2010	278	Small (subdivided into 4 groups according to the percentage of IAC filling)	RS	N/A	90%		N/A	Degree of IAC filling correlates w HP and FP
Phillips et al[13]	2010	40	<1 cm in CPA	MF 17 RS 23	N/A	N/A	Overall: 58% RS: 48% MF: 71%	N/A	Wave V intraop predicts HP. If yes, 78%, if no 41%
Sughrue et al[14]	2010	11,873	N/A	All	N/A	Overall regardless of size, approach, or age: 74% Approach: MF: 85% TL: 81% RS: 78% Size: <2 cm: 90% >2 cm: 67% Age: <65yrs: 71% >65yrs: 84%	N/A	N/A	Literature review of 79/295 studies on FP
Sameshima et al[15]	2010	125	<1.5 cm	MF 43 RS 82	GTR: 100%	100%	Early (2 wk): MF: 95% RS: 100% Late (8-12 mo): MF: 100% RS: 100%	MF: 77% RS: 73%	0%	Prefer RS due to other factors (longer operative time, more difficult exposure, and a higher incidence of temporal lobe brain edema and temporary facial weakness)

Study	Year	N	Tumor size	Approach						Comments
Sughrue et al[16]	2013	998	N/A	MF 286 RS 702	N/A	N/A	N/A	Overall: 52% MF: 63% RS: 47%	N/A	Review of 49/62 studies on HP. >1.5 cm and RS did worse (independently) with HP (on MVA)
Zhao et al[17]	2010	89	Large (>4 cm)	RS	GTR: 43% NTR: 39%	93%	Early: 40% Late (1 y): 54%	N/A	0%	
Chen et al[18]	2010	145	>3 cm: 119 <3 cm: 26	RS	GTR: 97%	91%	79%	N/A	0%	
Hillman et al[19]	2010	138	Average longest diameter: MF: 8 mm RS: 14 mm	MF 88 RS 50	N/A	N/A	MF: 88% RS: 90%	MF: 59% RS: 39%	N/A	- FN recovers quicker in RS than MF - HP more likely with MF
Samii et al[20]	2010	Group A (>4 cm): 50 Group B (<3.9 cm): 167	Mean tumor size: Grp A: 4.4 cm Grp B: 2.3 cm	RS	GTR: Grp A: 100% Grp B: 97.6%	Grp A: 92% Grp B: 98.8%	Grp A: 75% (HB I-III) Grp B: 91% (HB I-III)	Grp A: 33% (3/9) Grp B: 60%	Grp A: 0% Grp B: 0%	Retrospective review of 50 pts with >4 cm (Grp A) compared with a matched grp of 167 pts with VS <3.9 cm (Grp B).
Kameda et al[21]	2010	242	Mean tumor size: 2.1 cm	RS	N/A	N/A	N/A	N/A	N/A	Study evaluating the effect of RS resection of VS on tinnitus: 71% had it preop. Postop: 25% gone, 33% better, 32% no change, 10% worse. No diff if 8th N cut or not. New tinnitus in 9%.
Noudel et al[22]	2009	843	Intracanalicular	MF 529 RS 314	N/A	N/A	At 1 y: MF: 72-100% RS: 80-100%	MF: 38-100% RS: 13-100%	MF: RS: 0%	Review article comparing the HP and FP rates following resection of intracanalicular VS via MF (16 studies) and RS (19 studies) approaches.
Yang et al[23]	2008	110	<2 cm	RS	100%	91%	Early (1-2 mo): 81% Late (1-2 y): 91%	Among pts with class A or B hearing preop, 36% were class A or B, and 44% were class A,B or C postop	0%	

(continued on next page)

Table 1
(continued)

Authors	Year	N	Size	Surgery	Extent of Resection	FP (Anatomic Preservation)	FP (HB 1-2)	HP	Death	Comments
Cardoso et al[24]	2007	240	Hanover tumor extension classification: T1: 12, T2: 41, T3a: 21, T3b: 24, T4a: 63, T4b: 79	RS	GTR: 99%	85%	FP (HB I-III) in pts with preop facial function: 85% <3 cm: 100%	40% (in tumors up to 1.5 cm)	1.6%	
Samii et al[25]	2006	200	Hanover tumor extension classification: T1: 22, T2: 18, T3a: 28, T3b: 40, T4a: 72, T4b: 20	RS	GTR: 98%	98.5%	Overall: Early: 59% At last f/u: 81% T1, T2, T3: 100%	Overall: 51% T1: 57%% T2: 54% T3a: 42%	0%	

Abbreviations: FP, facial nerve preservation; GTR, gross total resection rate; HP, hearing preservation; MF, middle fossa approach; MVA, multivariate analysis; N/A, not available; NTR, near total resection rate; RS, retrosigmoid approach; VS, vestibular schwannoma.

The Hanover tumor extension classification system:

Class T1: intrameatal tumor

Class T2: intra- and extrameatal tumor

Class T3a: lesion filling the cerebello-pontine cistern

Class T3b: tumor reaching the brainstem

Class T4a: lesion compressing the brainstem

Class T4b: tumor severely dislocating the brainstem and compressing the fourth ventricle

Interposition grafts are used if the two ends of the facial nerve can be found but there is insufficient nerve length to allow tension-free primary anastomosis. Potential donors include the sural or greater auricular nerves due to their well tolerated sensory deficits and their comparable diameter to that of the facial nerve.

Complete hypoglossal-facial anastomosis is indicated after one year if there is no return of facial function in an anatomically preserved nerve or failure of recovery following primary repair or interposition grafting. The procedure may be performed earlier in situations that preclude primary or interposition graft repair such as unavailability of the proximal end of the facial nerve. Hypoglossal-facial anastomosis improves facial tone and symmetry and provides reasonably good voluntary function particularly around the mouth and midface with less satisfactory results around the eye. However, patients must undergo biofeedback and motor re-education to learn voluntary control, decrease synkinesis, and limit the facial grimacing that can occur with mastication. The resulting unilateral hypoglossal paralysis can cause problems with speech, mastication, and swallowing but is generally well tolerated. The technique consists of exposure of the extracranial facial and hypoglossal nerves. The facial nerve is dissected from the stylomastoid foramen to its terminal branches (pes anserinus) in the parotid gland. The hypoglossal nerve along with the descendens hypoglossi and ansa cervicalis are dissected as far proximally and distally as possible to maximize the length available for the anastomosis. The facial nerve is then sectioned as close to the stylomastoid foramen as possible while the hypoglossal nerve and descendens hypoglossi are divided as far distally as possible. A tension-free epineural end-to-end anastomosis is then performed by suturing the hypoglossal nerve trunk to the distal facial nerve stump. In an attempt to minimize the inevitable unilateral tongue paralysis, the descendens hypoglossi can be anastomosed to the distal stump of the hypoglossal nerve. Limitations of the complete hypoglossal-facial anastomosis include the inability to perform the procedure in patients with preexisting uni- or bilateral glossopharyngeal and vagal nerve or contralateral hypoglossal nerve injuries due to the potentially severe disability that would ensue from the added effect of hypoglossal paralysis. Furthemore the procedure cannot be performed bilaterally in patients with bilateral facial palsy. In these situations a *partial hypoglossal-facial anastomosis* can be performed although the results are not as satisfactory as a complete hypoglossal-facial anastomosis. The technique consists of splitting the hypoglossal nerve to a thickness that is comparable to that of the facial nerve. Part of the hypoglossal nerve is then anastomosed to the distal facial nerve stump while maintaining continuity of the remainder of the hypoglossal nerve.

Cochlear nerve

Injury to the cochlear function may occur during drilling if the labyrinth is violated or during tumor dissection as a result of transection or excessive traction on the nerve. Hearing loss may also occur if the internal auditory (labyrinthine) artery is sacrificed. The BAHA (Bone Anchored Hearing Aid) could be considered in patients with such unilateral complete deafness several months postop.

Lower cranial nerves

Inadvertent injury to the lower cranial nerves following resection of large tumors is a major cause of morbidity. These cranial nerves are very sensitive to manipulation, necessitating very gentle retraction and sharp dissection. Lower cranial nerve injury may result in dysphagia, dysarthria, dysphonia, and inadequate airway protection. Thus, patients should be started on an oral diet only after a formal evaluation of lower cranial nerve function has been performed.

Brain Stem and Vascular Injury

Brain stem injuries may result from either excessive retraction or vascular injury. The AICA lies in close relation to the VII/VIII nerve complex and is frequently incorporated in the tumor capsule. AICA injuries may result in significant morbidity due to brainstem and cranial nerve ischemia. Occlusion of the internal auditory (labyrinthine) branch of the AICA may result in hearing loss. Although uncommon, compromise of the PICA or its perforators may result in postoperative lateral medullary (Wallenberg) syndrome.

Cerebrospinal Fluid Leak

Cerebrospinal fluid leakage may occur through the wound or may present as rhinorrhea by passing through the perilabyrinthine air cells to the middle ear cleft and eustachian tube. Possible etiologies include inadequate wound or dural closure, an open air cell in the bone, or postoperative hydrocephalus. A head CT should be obtained to rule out hydrocephalus, pneumocephalus, or a pseudomeningocele. A thin-cut CT of the temporal bone may demonstrate a large open air cell in the petrous bone or fluid within the mastoid and give clues to a possible route of cerebrospinal fluid leakage. Initial management with head elevation, a pressure bandage in the presence of a pseudomeningiocele, and spinal fluid drainage either through repeated lumbar punctures or a lumbar drain may be sufficient for small leaks. On the other hand, large persistent leaks or the presence of pneumocephalus requires surgical repair. This may consist of waxing of any open air cells, possible packing of the middle ear if there is no hearing, and meticulous water-tight closure of the dura and wound. Troublesome leaks may require endoscopic obliteration of the eustachian tube as a last resort, with the inevitable subsequent conductive hearing loss. The presence of hydrocephalus requires placement of a shunt after confirming the absence of meningitis.

CONCLUSIONS ON RETROSIGMOID APPROACH

The retrosigmoid approach, as performed by experienced surgeons today, is the most versatile approach for the resection of acoustic neuromas. It is appropriate for small and large tumors, as well as deaf and hearing ears. Expertise in this surgery is very much experience dependent, as one incrementally learns new technical pearls in complication avoidance. The next frontier will be in any new technology that might facilitate facial and cochlear nerve preservation.

REFERENCES

1. Cushing H. Tumors of the nervus acusticus and the syndrome of the cerebellopontine angle. Philadelphia: Saunders; 1917.
2. Machinis TG, Fountas KN, Dimopoulos V, et al. History of acoustic neurinoma surgery. Neurosurg Focus 2005;18(4):e9.
3. Panse R. KlinischeundpathologischeMitteilungen.IV. Ein Glioms des Akustikus. Arch Ohrenheik 1904;61:251–5 [in German].
4. Cushing H. Further concerning the acoustic neuromas. Laryngoscope 1921;31: 209–28.
5. Cairns H. Acoustic neurinoma of the right cerebellopontine angle. Complete removal. Spontaneous recovery from post-operative facial palsy. Proc R Soc Med 1931;25:7–12.
6. Dandy WE. Results of removal of acoustic tumors by the unilateral approach. AMA Arch Surg 1941;42:1026–33.

7. McKenzie KG, Alexander E Jr. Acoustic neuroma. Clin Neurosurg 1954;2:21–36.
8. Olivecrona H. The removal of acoustic neurinomas. J Neurosurg 1967;26:100–3.
9. House WF. Surgical exposure of the internal auditory canal and its contents through the middle, cranial fossa. Laryngoscope 1961;71:1363–85.
10. Rhoton AL Jr. The cerebellopontine angle and posterior fossa cranial nerves by the retrosigmoid approach. Neurosurgery 2000;47(Suppl 3):S93–129.
11. Li JM, Yuan XR, Liu Q, et al. [Facial nerve preservation following microsurgical removal of large and huge acoustic neuroma]. Zhonghua Wai Ke Za Zhi 2011; 49(3):240–4.
12. Tringali S, Ferber-Viart C, Fuchsmann C, et al. Hearing preservation in retrosigmoid approach of small vestibular schwannomas: prognostic value of the degree of internal auditory canal filling. Otol Neurotol 2010;31(9):1469–72.
13. Phillips DJ, Kobylarz EJ, De Peralta ET, et al. Predictive factors of hearing preservation after surgical resection of small vestibular schwannomas. Otol Neurotol 2010;31(9):1463–8.
14. Sughrue ME, Yang I, Rutkowski MJ, et al. Preservation of facial nerve function after resection of vestibular schwannoma. Br J Neurosurg 2010;24(6):666–71.
15. Sameshima T, Fukushima T, McElveen JT Jr, et al. Critical assessment of operative approaches for hearing preservation in small acoustic neuroma surgery: retrosigmoid vs middle fossa approach. Neurosurgery 2010;67(3):640–4.
16. Sughrue ME, Yang I, Aranda D, et al. Hearing preservation rates after microsurgical resection of vestibular schwannoma. J Clin Neurosci 2010;17(9):1126–9.
17. Zhao X, Wang Z, Ji Y, et al. Long-term facial nerve function evaluation following surgery for large acoustic neuromas via retrosigmoid transmeatal approach. Acta Neurochir (Wien) 2010;152(10):1647–52.
18. Chen L, Chen LH, Ling F, et al. Removal of vestibular schwannoma and facial nerve preservation using small suboccipital retrosigmoid craniotomy. Chin Med J (Engl) 2010;123(3):274–80.
19. Hillman T, Chen DA, Arriaga MA, et al. Facial nerve function and hearing preservation acoustic tumor surgery: does the approach matter? Otolaryngol Head Neck Surg 2010;142(1):115–9.
20. Samii M, Gerganov VM, Samii A. Functional outcome after complete surgical removal of giant vestibular schwannomas. J Neurosurg 2010;112(4):860–7.
21. Kameda K, Shono T, Hashiguchi K, et al. Effect of tumor removal on tinnitus in patients with vestibular schwannoma. J Neurosurg 2010;112(1):152–7.
22. Noudel R, Gomis P, Duntze J, et al. Hearing preservation and facial nerve function after microsurgery for intracanalicular vestibular schwannomas: comparison of middle fossa and retrosigmoid approaches. Acta Neurochir (Wien) 2009; 151(8):935–44.
23. Yang J, Grayeli AB, Barylyak R, et al. Functional outcome of retrosigmoid approach in vestibular schwannoma surgery. Acta Otolaryngol 2008;128(8): 881–6.
24. Cardoso AC, Fernandes YB, Ramina R, et al. Acoustic neuroma (vestibular schwannoma): surgical results on 240 patients operated on dorsal decubitus position. Arq Neuropsiquiatr 2007;65(3A):605–9.
25. Samii M, Gerganov V, Samii A. Improved preservation of hearing and facial nerve function in vestibular schwannoma surgery via the retrosigmoid approach in a series of 200 patients. J Neurosurg 2006;105(4):527–35.

Translabyrinthine Approach:
Indications, Techniques, and Results

Moisés A. Arriaga, MD, MBA*, James Lin, MD

KEYWORDS

- Vestibular schwannoma • Translabyrinthine • Surgical complications
- Surgical outcomes • Surgical techniques • Benign tumor

Key Abbreviations: TRANSLABRYNTHINE APPROACH	
CPA	Cerebellopontine angle
IAC	Internal auditory canal
PTA	Pure tone average
SDS	Speech discrimination score

Otologists first described the translabyrinthine craniotomy as an approach to the cerebellopontine angle (CPA) at the beginning of the twentieth century; however, William F. House was the first surgeon to successfully perform the approach with regularity for vestibular schwannoma (VS) removal.[1] Although hearing is sacrificed in its traditional form, the translabyrinthine craniotomy allows the most direct access to the CPA, as well as exposure of the facial nerve from brainstem to stylomastoid foramen (**Figs. 1** and **2**). All drilling is extradural. The entire length of the internal auditory canal (IAC) from fundus to porus, as well as its connection to the CPA, is routinely exposed.

INDICATIONS FOR TRANSLABYRINTHINE APPROACH FOR VS

The translabyrinthine approach is used for VS when the hearing is poor or in cases in which hearing preservation would be unlikely. Advantages of the translabyrinthine approach are

- It is the most direct route to the CPA
- It exposes the IAC in its entirety
- The facial nerve can be found with typically undisturbed anatomy anterior to vertical crest (known as the Bill bar) at the fundus.

LSU Health Sciences Center New Orleans, Hearing and Balance Center, Our Lady of the Lake Regional Medical Center, 7777 Hennessey Boulevard, Suite 709, Baton Rouge, LA 70808, USA
* Corresponding author.
E-mail address: marria@lsuhsc.edu

Otolaryngol Clin N Am 45 (2012) 399–415
doi:10.1016/j.otc.2011.12.009
0030-6665/12/$ – see front matter © 2012 Elsevier Inc. All rights reserved.

oto.theclinics.com

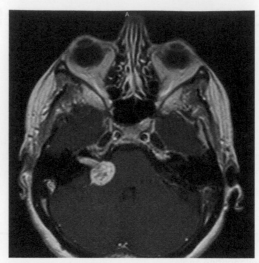

Fig. 1. Axial MRI of large VS with brainstem compression.

These factors allow for excellent tumor exposure and a reliable potential plane between tumor and facial nerve at the beginning of tumor dissection. The approach can also be used for facial nerve lesions of neoplastic or traumatic causes. The full-length exposure allows for decompression, involved facial nerve resection, translocation, and end-to-end anastomoses or nerve grafting (**Fig. 3**). The surgeon can extend the dissection through the stylomastoid foramen and into the parotid gland if required.

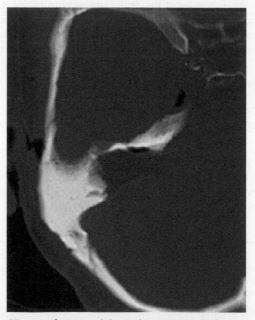

Fig. 2. Postoperative CT scan after translabyrinthine removal of tumor with abdominal fat medially and hydroxyapatite cement reconstruction of the mastoid defect.

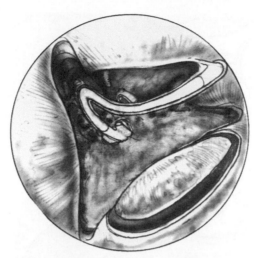

Fig. 3. Interposition facial nerve graft following translabyrinthine approach. The entire temporal course of the facial nerve is accessible through this exposure for transposition and repair.

The translabyrinthine approach can also be used for other tumors in the CPA. These include, but are not limited to, meningiomas, epidermoids, glomus tumors, and choroid plexus papillomas—so long as the determination is made that the potential for hearing preservation or hearing return is outweighed by the direct route of the approach. For tumors that are anterior to the IAC, the approach can be extended through removal of cochlea with or without facial nerve rerouting (**Fig. 4**). Removal of the cochlea allows better exposure of clival lesions, but requires multilayer closure of the external auditory canal (EAC).

The chosen approach for a given VS is highly variable based on the experience and background of the surgical team members. Tumor size and residual hearing are the most important factors influencing VS approach in centers that routinely use the translabyrinthine, retrosigmoid, and middle fossa craniotomies. Tumors larger than 2.5 cm tend to have poor likelihood of hearing preservation regardless of approach.[2] The translabyrinthine approach is recommended in cases in which the tumor is larger than 2.5 cm and hearing has progressed to a nonserviceable level.

The definition of nonserviceable varies by institution. Some centers adhere to a 50-50 rule in which the hearing is serviceable if the pure tone average is 50 dB or less, and the speech discrimination score is 50% to 100%. Other centers use the 30-70 rule in which hearing is serviceable if the pure tone average is 30 dB or less and the speech discrimination score is 70% to 100%. Use of the nonserviceable hearing cutoff assumes that hearing is not likely to improve after tumor removal. Hearing generally is not expected to improve through VS surgery.

TECHNIQUE
General Considerations

The translabyrinthine approach is performed under general endotracheal tube anesthesia without long-term muscle relaxation. Cranial nerve monitoring, especially the facial nerve, crucially depends on no paralysis and provides immediate feedback to the surgeon during tumor dissection, aids in facial nerve localization, and provides prognostic facial function information at the end of the case.

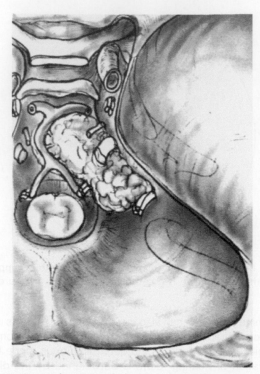

Fig. 4. CPA lesion anterior to the IAC and abutting the basilar artery.

After satisfactory anesthesia is induced, the patient receives an orogastric tube, a Foley catheter, recording needle electrodes into the facial musculature, and sequential compression devices to the lower extremities to help prevent deep venous thromboses.

The surgical side is then confirmed with the aid of the patient's audiogram and MRI films, and a postauricular shave using clippers is performed.

Within 1 hour of skin incision, the patient receives a dose of broad spectrum intravenous antibiotics with good cerebrospinal fluid (CSF) penetration; these antibiotics usually are continued for 24 hours perioperatively.

The operative sites at the ear, scalp, and neck, as well as the fat harvest site in the left, lower quadrant, are then outlined with adhesive drapes. Both areas are prepped and draped with towels and antibiotic-impregnated translucent adhesive drape.

Temporal Bone Exposure

One percent lidocaine with 1:100,000 epinephrine is injected into the postauricular region, extending into the temporal region, and an incision is made 2 to 4 cm behind the postauricular sulcus.

The larger the tumor, the more the retrosigmoid dura needs to be exposed to allow access, and the further posterior an incision is needed.

Simultaneous placement of an osseointegrated abutment for attachment of a hearing appliance is possible. In such cases, the incision is kept more anterior to prevent a soft tissue plane connection between the abutment site and the craniotomy site because this might lead to CSF wound leak through the abutment site, which cannot be water tight. The more anteriorly placed incision does make the posterior aspect of the craniotomy more difficult. Consequently, the authors prefer to place bone-anchored hearing devices at a secondary procedure after complete healing from the tumor resection.

Following a scalp incision, a musculoperiosteal incision is created such that it is staggered and minimizes any overlap with the scalp incision.

The bony EAC is identified with the use of the cautery and elevators.

Care is taken not to macerate the edges of soft tissue because a comprehensive, layered closure is essential to prevent CSF wound leak.

Emissary veins are often encountered with elevation of the pericranium posteriorly. This provides an estimate of the sigmoid sinus location and the bleeding is controlled with bone wax.

Temporalis muscle is harvested from underneath the temporalis fascia and saved for packing of the eustachian tube and middle ear.

Antibiotic is used in the irrigation throughout all stages of the procedure.

The microscope is used throughout the bone dissection, tumor removal, and closure steps.

The traditional arrangement has the operative surgeon positioned on the tumor side of the patient's head with the stereoscopic binocular microscope and an observer with binocular viewing of half the field on one side and a camera taking images from the opposite side. Modern operative microscopes can be arranged so that two operating surgeons can have simultaneous stereoscopic visualization permitting a "four-handed" technique. By avoiding a "beam splitter" and positioning the binocular eye-pieces at 180° from each other, the cosurgeons can sit opposite each other and truly operate as cosurgeons. Although this is not necessary for all parts of the procedure, the authors have found this strategy facilitates rapid debulking, safe hemostasis, and countertraction during facial nerve dissection. A particular advantage of the technique is that during difficult aspects of tumor dissection, both surgeons have simultaneous access for visualization and palpation of crucial structures as the surgery proceeds and specific steps are completed. This simultaneous access with the four-hand technique is a contrast to the usual side-arm view, which is not stereoscopic for the observer and is not ergonomically positioned for access to the surgical field.

A wide cortical mastoidectomy is performed with saucerization of the edges at least 2 cm superior to the middle fossa floor and posterior to the sigmoid sinus.

The mastoid antrum, lateral semicircular canal, and incus are identified and the bone is thinned over the sigmoid sinus.

Bone is removed from the middle and presigmoid posterior fossa dura. The sigmoid sinus is then decompressed with a bony island of bone (the Bill bar) left over its center to protect it as drilling proceeds medially (**Fig. 5**).

Bleeding along the sigmoid sinus may be encountered. This is readily controlled using patiently applied gelatin sponge or powder, or oxidized cellulose packing soaked in thrombin.

At this point, the bony EAC is thinned to remove air cells and the facial recess is opened using the incus and lateral semicircular canal as landmarks. It is helpful to identify the descending facial nerve through a thin layer of bone during this portion the procedure. The anterior limit of the more medial dissection is the descending facial nerve. The bone posterior to it can be more aggressively thinned if its location is recognized with certainty.

A labyrinthectomy is then performed and all three ampullae of the semicircular canals are identified leading to the vestibule. The vestibule marks a thin layer of bone that overlies the fundus of the IAC.

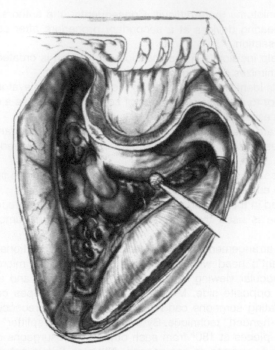

Fig. 5. Complete mastoidectomy with sigmoid sinus decompression (leaving a Bill bar) and skeletonizing the vertical segment of the facial nerve.

Traditional Labyrinthectomy

There are traditional and more time-efficient methods of performing the labyrinthectomy.

The traditional labyrinthectomy opens the semicircular canals methodically, beginning with the superior half of the lateral semicircular canal anterior to posterior.

The inferior half of the lateral semicircular canal provides a bony barrier that protects the mastoid (second) genu of the facial nerve.

The posterior dissection of the lateral semicircular canal leads one to the posterior semicircular canal, which is followed posterior, superiorly, and medially to the common crus.

The common crus is traced medially and anteriorly to the vestibule and then followed along the course of the superior semicircular canal, which proceeds superiorly, anteriorly, and laterally.

Bleeding from the subarcuate artery is often encountered while the superior semicircular canal is removed and it may be cauterized with a bipolar, occluded with bone wax, or controlled with a diamond burr.

Following the superior semicircular leads to its own ampulla first and then to the lateral canal ampulla, which lies inferior to that of the superior canal.

The inferior half of the posterior semicircular canal is followed with confidence posterior and sometimes medial to the already identified descending facial nerve to its ampulla.

At this point, the vestibule connecting all three ampullae should be fully exposed (**Fig. 6**). The labyrinthectomy is performed being mindful of a potential high-riding

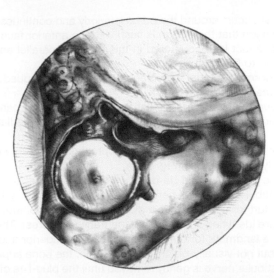

Fig. 6. Following labyrinthectomy, the ampullate ends of the three semicircular canals are opened and the vestibule is exposed. The latter is the landmark for the roof of the IAC.

jugular bulb, which may be encountered while the posterior semicircular canal is followed.

If the bulb is not identified during the labyrinthectomy, drilling is performed inferiorly at the level of the labyrinthectomy.

The bulb marks the inferior-most extent of medial dissection and it should be identified with a layer of bone overlying it.

Time-efficient Labyrinthectomy

The more time-efficient labyrinthectomy is begun along the medial-most aspect of the sinodural angle.

Bone removal begins here and continues with circular motion of the drill to remove all bone superiorly and posteriorly to the medial middle and posterior fossa dura.

Bony removal proceeds anteriorly to the descending facial nerve and inferiorly to the jugular bulb.

Care is taken to readily identify and preserve the vestibule connecting the three ampullae because these serve as landmarks for the fundus of the IAC and location of the Bill bar.

Steps Following Labyrinthectomy

After the labyrinthectomy is completed, the orientation of the IAC must be considered before performing further drilling. From porus to fundus, the IAC points parallel to the orientation of the EAC. There is typically a great deal of bone still overlying the porus.

Bony removal proceeds posteriorly along the posterior fossa dura down to the level of the porus of the IAC, which may be identified through bone by its darker color.

Bony removal continues laterally following the IAC's "blue line" up to the area of the vestibule.

At this point, the inferior trough is created between the inferior IAC and the identified jugular bulb.

Bone removal first occurs around the porus inferiorly and continues laterally, ideally drilling away bone such that the trough is flush with the anterior face of the IAC.

The cochlear aqueduct is encountered in this location, parallel and inferior to the IAC, which may lead to CSF leakage.

Drilling is not performed anterior and inferior to the cochlear aqueduct because this places cranial nerves IX, X, and XI at risk.

The superior trough is created in similar fashion with greater care taken laterally because the location of the facial nerve assumes a superior medial position in the lateral IAC.

At this point, the IAC should be uncovered approximately 270°, with the vestibule and bone still overlying the fundus (**Fig. 7**).

The drilling of the fundus should be done with great care because the landmarks delineating the vestibular and facial nerves are in very close proximity.

The vestibule is further opened with a diamond bur and the superior and inferior vestibular nerves are identified separated by the transverse crest. The superior canal ampulla serves as a landmark for the Bill bar, which lies superior and deep to it.

Using copious, but not visually-obstructive irrigation, the bone superior and medial to the superior vestibular nerve is gently removed until the blue-line of the facial nerve is identified coursing in anterior superior direction, and placed medial to the superior vestibular nerve.

The proximity of the facial nerve is typically announced by a brief burst of the facial nerve monitor at this point.

The triangular section of bone separating the superior vestibular nerve and the facial nerve at the fundus is the transverse crest (Bill bar).

At this point, the wound is copiously irrigated to remove all free bone dust from the incision edges, the retractors, and the craniotomy defect.

Before opening the dura, the eustachian tube is occluded to prevent postoperative CSF leakage through the nose.

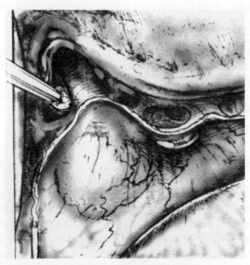

Fig. 7. The IAC is skeletonized by creating inferior and superior bone troughs. The orientation of the IAC is parallel to the orientation of the EAC. Accordingly, there is significant more bone removal required at the porus medially than at the fundus laterally.

First, the incus is removed with a hook and the tensor tympani tendon is cut to improve access to the eustachian tube and to facilitate complete packing of the anterior epitympanum.

The distal end of the eustachian tube is packed with alternating small pieces of oxidized cellulose and temporalis muscle.

The middle ear, facial recess, and antrum are then filled with more temporalis muscle with care not to disrupt the tympanic membrane. A tear in the tympanic membrane will likely result in CSF otorrhea and increase the risk of meningitis.

Opening the IAC

Attention is then turned back to the fundus of the IAC.

Using the Bill bar as the medial landmark, superior, then inferior, vestibular neurectomies are performed using a sharp hook (**Figs. 8** and **9**). The Bill bar is used to initiate the plane of dissection between the superior vestibular nerve and the facial nerve deep to it.

This plane is followed medially as nerve or tumor dissection proceeds.

Certain identification of the facial nerve in the IAC allows for removal of all its other contents because they serve no more purpose after labyrinthectomy.

Posterior Fossa Tumor Removal

After section of the eighth nerve, the posterior fossa dura is opened sharply.

The incisions should be made widely enough to encompass the tumor's dimensions, with room to spare.

Blood vessels running along the dura, as well as blood vessels adjacent and deep to the dura, must carefully be avoided.

The posterior fossa dura incision is then carefully continued along the porus and brought onto the IAC over the inferior vestibular nerve.

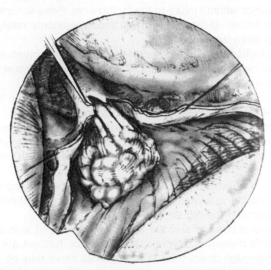

Fig. 8. The transverse crest separates the superior vestibular nerve from the inferior vestibular nerve. The Bill bar is a bone wedge just medial to the lateral aspect of the superior vestibular nerve that separates the facial nerve and superior vestibular nerve.

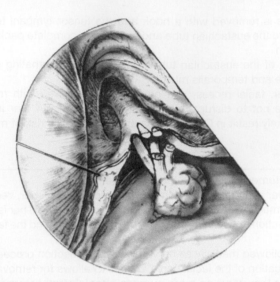

Fig. 9. The superior and inferior vestibular nerves are transected to begin dissection of the tumor from the facial nerve in the IAC.

For smaller tumors that are primarily intracanalicular, the facial nerve is identified both proximal and distal to the tumor with aid of the stimulator.

The plane between the tumor and facial nerve is further developed proximally and the tumor can typically be "shelled out."

If the plane between the tumor and the facial nerve is less clear, then one errs on the side of caution and removes tumor that is confirmed by appearance, texture, and electromyogram (EMG) stimulation to not be a stretched or distorted facial nerve. Increasingly, a philosophy of tumor management has evolved that emphasizes the reality that a VS is a benign disease process. If there is uncertainty regarding the ability to remove a small portion of tumor without injury to the facial nerve, these scraps of tumor are left behind. Long-term follow-up has shown that these remnants rarely grow, perhaps because they have been devitalized.

Larger tumors will often stretch and distort the facial nerve, creating a difficult plane between tumor and nerve. With such tumors, the most urgent issue that needs to be dealt with is the brainstem compression.

After the posterior fossa dura is opened, the plane between the tumor and brainstem may be developed and preserved with cottonoid pledgets.

By remaining directly on the tumor surface, one may avoid blood vessels in the CPA.

Given the anatomic relationship of the vestibular nerves to the facial nerve, the facial nerve is typically deflected anteriorly by tumor, but rarely may be located superior or inferior.

If the facial nerve is deflected posteriorly, one might question the diagnosis of VS.

After stimulation confirms absence of facial nerve, the posterolateral surface of the capsule is cauterized with the bipolar surface.

The tumor capsule is opened and the tumor is eviscerated with a combination of scissors, an ultrasonic dissector, a mechanical dissector, forceps, suction, and bipolar cautery (**Fig. 10**). Although direct trauma to the facial nerve may be avoided through this technique, indirect traction injury can still occur with excessive tumor manipulation. By staying within the tumor capsule, one avoids damaging the facial nerve and other neurovascular structures within the CPA.

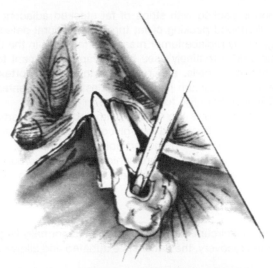

Fig. 10. Internal decompression of the tumor in the CPA is necessary to complete dissection of the tumor capsule from the facial nerve, brainstem, and other critical structures.

After debulking the tumor contents, the capsule that is closest the more medial neurovascular structures is more easily manipulated and peeled from vital underlying structures.

The brainstem side of the tumor capsule is then carefully deflected distally in an attempt to identify the facial nerve proximally with the aid of the stimulator.

Typically, the eighth nerve is transected close to the brainstem root entry zone, and the facial nerve is identified just anterior and superior to an intervening branch of the anterior inferior cerebellar artery.

The lower cranial nerves may be stretched inferiorly if the tumor is of great length and stimulation of these nerves may lead to change in pulse or blood pressure.

Once the facial nerve is identified on both proximal and distal ends of the tumor, dissection may proceed in a proximal to distal fashion or vice versa.

As the nerve typically withstands stretching by slow tumor growth without obvious paresis, its fibers may be flattened and spread out over the tumor surface making it difficult stay in the plane of dissection.

The facial nerve monitor provides direct feedback to the surgeon regarding facial nerve irritation and, with probe stimulation, helps the surgeon identify areas safe to resect.

The most urgent goal of decompressing the brainstem should be accomplished by this point.

For prognostic information, the facial nerve is stimulated using as low a current as possible, with the minimal stimulus level required at the brainstem to elicit a response recorded. Stimulation at a level of 0.05 µA with a result of greater than 240 µV predicts a 98% probability of a House-Brackmann grade I or II one year after surgery.[3]

The operative field is then carefully irrigated with warmed antibiotic saline.

All remaining blood clots and bone dust are washed away. Any remaining bleeding should be controlled using a judicious combination of bipolar cautery, oxidized cellulose packing, and thrombin gelatin sponge or powder.

Subcutaneous fat is then harvested from the left, lower quadrant of the abdomen.

The donor site is closed in layers over a Penrose or suction drain at the discretion of the surgeon.

The dural opening is packed with strips of fat stacked adjacent one to another, creating a dumbbell-shaped packing of fat through the dural defect. Care must be taken not to iatrogenically replace tumor mass with fat mass in the CPA.

One of the authors (MA) routinely uses hydroxyapatite cement to hold the fat in place, seal the mastoid air cells, and recontour the lateral cortex surface. Using hydroxyapatite cement or titanium plate cranioplasty, some centers have lowered the incidence of CSF leak from 5% to 12% to 1% to 4%.[4,5]

The musculoperiosteal layer is then reapproximated in as watertight a fashion as possible with interrupted 2–0 undyed polyglycolic sutures, and the scalp is then closed with inverted, interrupted 3–0 undyed polyglycolic sutures.

The skin is closed with a running suture, which can be absorbable or nonabsorbable, and sterile pressure dressings are placed along both scalp (mastoid type) and abdominal incisions.

Postoperative Care

Unless there are unusual circumstances, such as an abnormally large tumor, or prolonged or complicated recovery, the patient is extubated and allowed to recover after the procedure.

Facial nerve function is assessed immediately after the patient is able to follow commands.

The mastoid dressing stays in place for 2 to 3 days if reconstruction is with fat alone. Alternatively, if a cranioplasty is performed, the mastoid dressing can be removed the day after surgery.

Perioperative intravenous antibiotics are continued for 24 hours.

The patient typically stays in the intensive care unit overnight while receiving hourly neurologic examinations.

The day after surgery, the patient sits in a chair and is encouraged to walk with the aid of a physical therapist.

The Foley catheter is discontinued and the diet is slowly progressed to the same as preoperative.

By minimizing the use of antinausea medications and starting vestibule-ocular reflex exercises on the first postoperative day, vestibular compensation is maximized and hospital discharge is expedited.

In the case of postoperative facial weakness, proper eye care is paramount. The patient receives artificial tears every 2 hours to the affected eye while awake and a more viscous eye lubricant before going to sleep. The patient may be provided a moisture chamber to prevent drying of the eye and, once properly instructed, may tape the eye shut at night. Involvement of an ophthalmologist for examinations and care is helpful to decrease the risk of permanent corneal damage.

Complications of VS Surgery

Facial nerve

Facial nerve function is one of the primary outcome measures in VS surgery. Intraoperative injury can be related to

- traction
- blunt trauma
- cautery
- transection.

Positive probe stimulation at the brainstem root exit zone or paresis on postoperative examination implies continuity of the nerve and portends a good prognosis. Lack of response to stimulation at elevated current levels suggests poor recovery. Obvious transection means immediate paralysis. If transection does occur during surgery and the proximal and distal ends of the nerve can be identified, primary anastomosis is attempted. Approximation of the facial nerve ends in the CPA is difficult and usually only one suture may be passed.

Alternatively, an absorbable implant nerve guide tubule may be used to coapt the nerve endings.

Extra length along the distal nerve may be obtained by drilling away the restrictive fallopian canal. This may compromise the blood supply.

A greater auricular nerve graft may also be harvested and used as an interposition graft.

A House-Brackmann grade III is the best possible outcome after repair of a severed facial nerve.

If primary anastomosis yields minimal return of function after 6 to 12 months, the patient may undergo EMG testing to determine if any evidence of nerve regeneration is underway. If the EMG reveals poor prognostic information or if the primary anastomosis of the severed nerve was not possible during tumor removal, some variation of hypoglossal-facial (XII-VII) anastomosis can be performed.

Bleeding

Different potential sources of bleeding are encountered during the approach versus tumor removal. During the early drilling stages, the sigmoid sinus can lead to dramatic blood loss particularly with a large, dominant sinus.

Small tears in the sinus can be controlled with patient application of thrombin-soaked gelatin sponges.

Larger tears may require large pieces of oxidized cellulose and pledgets applied with a higher degree of pressure. Control of these larger rents in the sinus increase the likelihood of ipsilateral venous outflow compromise.

More medial drilling along the sinodural angle raises the risk of tearing the superior petrosal sinus. This angle of intersection of the posterior fossa dura and tentorium makes the sinodural intersection a difficult area to achieve full bony decompression and places the superior petrosal sinus at greater risk.

Bleeding from the superior petrosal sinus also can be controlled with topical hemostatic agents, but one must be aware of the anatomic variant where the vein of Labbé drains into this sinus.

Drilling along the inferior trough of the IAC can place the dome of the jugular bulb at risk, particularly when the bulb is elevated. Jugular bulb tears can be controlled similarly to those of sigmoid sinus tears, although in rare instances ligation of the jugular vein in the neck with extraluminal packing of the sigmoid sinus may be required.

Bleeding during tumor dissection is avoided by careful identification and isolation of vessels with mobilization away from the tumor, if possible, and bipolar cautery if they feed the tumor. Vessels are cauterized only if necessary and as to close their entrance to tumor as possible.

Diffuse bleeding in the CPA or within the tumor is controlled with judicious use of bipolar cautery, laser coagulation, or topical hemostatic agents.

After tumor dissection, careful observation for bleeding after irrigation of the operative bed is imperative to decrease the likelihood of postoperative compressive CPA hematoma. Anesthesia may be asked to apply Valsalva maneuver or temporarily elevate blood pressure to allow potential bleeders to declare themselves.

CPA hematoma is a potentially fatal complication that leads to increased intracranial pressure and brainstem compression. Patients may have decreased level of consciousness and/or dilation of pupils. If onset of these symptoms is rapid and the patient becomes unstable, opening the incision for removal of the cranioplasty, abdominal fat, and blood clot at the bedside may be necessary. A more stable patient may undergo noncontrasted head CT scan with removal of the clot in the operating room under more sterile, controlled conditions. After a bedside or intraoperative removal of a CPA hematoma, a diligent search for and control of the offending vessels is performed in the operating room.

CSF Leak

The rates of CSF leak after translabyrinthine craniotomy have dropped over the past few decades. CSF otorhinorrhea is more common than wound leak. As mentioned above, cranioplasty with hydroxyapatite cement or titanium mesh presumably bolsters the fat packing and drops the rate of leak to 1% to 5%. There are also reports of less than 1% leak rates without the use of cranioplasty and relying on "meticulous" closure techniques.[6–8] Leaks through the wound are very rare with carefully layered, watertight closures.

Treatment of postoperative CSF rhinorrhea entails initial bed rest and maintenance of the pressure dressing.

With recalcitrant leaks, lumbar drainage may be performed for 3 to 5 days.

Wound re-exploration and closure of the ear canal allows more direct visualization and thorough packing of the eustachian tube and middle ear space for better control of CSF rhinorrhea.

Wound leaks are typically controlled with deep figure-eight sutures and continued pressure dressing.

More recently, transnasal endoscopic eustachian tube closure has been described as an alternative to exploration of the original surgical site.

A special mention should be given to patients with postoperative subcutaneous CSF collections or "pseudomeningoceles." If they are neither tense nor leaking through the wound, observation with pressure dressing may be the best option because they typically resolve with time. Attempt at aspiration risks introducing bacterial contaminants into a sterile craniotomy wound.

Meningitis

A recent review of literature places the risk of meningitis after translabyrinthine craniotomy at 0% to 10%.[7]

If a patient presents postoperatively with any combination of high fevers, stiff neck, obtundation, and excruciating headache, a head CT scan and lumbar puncture are performed.

If the clinical presentation is highly suggestive of meningitis, intravenous antibiotics with good CSF penetration are initiated immediately as disease progression may be rapid.

The duration and type of antibiotic may be tailored to the cultures of the lumbar puncture, but often no bacterial growth will arise from the CSF given early administration of antibiotics.

The patient may be followed clinically for improvement and typically receives a combination of intravenous and oral antibiotics for no less than 2 weeks.

Corticosteroids may also be initiated to decrease the inflammatory component of this complication and is the primary treatment modality for aseptic meningitis.

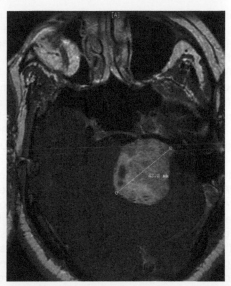

Fig. 11. MRI of a giant VS showing that opening a retrosigmoid dural opening risks cerebellar herniation before reaching the CPA cistern for draining CSF. In contrast, presigmoid exposure tends to deliver tumor into the wound rather than cerebellum until CSF drainage is accomplished. Thus, tumor decompression can proceed expeditiously.

SUMMARY

Over the past decade, outcomes of the translabyrinthine approach to VS have focused largely on facial nerve function after removal of large (>3 cm) tumors. A relatively recent paper reviewed 1 year postoperative facial nerve function results on 512 patients undergoing translabyrinthine craniotomy for unilateral, sporadic VS.[4] In that study, average tumor size was 2.4 cm, total tumor removal was achieved in 94.5% of cases, and anatomic preservation of the facial nerve was accomplished in 97.5% of cases. One-year House-Brackmann grade I–II was accomplished in 81%, IIII–V in 15%, and V–VI in 4%. For patients with tumors larger than 3.5 cm, the 1-year House-Brackmann grade I–II dropped to 53% while the grade V–VI rose to 17%.

A 2007 report reviewed results on VS resection outcomes, of which 231 were approached through a purely translabyrinthine approach. Of these 231 patients, 88% had a "favorable" facial nerve outcome (House-Brackmann grade I–III) at final follow-up. Nineteen of the 231 patients had tumors larger than 3 cm. Of these, 16 (84%) had House-Brackmann grade I–III at final follow-up.[9]

A study from 2005 examined outcomes of tumors larger than 3 cm removed through translabyrinthine, retrosigmoid, or combined approaches. Twenty-five of these patients underwent tumor removal through translabyrinthine craniotomy alone. After exclusion of patients with preoperative weakness, the House-Brackmann grade I to II was obtained in 78% of tumors at least 6 months postoperatively.[10]

Another recent study examined 110 tumors larger than 4 cm removed mostly through their extended translabyrinthine approach with transapical extension with a minority removed through either transotic or transcochlear approaches. The results reveal that complete tumor removal was achieved in 91.8% of cases; some of which required staged operations. The facial nerve was maintained anatomically intact in 76.4% of cases. Of the 88 patients who had at least 12 months of follow-up, House-Brackmann grade I was achieved in 7.9% of cases, grade II in 7.9%, grade III in 46.6%, grade IV in 9.1%, grade V in 3.4%, and grade VI in 25%. By grouping these percentages, grade I–III results were obtained in 62.4% of cases and grade IV–VI in 37.6%.[11]

In keeping with the theme of outcomes from large VS removal, Patni and Kartush[12] described removal of 34 tumors larger than 3 cm (average size 4.4 cm) in 2 to 3 stages with most (31) cases of tumors removed in two stages. While making note that the initial stage of tumor removal occurred through a retrosigmoid approach while only the second stage occurred through a translabyrinthine approach, they were able to achieve total or near-total tumor removal in all patients and 94% of patients had a House-Brackmann grade I with at least 11 months of follow-up, while one patient had a grade III and another had a grade VI long-term.

Finally, a specific advantage of the translabyrinthine approach over the retrosigmoid approach in large CPA lesions is that the presigmoid dural opening facilitates CSF drainage from the CPA cistern. This necessary step for posterior fossa relaxation in large tumors minimizes the risk of cerebellar herniation through the dural opening because the tumor is directly beneath the presigmoid dural incision, unlike the interposed cerebellum in the retrosigmoid approach. **Fig. 11** depicts a problematic relationship between a giant VS, the cerebellum, and the sigmoid sinus in which cerebellar herniation into the retrosigmoid defect can pose a problem and decrease visualization of the tumor.

REFERENCES

1. Nguyen-Huynh AT, Jackler RK, Pfister M, et al. The aborted early history of the translabyrinthine approach: a victim of suppression or technical prematurity? Otol Neurotol 2007;28(2):269–79.
2. Yates PD, Jackler RK, Satar B, et al. Is it worthwhile to attempt hearing preservation in larger acoustic neuromas? Otol Neurotol 2003;24(3):460–4.
3. Neff BA, Ting J, Dickinson SL, et al. Facial nerve monitoring parameters as a predictor of postoperative facial nerve outcomes after vestibular schwannoma resection. Otol Neurotol 2005;26(4):728–32.
4. Brackmann DE, Cullen RD, Fisher LM. Facial nerve function after translabyrinthine vestibular schwannoma surgery. Otolaryngol Head Neck Surg 2007; 136(5):773–7.
5. Arriaga MA, Chen DA, Burke EL. Hydroxyapatite cement cranioplasty in translabyrinthine acoustic neuroma surgery-update. Otol Neurotol 2007;28(4):538–40.
6. Goddard JC, Oliver ER, Lambert PR. Prevention of cerebrospinal fluid leak after translabyrinthine resection of vestibular schwannoma. Otol Neurotol 2010;31(3): 473–7.
7. Merkus P, Taibah A, Sequino G, et al. Less than 1% cerebrospinal fluid leakage in 1,803 translabyrinthine vestibular schwannoma surgery cases. Otol Neurotol 2010;31(2):276–83.
8. Bellachew T, Eter E, Telischi FF, et al. Management of recalcitrant CSF rhinorrhea after acoustic tumor removal via an endoscopic endonasal eustachian tube closure. 20th Annual North American Skull Base Society. New Orleans (LA), 2009.
9. Jacob A, Robinson LL, Bortman JS, et al. Nerve of origin, tumor size, hearing preservation, and facial nerve outcomes in 359 vestibular schwannoma resections at a tertiary care academic center. Laryngoscope 2007;117(12):2087–92.
10. Anderson DE, Leonetti J, Wind JJ, et al. Resection of large vestibular schwannomas: facial nerve preservation in the context of surgical approach and patient-assessed outcome. J Neurosurg 2005;102(4):643–9.

11. Angeli RD, Piccirillo E, Di Trapani G, et al. Enlarged translabyrinthine approach with transapical extension in the management of giant vestibular schwannomas: personal experience and review of literature. Otol Neurotol 2011;32(1): 125–31.
12. Patni AH, Kartush JM. Staged resection of large acoustic neuromas. Otolaryngol Head Neck Surg 2005;132(1):11–9.

Middle Fossa Approach:
Indications, Technique, and Results

Simon Angeli, MD[a,b],*

KEYWORDS

- Vestibular schwannoma • Middle fossa • Surgical technique

Key Abbreviations: MIDDLE FOSSA APPROACH	
ABR	Auditory brainstem response
CNAP	cochlear nerve action potentials
CSF	Cerebral spinal fluid
GSPN	Greater superficial petrosal nerve
IAC	Internal auditory canal
MFC	Middle fossa craniotomy
PTA	Pure tone threshold average
VEMP	Vestibular evoked myogenic potentials
WRS	Word recognition score

MIDDLE FOSSA CRANIOTOMY

The middle fossa craniotomy (MFC) approach for removal of vestibular schwannomas, also known as the *transtemporal-supralabyrinthine approach*, was popularized by House[1] and consists of the supralabyrinthine dissection of the internal auditory canal (IAC). House introduced revolutionary concepts, including many of the principles of skull base surgery that are now taken for granted, such as the use of the operating microscope, continuous suction irrigation, diamond stone burs, and a multidisciplinary team approach.

The MFC had been used for other indications, and Hartley[2] has been credited with the first description of this approach for the surgical treatment of trigeminal neuralgia. Over the years this approach has been used for the treatment of other neurotologic conditions, such as debridement of inflammatory lesions of the petrous apex, facial

The author has no financial disclosures in relation to this work.

No external funding was used for the creation of this work.

[a] Neurotological Skull Base Surgery, Department of Otolaryngology, University of Miami Miller School of Medicine, 1120 Northwest 14 Street, Miami, FL 33136, USA

[b] Department of Otolaryngology, University of Miami Ear Institute, 1120 Northwest 14 Street, Suite 500, Miami, FL 33136, USA

* University of Miami Ear Institute, 1120 Northwest 14 Street, Suite 500, Miami, FL 33136.

E-mail address: sangeli@med.miami.edu

Otolaryngol Clin N Am 45 (2012) 417–438

doi:10.1016/j.otc.2011.12.010

oto.theclinics.com

nerve decompression and grafting, repair of meningoceles, repair of semicircular canal dehiscence, and vestibular nerve sectioning. Kawase and colleagues[3] described an extended middle fossa approach that included dissection of the petrous apex for the exposure of aneurysms of the basilar artery, and this modification has helped expand the indications of this technique for the treatment of selected petro-clival tumors.

INDICATIONS FOR SURGERY

With the current increase in the use of MRI, the identification of small (<1.5 cm) tumors in patients with normal or near-normal hearing also has been on the rise. Today's skull base surgeons face the dilemma of selecting among three different therapy options for small and minimally symptomatic tumors: microsurgical removal, stereotactic radiation, and observation. During the initial evaluation of patients, surgeons must consider several audiometric, tumor, and patient factors to determine the risk of intracranial surgery, chances of function preservation, and long-term quality-of-life issues. MFC should be offered only for patients who have the best chance of serviceable hearing preservation, and when the risk/benefit analysis is favorable and accepted by the informed patient.

Audiometric Factors

Preservation of serviceable hearing
The goal of MFC is to achieve tumor removal and preserve auditory function that will be useful to the patient long-term. Useful, or "serviceable," hearing can only be preserved if it is present preoperatively. The definition of *serviceable hearing* must be individualized, because it depends on several factors, such as audiometric values of the ipsilateral and contralateral ears, progression of hearing loss, patient preference, and available strategies of hearing loss habilitation. Preservation of binaural hearing is important for sound localization and speech understanding in noise; for a patient to benefit from binaural hearing, the interaural average four-frequency (0.5, 1.0, 2.0, and 3.0 kHz) hearing threshold should be less than 20 dB, and the interaural word discrimination score should be less than 20%.[4] The determination of serviceable hearing in a patient with a tumor in the only hearing ear or in patients with bilateral tumors is obviously very different; some patients would choose to keep their hearing at any level even if it only provides sound awareness. The surgeon's must ensure that the patient has appropriate expectations, habilitation options are available, and the overall quality of life is not placed at risk in exchange for the promise of some measurable auditory function.

From the audiometric standpoint, hearing is characterized by the combination of the four-frequency pure-tone threshold average (PTA) and the word recognition score test (WRS). What is considered serviceable hearing and a definition of success in hearing preservation in some centers is PTA and WRS values of at least 30 dB and 70%, respectively, and in other centers at least 50 dB and 50%, respectively. Hearing aid benefit is limited below the 50/50 level. Because some hearing may be lost immediately or gradually after surgery, and better preoperative hearing has been associated with better chances of early and long-term hearing preservation,[5] it seems intuitive that hearing preservation surgery should be offered only to patients with hearing well above the 50/50 level. The 50/50 level of hearing represents the minimum serviceable hearing and, if preserved at or above this level, allows patients the use of amplification if needed.

Audiologic prognostic parameters beyond preoperative hearing function
Several prognostic signs for hearing preservation have been studied but, except for good preoperative hearing, most of these lack sufficient sensitivity and specificity to be reliable.

Auditory brainstem response test The morphology and latency of the waveforms of the auditory brainstem response (ABR) test have been used for prognosis of hearing preservation. The absence of a response is associated with a low chance of hearing preservation, whereas a measurable response has no prognostic significance. Shelton and colleagues[6] reported that hearing was preserved in 78% of patients with an inter-aural wave V latency difference of less than 0.4 ms, and in only 50% of those with no measurable ABR response. More recently, Brackmann and colleagues[7] also showed a significant difference between the mean latency of the interaural wave V latency for patients with preserved hearing compared with those who lost their hearing. The prognostic significance of ABR has been confirmed by other studies, whereas a few have found no relationship.[8,9]

Tumor location It is generally accepted that the chances of hearing preservation are better in tumors arising from the superior vestibular nerve as opposed to those of the inferior vestibular nerve. The inferior vestibular nerve shares the inferior compartment of the IAC with the cochlear nerve, and hence tumor adhesion to the cochlear nerve is more likely. In addition, the MFC approach allows the unroofing of the IAC and a direct view of tumors in the superior compartment, whereas the transverse crest of the IAC may obstruct the view to the lateral inferior compartment. Greater tumor adhesion to the cochlear nerve and blind surgical dissection in the inferior compartment carry a risk of injury to the cochlear nerve fibers and the vascular supply to the labyrinth. The preoperative identification of the nerve of origin is therefore an important prognostic consideration. The nerve of origin of small intracanalicular tumors may be identified with MRI (**Fig. 1**); however, this may not be possible for larger tumors.

Vestibular tests for nerve of origin Two vestibular tests have been used for the preoperative identification of the nerve of origin. The caloric test of electronystagmography assesses the function of the lateral semicircular canal, which is innervated by the superior vestibular nerve. Low caloric responses represent involvement of the superior vestibular nerve, whereas normal caloric function is considered to represent sparing of this nerve and inferior vestibular nerve involvement. Consequently, hearing preservation was reported in 64% of patients with a hypoactive response and in only 45% of

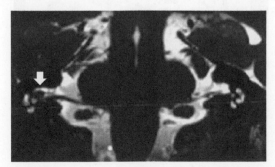

Fig. 1. Constructive interference in the steady state T2 sequence coronal view showing an intracanalicular vestibular schwannoma originating from the right superior vestibular nerve (*white arrow*).

those with normal caloric responses.[6] Another vestibular test that indicates involvement of the inferior vestibular nerve and hence may have some prognostic usefulness is the vestibular-evoked myogenic potential (VEMP) test. VEMP testing reflects function of the saccular branch of the inferior vestibular nerve, and absent responses may represent tumor involvement of this nerve. However, the prognostic significance of the VEMP in acoustic neuroma surgery has not been evaluated in large series.

Tumor Factors

High-resolution, thin-cut MRI with and without gadolinium provides critical information for selection of the optimal surgical approach. The medial extension of the tumor into the cerebellopontine angle and the depth to which the tumor occupies the fundus of the IAC are important parameters for approach selection and prognosis of hearing preservation. The MFC approach is best suited for small intracanalicular tumors with less than 1 cm extension into the cerebellopontine angle that do not contact the brainstem (**Fig. 2**). The standard MFC offers only limited exposure of the posterior cranial fossa for tumor dissection and intraoperative hemostasis. Tumors of the cerebellopontine angle and intracanalicular tumors with more than 1 cm of medial extension into the cerebellopontine angle are more suitable for a retrosigmoid craniotomy approach.

The degree of lateral extension of the tumor into the fundus of the IAC is best seen on T2-weighted sequences of MRI, which can show the bright signal of cerebrospinal fluid (CSF) lateral to the tumor at the fundus (**Fig. 3**). One to 2 mm of room between the tumor and the fundus of the IAC has been associated with a greater chance of hearing preservation. A lower rate of hearing preservation in tumors that completely fill the IAC compared with cases in which the lateral end of the canal seems uninvolved has been reported.[10]

Given the anatomic variability of the petrous bone, information about the degree of pneumatization and amount of bone overlying the superior semicircular canal is helpful when planning an MFC. This fact is shown best with a high-resolution CT with images in the plane of (Poschel) or perpendicular to (Stenver) the superior semicircular canals (**Fig. 4**).

Patient Factors

The MFC approach involves retraction of the temporal lobe for exposure of the superior petrous bone. Supratentorial craniotomy is associated with higher morbidity in

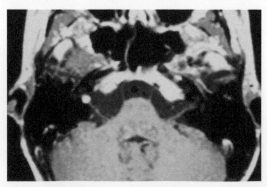

Fig. 2. MRI, axial view, T1-weighted sequence after intravenous gadolinium, showing a homogenously enhancing lesion near the fundus of the right internal auditory canal. This is a vestibular schwannoma.

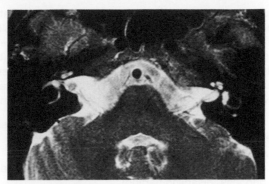

Fig. 3. TS-weighted image, axial view, showing a space occupying lesion in the mid-portion of the right internal auditory canal, and a bright signal (cerebrospinal fluid) filling the fundus.

elderly patients (older than 69 years of age). These patients have a dura mater that is thinner and more adherent to the skull than younger patients. Similarly, the rate of medical comorbidities (eg, blood dyscrasia, cerebrovascular disease) increases with age. A recent multicenter, prospective study of complications after craniotomy for meningiomas showed that even after carefully controlling preoperative comorbidities, elderly patients have a poorer outcome than younger patients.[11] Prognostic factors of increased morbidity and mortality after craniotomy include[12]:

- Age older than 69 years
- Tumor location in the skull base
- Peritumoral brain edema
- American Society of Anesthesiologists (ASA) class greater than II
- Karnofsky performance scale score less than 60

Summary of Patient Selection for Middle Fossa Surgery

The benefits, postoperative care, results, potential complications, and alternatives of the MFC should be thoroughly discussed with the patient. Small intracanalicular vestibular schwannomas can be managed with MFC, stereotactic radiation, or observation; treatment should be selected only after the patient has had the opportunity to consider the pros and cons of each modality. The other surgical methods are discussed in other articles in this issue, and the treatment must be individualized. Newly diagnosed patients may benefit from an initial period of observation, with periodic scanning. Because tumor growth and function deterioration is highly variable, the

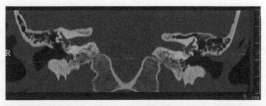

Fig. 4. Thin-cut CT of the temporal bone, coronal cuts, showing the relationship between the arcuate eminence (AE) and the superior semicircular canal (SSC), and the variability of the profile of the AE in the same patient. Right ear: "prominent" nonpneumatized AE. Left ear: flat AE with air cells above SSC.

demonstration of tumor growth through imaging or clinical deterioration supports the need for intervention. The indications of the MFC in cases of unilateral vestibular schwannomas are shown in the following sections. Treatment selection in patients with tumors in the only hearing ear and in neurofibromatosis type 2 (bilateral acoustic tumors) is not as straightforward and is discussed separately in the section *Surgery in the Only Hearing Ear and in Neurofibromatosis Type 2*. In general terms, the MFC is indicated for removal of unilateral vestibular schwannomas in patients with

1. Intracanalicular tumors extending less than 1 cm into the cerebellopontine angle, without brainstem contact
2. Good hearing (better than or near 30 dB PTA and 70% WRS)
3. Imaging (MRI) evidence of tumor growth and/or functional deterioration (eg, progressive hearing loss, disabling vertigo)
4. No contraindications for a supratentorial craniotomy (ie, age >69 years, ASA class >II, and Karnofsky Performance Scale score <60)

SURGICAL TECHNIQUE

The basic steps of specific perioperative, intraoperative, and postoperative techniques are generally accepted but, as is true for most surgical procedures, many modifications and variations exist in the literature.

Patient Preparation

To avoid wrong-side surgery, the ear of the side of the tumor is marked with indelible ink while the patient is awake in the preanesthesia holding area. The surgery is performed under general endotracheal anesthesia with direct monitoring of the arterial blood pressure, heart rate, oxygen saturation, blood carbon dioxide concentration, and urinary output. Only short-acting neuromuscular blockade is used at induction to allow the use of the facial nerve electromyography monitoring system.

The operating table is rotated 180° from the anesthesiologist. The patient is placed supine with the ipsilateral shoulder elevated and the head rotated 45° to the side opposite the tumor. The neck is slightly extended, with the vertex of the head directed toward the floor. It is not necessary to use an external head-fixation device. The patient's body is firmly strapped to the table and padded to prevent sliding and pressure injuries. The operating table must allow inclination in all of the planes. The head is shaved from the vertex to 6 cm behind the pinna. A lumbar drain is placed to help relax the brain and allow safe elevation of the temporal lobe.[13]

For intraoperative facial nerve monitoring, bipolar needle electrodes are inserted percutaneously into the lateral orbicularis oris and oculi muscles, and the ground and stimulating electrodes are inserted into the ipsilateral deltoid area, after which a baseline recording of the electromyographic activity of the facial muscles is obtained and the electrodes impedances recorded. Earphones are inserted and recording electrodes placed for far-field ABR, and the pinna and ear canal are covered with plastic drapes. The electrode for direct eight-nerve recording and the stimulating facial nerve probe are kept sterile and connected to the monitoring systems once the patient is draped. A standard iodine (or similar) scrub is performed and the field covered with sterile drapes.

The authors routinely use intravenous antibiotic prophylaxis for 24 hours. Intravenous mannitol (20% solution, 1 g/kg of body weight) and furosemide (10 mg) are given at the start of the surgery to facilitate temporal lobe retraction. Dexamethasone (10 mg every 12 hours) is given preoperatively and continued for 2 days to prevent brain and nerve edema.

The operating microscope is draped and positioned at the side of the operating table opposite to the side of the position of the instrument nurse. The surgeon sits at the head of the table. A high-speed drill with an assortment of cutting and diamond burs, and a suction-irrigation system are set up. The pedals for the drill and bipolar electrocautery should be within comfortable reach, and the facial nerve monitor should be easily visible and audible to the surgeon. The audiologist monitors the ABR and direct eight-nerve recording systems.

Craniotomy

The incision is marked and infiltrated with 1% lidocaine and 1:100,000 epinephrine solution. The incision begins caudally at the root of the zygoma in front of the tragus, extends superiorly and posteriorly around the superior auricular crease, and then curves cephalad and anteriorly, forming a curve of at least 8 cm in diameter behind the hairline (**Fig. 5**). Skin and subcutaneous tissue are incised; branches of the superficial temporal vessels are cauterized or suture ligated; the anteriorly based skin and subcutaneous tissue flap is elevated to expose the temporalis muscle. A 4 × 4–cm graft of temporalis muscle fascia is harvested and set aside for later use. The temporalis muscle is then incised with the monopolar electrocautery to form an inferiorly based flap, which is then elevated with a wide periosteal elevator to expose the squamous portion of the temporal bone, the temporoparietal suture line, and the root of the zygoma. The soft tissue flaps are retracted with fishhooks or self-retaining retractors, and covered with saline moist gauzes to prevent tissue dehydration. The craniotomy is marked as a 5 × 5–cm square centered at the root of the zygoma (1 cm in front of the external ear canal), with its inferior border at the level of the floor of the middle cranial fossa (**Fig. 6**).

If plating of the craniotomy bone flap is planned, titanium miniplates are placed at this point and then removed to mark the holes for the screws. Drilling of the craniotomy begins with a 4-mm cutting bur. To prevent dural injury, a 3- or 4-mm diamond bur is used once the outer cortex is drilled, and the inner cortex is skeletonized until the

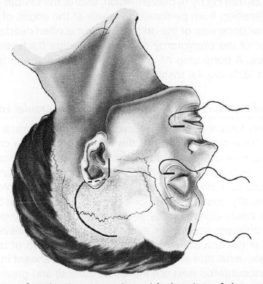

Fig. 5. Surgeon's view of patient's preparation with drawing of the surgical incision.

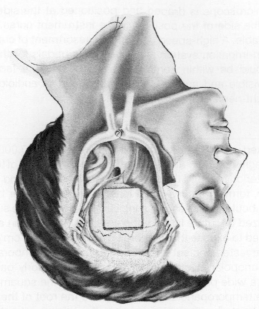

Fig. 6. Surgeon's view of the retracted soft tissue flaps and the marking of the craniotomy.

vessels and dura are visible through a very thin layer of bone. Using a curved blunt periosteal elevator, the thin bone is cracked and the dura is separated from the bone flap in a cephalad-to-caudal direction. The bone flap is then kept covered with a saline-moistened gauze until it is needed for the repair of the craniotomy at the end of the procedure. Care is taken to prevent perforating the dura or cracking the bone flap.

At this point, to facilitate brain retraction if the brain seems tense, additional doses of intravenous mannitol and furosemide are administered, the blood carbon dioxide level is lowered to 27 to 28 mm Hg by hyperventilation, and/or the lumbar drain is opened to drain some CSF. Bleeding from perforating vessels at the edges of the craniotomy is controlled with either bone wax or the drill. A Rongeur is often needed to remove bone at the inferior edge of the craniotomy to make this edge flush with the floor of the middle cranial fossa. A bone chip of at least 10 mm in diameter is saved for repair of the floor of the middle cranial fossa.

Dural Elevation and Exposure of the Floor of the Middle Cranial Fossa

Under magnification with the operating microscope, the dura is circumferentially elevated from the bone edges and from the floor of the middle cranial fossa using a blunt elevator, such as the Penfield or Roton dissectors. The first landmark is the middle meningeal artery as it emerges from the foramen spinosum. Small bleeding vessels on the dura can be cauterized with the irrigating-bipolar electrocautery. Venous bleeding usually occurs at the posterior and anterior ends of the dural elevation, which can be easily controlled by packing with sheets of oxidized cellulose or powdered bovine collagen soaked in thrombin. With further elevation of the dura, the next landmark is the arcuate eminence, a round elevation of bone overlying the superior semicircular canal (the arcuate eminence may be absent in 15% of patients).

The structures encountered next are the lesser (lateral) and greater (medial) superficial petrosal nerves. Dural elevation at the floor of the middle cranial fossa proceeds along the posterior-anterior direction while moving medially to avoid avulsion of the greater superficial petrosal nerve (GSPN) or a dehiscent geniculate ganglion. The authors try to preserve the GSPN whenever possible to avoid postoperative "dry eye" from impaired lacrimation. In rare cases, sacrifice of this structure may be necessary to prevent traction injury to the geniculate ganglion. The GSPN marks the lateral margin of the underlying horizontal segment of the petrous internal carotid artery. The geniculate ganglion, petrous carotid artery, or even superior semicircular canal can be dehiscent and at risk of injury. Medially, the petrous ridge is identified and the superior petrosal sinus is carefully elevated of its trough. A self-retaining retractor, such as the House-Urban or the Fisch middle fossa retractor, is positioned and secured in place along the vertical edges of the craniotomy. The blade of the retractor is positioned under the lip of the petrous ridge at the anticipated location of the IAC, centered along a line extending medially from the external auditory canal. Appropriate placement of the retractor affords adequate exposure of the floor of the middle cranial fossa without excessive brain retraction (**Fig. 7**). After controlling excess oozing, the superficial landmarks are identified under magnification (**Fig. 8**).

It is important for surgeons to be knowledgeable of the regional anatomy and its variations. Visualization of some of the anatomic landmarks depends partly on the degree of pneumatization of the petrous bone. The foramen spinosum, the petrous ridge and the GSPN are constant and visible landmarks. The superior semicircular canal can be dehiscent but more commonly is bony-covered and within the arcuate eminence. The profile of the arcuate eminence is highly variable and dependent on race and the degree of pneumatization of the bone surrounding the superior semicircular canal (see **Fig. 4**).[14] Similarly, the tegmen tympani can be porous and the head of the malleus and body of incus can be visible, facilitating the orientation.

Dissection of the IAC

Dissection of the IAC requires high-magnification, drilling with diamond burs of 4 to 0.5 mm in size, and an adequate suction-irrigation system. Given the anatomic variability

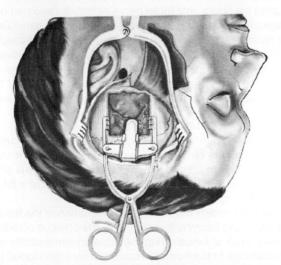

Fig. 7. Surgeon's view of the floor of the middle fossa after placing the middle fossa retractor.

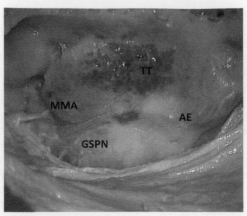

Fig. 8. Right temporal bone. Middle fossa craniotomy approach, exposure of the petrous bone after elevation of the dura. Note the 120° angle formed between the axis of the GSPN and the profile of the superior semicircular canal in the AE. AE, arcuate eminence; GSPN, greater superficial petrosal nerve; MMA, middle meningeal artery exiting the foramen spinosum; TT, tegmen tympani.

of the petrous bone, the surgeon performing the MFC should be familiar with the many different approaches that have been described to reach the IAC.

House approach to dissection of IAC
House[1] described the route to the IAC by following the GSPN to the geniculate ganglion and then to the labyrinthine segment of the facial nerve. Subsequently, Bill's bar (the vertical crest at the fundus of the IAC) and the superior vestibular nerve are identified, and then lateral-to-medial bone removal uncovers the entire IAC up to the porus acusticus.

The advantage of this technique is that the GSPN is a constant landmark; when doubt exists, the electrical stimulator can be used to identify the GSPN through anti-dromically stimulating the fibers until facial nerve activity is recorded on the monitor.[15]

The disadvantage of the classic House technique is that the geniculate ganglion and distal labyrinthine facial nerve are exposed to drilling, and that dissection of the labyrinthine segment of the facial nerve carries a risk of injury to the cochlea and the ampullated end of the superior semicircular canal. The basal turn of the cochlea lies an average distance of 0.6 mm anterior to the labyrinthine segment of the facial nerve; therefore, the authors use a 0.5-mm diamond bur when exposing the nerve at this level.

Fisch approach to dissection of IAC
Fisch[16] described the technique of blue-lining the superior semicircular canal through drilling the bone of the arcuate eminence. The arcuate eminence is used as the landmark to locate the superior semicircular canal, but the profile of the arcuate eminence is highly variable. The axis of the IAC lies along a line located at a 60° angle from the axis of the superior semicircular canal.

Although this technique avoids the retrograde dissection of the facial nerve through the geniculate ganglion and labyrinthine segment, the obvious disadvantage of blue-lining is that it carries a risk of fenestrating the superior semicircular canal. This technique can pose a challenge to the novice because, in well-developed temporal bones, drilling of the arcuate eminence is performed in a blind fashion until the semicircular canal is found, or air cells in the arcuate eminence can be taken for the canal lumen.

A congenital superior semicircular canal dehiscence can be found in approximately 1% of temporal bones[17] and this finding helps identify the location of the canal within the arcuate eminence before drilling.

García-Ibañez approach to dissection of IAC
The GSPN and the axis of the superior semicircular canal form a 120 angle and the IAC axis bisects this angle (see **Fig. 8**). García-Ibañez and García-Ibañez[18] described a technique whereby bone removal begins at the most medial aspect of the petrous ridge in the plane of this bisectrix and proceeds in a medial-to-lateral direction (**Fig. 9**). Bone anterior and posterior to the IAC at the level of the porus acusticus is removed down to the dura of the posterior cranial fossa. In this manner the IAC is skeletonized 270° in its medial half to allow for easier tumor removal.[19] A high-riding jugular bulb reaching the level of the IAC can be found and care is taken to avoid inadvertent injury to this vessel when drilling posterior to the IAC. As the bone removal proceeds laterally, the skeletonization of the IAC progressively narrows to 90° at the level of the fundus to avoid injury to the cochlea or superior semicircular canal ampulla. Drilling at the fundus is done with 1- or 0.5-mm diamond burs until the labyrinthine facial nerve, vertical crest (Bill's bar), and superior vestibular nerve are clearly visible through the thinned bone. The last flecks of bone are removed with a 1-mm angled elevator.

Exposure of Superior Semicircular Canal and Middle Ear Approach

Other techniques of IAC dissection are possible through the MFC. Through illuminating the arcuate eminence and petrous bone using a fiberoptic endoscope, or removing bone covering the tympanic tegmen, the superior semicircular canal and the contents of the middle ear are identified with transillumination or direct visualization, respectively. Locating the position of the head of the malleus, the body of the incus, and the cochleariform process helps define the approximate position of the IAC fundus. The labyrinthine facial nerve is expected along a line drawn medially from the cochleariform process (**Fig. 10**). At the end of the procedure, a tegmen defect is repaired with a bone graft. This approach can be useful when the landmarks are obscured by previous trauma or surgery. **Table 1** provides a summary of approaches.

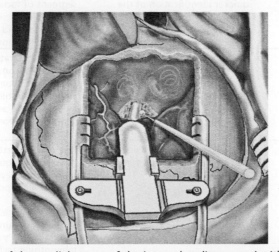

Fig. 9. Dissection of the medial aspect of the internal auditory canal with a diamond bur.

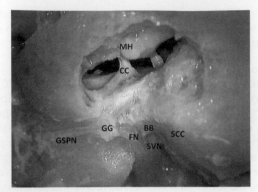

Fig. 10. Right temporal bone. Middle fossa craniotomy approach, exposure of the petrous bone after elevation of the dura. The facial nerve and internal auditory canal have been exposed. Exposure of the middle ear after removal of the tegmen tympani. BB, Bill's bar; CC, cochleariform process; FN, (labyrinthine segment of) facial nerve; GG, geniculate ganglion; GSPN, greater superficial petrosal nerve; MH, malleus head; SSC, superior semicircular canal; SVN, superior vestibular nerve.

Tumor Removal Through the IAC

The dura of the IAC is opened longitudinally along its posterior border with a microsurgical blade or hook. The dural flaps are reflected and the content of the IAC is exposed. The separation between the facial nerve and the superior vestibular nerve

Table 1		
Dissection of internal auditory canal approaches, advantages, disadvantages		
Surgical Approach	**Advantages**	**Disadvantages**
House	• GSPN is a constant landmark • The labyrinthine facial nerve is found early during the dissection and allows for quicker identification of the fundus of the IAC	• Geniculate ganglion and distal labyrinthine facial nerve are exposed to drilling • Dissection of labyrinthine segment of facial nerve carries risk of injury to cochlea and the ampullated end of the superior semicircular canal
Fisch	• Avoids retrograde dissection of the facial nerve through geniculate ganglion and labyrinthine segment	• Risk of fenestrating the superior semicircular canal • Drilling of arcuate eminence is performed in blind fashion and air cells in the arcuate eminence can be taken for the canal lumen
García-Ibañez	• IAC is skeletonized in its medial half to allow for easier tumor removal	• Risk of inadvertent injury to high-riding jugular bulb reaching the level of the IAC when drilling posterior to the IAC • Exposure of the fundus of the IAC is limited unless dissection is carried laterally toward the labyrinthine facial nerve

at the fundus, and the intervening vertical crest (Bill's bar) are identified. The facial nerve stimulating probe, starting at a stimulus level of 0.025 mA and increasing in 0.025- to 0.05-mA increments, is used to positively identify the facial nerve. Repeated stimulation of the facial nerve is an important tool during the dissection of the nerve from the tumor and from the vestibular nerve; in contrast to the facial nerve, the other two structures fail to elicit activity in the facial nerve monitor when electrically stimulated.

The vestibular and facial nerves are stimulated once more before sectioning the vestibular nerve in the cerebellopontine angle before tumor removal. The facial nerve is stimulated proximally to the tumor and the threshold response is recorded; a threshold of 0.5 mA or less and a response amplitude of 240 μV or more predict a good postoperative facial nerve function.[20] Continuous facial nerve electromyographic activity is recorded and the occurrence of train activity (continuous audible high-frequency activity) prompts the surgeon to stop all manipulation of the nerve until this activity ceases. Train activity has been correlated with postoperative facial paresis.[21]

A recording electrode is then placed between the dura and the cochlear nerve in the inferior-anterior aspect of the IAC for monitoring cochlear nerve action potentials (CNAP) in real time. This is a Teflon-coated multistrand silver wire electrode with a cotton whisk attached to the wire. The cotton whisk is secured with the help of a bovine collagen sponge to maintain contact with the nerve. CNAP or near-field ABR recordings are obtained and provide feedback about the integrity of the cochlea and auditory function during the dissection (**Fig. 11**). Before this point, the audiologist has been monitoring the hearing with ABR.

The authors recommend the use of high magnification (×25 or ×40) at this point to ensure accurate identification of the plane between the tumor and the facial nerve. The tumor is separated from the facial nerve starting at the fundus to the level of the porus acousticus using sharp dissection. The tumor can be gently rolled from medial-to-lateral or from anterior-to-posterior and carefully separated from the facial nerve

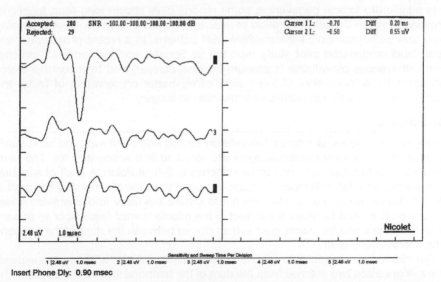

Fig. 11. Direct measurement of the cochlear nerve action potential (CNAP). Responses after removal of a 1-cm intracanalicular acoustic tumor via a middle fossa craniotomy. Db, decibels; Dly, delay; L, left; ms and msec, millisecond; SNR, signal to noise ratio; uV, microvolt.

and the delicate fibers of the cochlear nerve and labyrinthine artery using a 2-mm hook. Sectioning the superior vestibular nerve at the level of the fundus allows some slack for tumor mobilization. In tumors of the superior vestibular nerve, the authors prefer not to section the inferior vestibular nerve to avoid dissection in the inferior compartment of the IAC (inferior to the falciform or transverse crest), which may compromise the cochlear nerve and delicate fibers of the labyrinthine artery. This selective sectioning of the superior division instead of the traditional technique of sectioning both vestibular nerve divisions results in preservation of some vestibular nerve fibers. Traditionally, the preservation of vestibular nerve fibers was thought to increase the risk for tumor recurrence or postoperative vestibular symptoms; despite these risks, this selective neurectomy of only the superior vestibular nerve has been advocated to maximize chances of hearing preservation.[22]

Removal of Tumors with Extrameatal Component

In tumors that have an extrameatal component, the authors carefully create a plane between the tumor's pseudocapsule and the structures of the cerebellopontine angle. They separate the tumor from the anterior-inferior cerebellar artery and its branches to avoid inadvertent injury. Bleeding into the posterior cranial fossa is difficult to control from this approach and is best avoided. Larger tumors may be debulked from within using a combination of bipolar cauterization, forceps, suction, and the ultrasonic dissector. Cauterization is always performed away from the facial and cochlear nerves. When the tumor has been separated from the facial nerve, the vestibular nerve is cut distal to its emergence from the main trunk of the eighth cranial nerve and removed along with the tumor. During dissection of the IAC and tumor removal, the audiologist should monitor auditory function with either CNAP or ABR. The surgeon should be warned when the waveform amplitudes decrease/disappear or when the latency of wave V exceeds 0.5 ms from baseline. Tumor manipulation is stopped and papaverine is applied topically to the cochlear nerve for several minutes until the response recovers.

In addition to topical papaverine, some reports have shown long-term functional preservation with the administration of vasoactive agents to patients who develop reversible pathognomonic intraoperative ABR patterns. In a recent prospective and open-label randomized pilot study reported by Scheller and colleagues,[23] prophylactic intravenous nimodipine (a calcium channel blocker) and hydroxyethyl starch (an agent for hemodilution) showed significantly better preservation of facial and cochlear nerve function in vestibular schwannoma surgery.

Wound Closure

During wound closure, all exposed air cells are sealed with bone wax, and hemostasis is secured. All cottonoid neuropledgets are removed and accounted for. The dural flaps are approximated with one or two stitches of 6-0 neurolon. A graft of subcutaneous abdominal fat or temporalis muscle is used to obliterate the IAC; the graft is placed into the bone defect with care not to disturb the facial and cochlear nerves. A bone graft is used to repair the defect in the middle cranial fossa floor to prevent brain herniation, and the fascia graft is then placed between the dura of the temporal lobe and the bone graft.

The middle fossa retractor is removed and the temporal lobe is allowed to expand. The authors place two stitches from the dura of the temporal lobe to the edges of the temporalis muscle incision to prevent compression of the brain by an epidural hematoma. A Penrose drain is placed along the floor of the middle cranial fossa and sutured to the skin. The wound and soft tissue flaps are thoroughly irrigated with antibiotic solution to remove all bone dust and blood debris. The craniotomy bone flap is replaced and secured with miniplates. The temporalis muscle and the subcutaneous tissue flaps are sutured in layers with interrupted absorbable sutures. A running 4-0 nylon suture is used for the skin closure. A sterile pressure dressing is applied after removal of the probes inside of the external ear canal.

POSTOPERATIVE CARE

During postoperative care, the patient is monitored in the neurosurgical intensive care unit for at least 24 hours. High-blood pressure is controlled to prevent an intracranial hemorrhage. Neurologic checks, including facial nerve function, are performed as soon as the patient recovers from general anesthesia and repeated hourly for the first 24 hours to identify any neurologic complication.

The lumbar drain is either removed at the end of surgery in the operating room or left clamped and removed after several days if there is no sign of a CSF leak. Sequential compression stockings are used for prophylaxis of deep venous thrombosis. Dexamethasone is continued for 48 hours, or extended for 7 days if facial paresis or signs of brain swelling ensue. Prophylaxis against gastric bleeding is given.

Analgesia is secured with nonnarcotic medications except codeine. Droperidol or ondansetron is used for nausea and vomiting. On the first postoperative day, the Penrose drain, bladder catheter, arterial line, and electrocardiogram leads are removed and the patient is transferred to the skull base surgery/neurosurgical ward. A hemoglobin level can be obtained if significant intraoperative bleeding occurred. When nausea resolves, a liquid diet is started and advanced as tolerated. A reservoir test (head tilt test) is performed and repeated daily; if no CSF rhinorrhea is present, the patient is allowed to sit down and then progressively encouraged to walk with assistance. During the postoperative hospitalization, an MRI scan is typically obtained to assess completeness of tumor removal and as a baseline for monitoring the patient for recurrence. Between the third and fifth postoperative day, the dressing is removed and the patient discharged if tolerating a regular diet, is ambulating, and has no CSF rhinorrhea. The patient is instructed on wound care, daily temperature checks, activity, analgesia, and CSF leak prophylaxis. The patient is seen in the clinic 2 weeks after surgery to remove the sutures, and 6 weeks after surgery to assess the hearing with an audiogram.

COMPLICATIONS
Epidural Hematoma, Severe Brain Swelling, Pneumoencephalus

Life-threatening intracranial complications such as epidural hematoma, severe brain swelling, and pneumoencephalus are uncommon. Patients with these complications show signs of increased intracranial pressure, such as elevated blood pressure, bradycardia, and a deteriorating level of consciousness. If a hematoma is suspected, the dressing is immediately removed, the wound is opened, and the hematoma evacuated at the bedside before obtaining any imaging studies to avoid delay and irreversible neurologic injury. The patient is then taken to surgery to secure hemostasis and repack the wound. To prevent this complication, the authors recommend meticulous hemostasis before wound closure and leaving a Penrose drain in the wound for the first 24 hours.

Temporal Lobe Injury

Postoperative seizures, aphasia, and auditory hallucinations are, fortunately, rare and suggest a temporal lobe injury. The treatment is medical and includes measures to reduce brain swelling and antiseizure medications.

CSF Leak

If the patient develops a CSF leak, the lumbar drain is opened to drain 10 to 15 mL of CSF per hour for 4 to 5 days. The patient is placed on strict bed rest, with the head elevated 30°, and with total fluid restriction of 2000 to 2400 mL/d. The drain is clamped on the morning of postoperative day six and a reservoir test with jugular vein compression is performed. If the test is negative, the drain is removed and the patient observed for 24 hours. If CSF rhinorrhea occurs, revision surgery to close the leak is indicated. The surgical approach depends on the hearing status. If hearing is present, the MFC wound is revised. Additional fat, fascia, or muscle is packed into the IAC defect. Any air cells that are encountered are firmly waxed. If hearing is absent, endoscopic endonasal obliteration of the Eustachian tube should be considered as a first step; in recalcitrant cases, a combination of wound revision, subtotal petrosectomy, dural closure, and Eustachian tube obliteration may be needed. The lumbar drain is used for an additional 5 days postoperatively.

Meningitis

Headaches, photophobia, neck stiffness, and fever are signs of meningitis. Meningitis can be chemical (sterile) or bacterial, and can occur with or without a CSF leak. A sample of CSF can be obtained from the lumbar drain for chemistry and cultures. Chemical meningitis occurs from the presence of blood or debris in the subarachnoid space and is usually managed successfully with a few additional doses of intravenous dexamethasone. Culture-guided antibiotic therapy is recommended for bacterial meningitis.

Wound Complications

Other reported complications include those related to the wound (eg, seroma, bleeding, and infection), cystitis, deep venous thrombosis, bronchopneumonia, and cardiopulmonary and cerebrovascular problems.

Mortality

Mortality from acoustic neuroma surgery is mainly associated with the treatment of large tumors and has fallen to a level lower than 0.2% in most major centers. Because only small tumors are amenable for MFC, serious medical complications with this technique are usually related to the age and health status of the patient; hence the importance of considering these factors before recommending MFC for small tumors.

RESULTS
Results of Facial Nerve Function

Facial nerve paresis can be noted in the immediate postoperative period or can develop in a delayed fashion several days after surgery. If facial weakness occurs, immediate treatment is required to prevent exposure keratitis. The treatment includes a combination of systemic steroids, artificial tears, moisture chambers, and soft contact lenses. If the paralysis is anticipated to persist beyond 6 months, insertion of a gold weight may be necessary. Delayed facial paresis is thought to be caused by either progressive swelling with facial nerve entrapment or Herpes simplex virus reactivation. Decompression of the meatal foramen segment of the facial nerve has been proposed to prevent injury from entrapment, and routine perioperative use of antivirals seems to prevent virus reactivation.

Tumor size is perhaps the most important prognostic factor of postoperative facial nerve outcome. Facial nerve outcome after the MFC is very good because this approach is mainly performed to remove small (<2 cm) tumors. Arriaga and colleagues[24] reported a follow-up (1 year) rate of 96% good facial function (House-Brackmann grades I or II) in tumors 1.5 cm or smaller and removed using the MFC approach. A more recent review from the same center showed good facial function in 94.5% of 271 tumors smaller than 1 cm removed using the MFC approach.[25] Similarly, another group reported rates of good facial function in 94% of 64 intracanalicular tumors and 98% of 42 tumors with 1 to 9 mm cerebellopontine extension.[26]

Results of Hearing Preservation

Hearing preservation is commonly defined as the preservation of postoperative hearing within the serviceable hearing range of at least 50 dB PTA and 50% WRS (50/50 rule). This definition encompasses classes A and B of the American Academy of Otolaryngology-Head and Neck Surgery system,[27] and classes 1 and 2 of the Gardner-Robertson system.[28] Both are based on the four-frequency PTA and the best WRS. Using these criteria in a recent series of MFC, Brackmann and colleagues[7] reported that 59% of 333 patients had serviceable hearing, and 50% retained postoperative hearing at or near preoperative levels. Satar and colleagues[26] reported rates of functional hearing preservation in intracanalicular tumors and in those with up to 9 mm extension into the cerebellopontine angle of 62% and 63%, respectively. Furthermore, 70% of patients with immediate postoperative serviceable hearing maintained serviceable hearing at more than 5 years after surgery.[5] In a recent series of MFC, Hilton and colleagues[29] showed that only 5 of 44 patients with preserved hearing after MFC surgery had degradation of their hearing to the nonserviceable range in 4 years (mean follow-up). Two of the five patients with hearing degradation in their series had tumor recurrences, illustrating the importance of surveillance for tumor recurrence when functional degradation occurs.

The results of the MFC surgery should be compared with the results of alternative therapies, such as observation and stereotactic radiation. Comparing hearing outcomes between treatment modalities (ie, MFC approach, retrosigmoid approach, stereotactic radiation, observation) is more meaningful when controlling for important prognostic variables such as tumor location and size, and preoperative hearing. Staecker and colleagues[30] reported a hearing preservation rate of 57% in mainly intracanalicular tumors removed using the MFC approach and 47% in similar tumors removed using the retrosigmoid approach. In a recent review of published series of intracanalicular schwannomas, Noudel and colleagues[31] reported a rate of preservation of hearing within the 50/50 rule of 62% for the MFC approach and 58% for the retrosigmoid approach.

Randomized control trials comparing MFC surgery and stereotactic radiation are lacking. However, case series[32–34] of different radiation modalities and tumor sizes report tumor control rates of 90% to 98%, and facial nerve dysfunction rates of less than 5%. Niranjan and colleagues[35] recently published a series of 96 intracanalicular acoustic tumors treated with gamma knife therapy. Using the 50/50 rule with a mean follow-up of 3.5 years, their rate of hearing preservation after radiation treatment was 61%. Other groups have reported on the long-term hearing results after gamma knife radiation and noted an ongoing deterioration of hearing over time, with an actuarial rate of keeping the same Gardner and Robertson class declining to 44% after 10 years.[36] This hearing decline seems unrelated to tumor growth, which argues against a protective effect of radiosurgery on hearing. The results from radiosurgery studies should be compared with series of acoustic neuromas managed expectantly, because many of these small tumors do not exhibit significant growth or functional deterioration after prolonged periods of observation.

Pennings and colleagues[37] recently reported on the natural history of intracanalicular vestibular schwannomas and showed in some patients a deterioration of both the PTA and the WRS after 3.6 years, with 74% maintaining good hearing (above the 50/50 cut-off). In this series, hearing deteriorated significantly in 26% of patients during this short follow-up period, and this deterioration occurred irrespective of any radiologic evidence of tumor growth[37] **(Table 2)**.

Quality of Life

Several studies have examined the quality of life of patients with acoustic neuroma. Baumann and colleagues[38] used the SF-36 Health Survey in German patients who underwent MFC surgery. They showed that impairments could not be eliminated by surgery. On the contrary, in addition to any hearing loss, vertigo, and facial paresis after surgery, some patients also experienced trigeminal neuralgia and psychological and psychosomatic disorders, such as depression, anxiety, and sleeping problems.[38] Mental, psychological, and physical impairments have also been shown in untreated patients undergoing conservative management (wait-and-scan approach). A recent study showed that untreated patients scored lower in physical domains than the general population, and analyses have shown that the dizziness handicap and age (and not hearing loss) were the strongest predictors of disability in these patients.[39] The facts that dizziness negatively affects the quality of life of patients with untreated acoustic neuromas, and that balance disturbances generally improve after microsurgical removal of small tumors, support surgical intervention for patients with disabling imbalance. When discussing treatment options with a patient who has a small tumor and is minimally symptomatic, the surgeon should insure that the patient clearly understands that presurgical impairments (other than dizziness) are not likely to improve, and that there is the risk of additional physical, mental and psychological impairments after surgery. Moreover, patients should be directed to seek contact with support groups before they undergo surgery.

Table 2
Hearing preservation after surgery, radiotherapy, and observation

Study	N	Outcomes for Serviceable Hearing
Brackmann et al,[7] 2000	333	MFC: 59% serviceable hearing 50% postoperative hearing near preoperative hearing levels
Satar et al,[26] 2002		MFC: 62%–63% functional hearing preservation 70% of the 62%–63% maintained serviceable hearing 5 y after surgery
Hilton et al,[29] 2011	44	MFC: 5 patients with degradation to nonhearing 4 y after surgery; 2 of 5 because of tumor recurrence
Staecker et al,[30] 2000		MFC: 57% Retrosigmoid: 47%
Noudel et al,[31] 2009		MFC: 62% Retrosigmoid: 58%
Niranjan et al,[35] 2008	96	Gamma knife: 61% at mean 3.5 y
Chopra et al,[36]		Gamma knife: 44% after 10 y
Pennings et al,[37] 2011		Observation: 74% at 3.6 y 26% had significant hearing deterioration at 3.6 y

SURGERY IN THE ONLY HEARING EAR AND IN NEUROFIBROMATOSIS TYPE 2

Patients with bilateral acoustic tumors (neurofibromatosis type 2 [NF2]) face a tremendous challenge when trying to reconcile the treatment of their tumor-related manifestations and the preservation of neurologic function. A comprehensive discussion of NF2 is beyond the scope of this presentation, but it is commonly accepted that outcomes after surgery and radiotherapy are worse in NF2 than in sporadic unilateral vestibular schwannoma. NF2 acoustic tumors behave in a more aggressive manner than their unilateral counterparts. Histologically, these tumors are multifocal and tend to infiltrate sensory fibers, and concerns are increasing about their increased susceptibility to malignant degeneration after radiotherapy.[40] These facts have a significant impact on the treatment selection and results of hearing preservation. The objective of contemporary management of NF2 is preservation of function. Patients with NF2 should be informed of all of the available treatment options and treated only in experienced multidisciplinary centers. Microsurgery, radiation, and observation have been the available options, but medical therapy is emerging as an alternative. In a recent publication, treatment with the angiogenesis inhibitor bevacizumab resulted in temporary tumor shrinkage, improved hearing, and alleviation of other symptoms of brainstem compression.[41]

In terms of the MFC, Brackmann and colleagues[42] reported on their experience with this approach for removal of NF2 tumors and showed hearing results within 15 dB of preoperative levels in 48% of patients. Similarly, this same group reported on the technique of MFC decompression of the IAC (instead of tumor removal) to prolong function in patients with impending or progressive hearing loss in their only hearing ear.[43] One of the possible explanations for the hearing loss in patients with acoustic tumors is the increase in pressure inside the IAC that occurs with tumor growth. Through decompressing the IAC, the resulting increase in the volume of the IAC may lead to a decrease in the pressure that the tumor exerts on the nerve fibers and vascular channels.

The reported results on successful hearing preservation after MFC tumor removal and IAC decompression argue in favor for an early proactive management in selected patients with NF2. Hearing preservation surgery in NF2 should only be attempted in patients who have a realistic chance of successful preservation of hearing or at least an intact cochlear nerve; patients with intact cochlear nerves may still be suitable for cochlear implant habilitation.

SUMMARY ON MICROSURGERY FOR VESTIBULAR SCHWANNOMA

The microsurgical removal of acoustic neuromas via an MFC approach is indicated in cases of intracanalicular tumors to preserve serviceable hearing. Alternative modalities (stereotactic radiation and observation) are equally considered before a joint decision with the patient is reached. Microsurgery (ie, MFC) offers the opportunity of total tumor resection with acceptable surgical risks. Results of MFC compare favorably with other modalities, with serviceable hearing preservation in more than 60% of cases and good postoperative facial nerve function in more than 95%. The morbidity is acceptable and the most common complications include facial weakness and cerebrospinal fluid leak in approximately 5% of cases.

The preoperative evaluation is geared toward the identification of the best candidates for long-term serviceable hearing preservation. Serious consideration should be given to the discussion of the expected surgical benefits and risks, keeping in mind that the main objective is the maintenance of the patients' short- and long-term quality of life.

REFERENCES

1. House WF. Surgical exposure of the internal auditory canal and its content through the middle cranial fossa. Laryngoscope 1961;71:1363–85.
2. Hartley F. Intracranial neurectomy of the second and third divisions of the fifth nerve: a new method. N Y Med J 1892;55:317–9.
3. Kawase R, Toya S, Shiobara R, et al. Transpetrosal approach for aneurysm of the lower basilar artery. J Neurosurg 1985;63:857–61.
4. Hall JW III, Derlacki EL. Binaural hearing after middle ear surgery. Masking-level difference for interaural time and amplitude cues. Audiology 1988;27:89–98.
5. Friedman RA, Kesser B, Brackmann DE, et al. Long-term hearing preservation after middle fossa removal of vestibular schwannoma. Otolaryngol Head Neck Surg 2003;129:660–5.
6. Shelton C, Brackmann DE, House WF, et al. Acoustic tumor surgery. Prognostic factors in hearing conversation. Arch Otolaryngol Head Neck Surg 1989;115:1213–6.
7. Brackmann DE, Owens RM, Friedman RA, et al. Prognostic factors for hearing preservation in vestibular schwannoma surgery. Am J Otol 2000;21:417–24.
8. Ferber-Viart C, Laoust L, Boulud B, et al. Acuteness of preoperative factors to predict hearing preservation in acoustic neuroma surgery. Laryngoscope 2000; 110:145–50.
9. Jaisinghani VJ, Levine SC, Nussbaum E, et al. Hearing preservation after acoustic neuroma surgery. Skull Base Surg 2000;10:141–7.
10. Mohr G, Sade B, Dufour JJ, et al. Preservation of hearing in patients undergoing microsurgery for vestibular schwannoma: degree of meatal filling. J Neurosurg 2005;102:1–5.
11. Patil CG, Veeravagu A, Lad SP, et al. Craniotomy for resection of meningioma in the elderly: a multicentre, prospective analysis from the National Surgical Quality Improvement Program. J Neurol Neurosurg Psychiatry 2010;81:502–5.
12. Sacko O, Sesay M, Roux FE, et al. Intracranial meningioma surgery in the ninth decade of life. Neurosurgery 2007;61(5):950–4.
13. Telischi FF, Landy H, Balkany TJ. Reducing temporal lobe retraction with the middle fossa approach using a lumbar drain. Laryngoscope 1995;105:219–20.
14. Low WK. Middle cranial fossa approach to the internal auditory meatus: a Chinese temporal bone study. ORL J Otorhinolaryngol Relat Spec 1999;61:142–5.
15. Arriaga M, Haid R, Masel D. Antidromic stimulation of the greater superficial petrosal nerve in middle fossa surgery. Laryngoscope 1995;105:102–5.
16. Fisch U. Transtemporal surgery of the internal auditory canal: report of 92 cases, technique indications, and results. Adv Otorhinolaryngol 1970;17:203–40.
17. Carey JP, Minor LB, Nager GT. Dehiscence or thinning of bone overlying the superior semicircular canal in a temporal bone survey. Arch Otolaryngol Head Neck Surg 2000;126:137–47.
18. García-Ibañez E, García-Ibañez JL. Middle fossa vestibular neurectomy: a report of 383 cases. Arch Otolaryngol Head Neck Surg 1980;88:486–90.
19. Wigand ME, Haid T, Berg M, et al. Extended middle cranial fossa approach for acoustic neuroma surgery. Skull Base Surg 1991;1(3):183–7.
20. Neff BA, Ting J, Dickinson SL, et al. Facial nerve monitoring parameters as a predictor of postoperative facial nerve outcomes after vestibular schwannoma resection. Otol Neurotol 2005;26:728–32.
21. Romstock J, Strauss C, Fahlbusch R. Continuous electromyography monitoring of motor cranial nerves during cerebellopontine angle surgery. J Neurosurg 2000;93:586–93.

22. Brackmann DE, House JR III, Hitselberger WE. Technical modifications to the middle fossa craniotomy approach in removal of acoustic neuromas. Am J Otol 1994;15(5):614-9.
23. Scheller C, Richter HP, Engelhardt M, et al. The influence of prophylactic vasoactive treatment on cochlear and facial nerve functions after vestibular schwannoma surgery: a prospective and open-label randomized pilot study. Neurosurgery 2007;61:92-8.
24. Arriaga MA, Luxford WM, Berliner KI. Facial nerve function following middle fossa and translabyrinthine acoustic tumor surgery: a comparison. Am J Otol 1994;15:620-4.
25. Fayad JN, Brackmann DE. Treatment of small acoustic tumors (vestibular schwannomas). Neurosurg Q 2005;15:127-37.
26. Satar B, Jackler RK, Oghalai J, et al. Risk-benefit analysis of using the middle fossa approach for acoustic neuromas with >10 mm cerebellopontine angle component. Laryngoscope 2002;112:1500-6.
27. Monsell EM, Balkany TA, Gates GA, et al. Committee on Hearing and Equilibrium guidelines for the evaluation of hearing preservation in acoustic neuroma (vestibular schwannoma). American Academy of Otolaryngology-Head and Neck Surgery Foundation, INC. Otolaryngol Head Neck Surg 1995;113:179-80.
28. Gardner G, Robertson JH. Hearing preservation in unilateral acoustic neuroma surgery. Ann Otol Rhinol Laryngol 1988;97:55-66.
29. Hilton CW, Haines SJ, Agrawal A, et al. Late failure rate of hearing preservation after middle fossa approach for resection of vestibular schwannoma. Otol Neurotol 2011;32(1):132-5.
30. Staecker H, Nadol JB Jr, Ojeman R, et al. Hearing preservation in acoustic neuroma surgery: middle fossa versus retrosigmoid approach. Am J Otol 2000;21:399-404.
31. Noudel R, Gomis P, Duntze J, et al. Hearing preservation and facial nerve function after microsurgery for intracanalicular vestibular schwannomas: comparison of middle fossa and retrosigmoid approaches. Acta Neurochir 2009;151(8):935-44.
32. Chang SD, Gibbs IC, Sakamoto GT, et al. Staged stereotactic irradiation for acoustic neuroma. Neurosurgery 2005;56:1254-61.
33. Lunsford LD, Niranjan A, Flickinger JC, et al. Radiosurgery of vestibular schwannomas: summary of experience in 829 cases. J Neurosurg 2005;102(Suppl):195-9.
34. Friedman WA, Bradshaw P, Myers A, et al. Linear accelerator radiosurgery for vestibular schwannomas. J Neurosurg 2006;105:657-61.
35. Niranjan A, Mathieu D, Flickinger JC, et al. Hearing preservation after intracanalicular vestibular schwannoma radiosurgery. Neurosurgery 2008;63(6):1054-63.
36. Chopra R, Kondziolka D, Niranjan A, et al. Long-term follow-up of acoustic schwannomas radiosurgery with marginal tumor doses of 12 to 13 Gy. Int J Radiat Oncol Biol Phys 2007;68(3):845-51.
37. Pennings RJ, Morris DP, Clarke L, et al. Natural history of hearing deterioration in intracanalicular vestibular schwannoma. Neurosurgery 2011;68(1):68-77.
38. Baumann I, Polligkeit J, Blumenstock G, et al. Quality of life after unilateral acoustic neuroma surgery via middle cranial fossa approach. Acta Otolaryngol 2005;125:585-91.
39. Lloyd SK, Kasbekar AV, Baguley DM, et al. Audiovestibular factors influencing quality of life in patients with conservatively managed sporadic vestibular schwannoma. Otol Neurotol 2010;31(6):968-76.
40. Baser ME, Evans DG, Jackler RK, et al. Malignant peripheral nerve sheath tumors, radiotherapy, and neurofibromatosis 2. Br J Cancer 2000;82:998.

41. Plotkin S, Stemmer-Rachamimov A, Barker F, et al. Hearing improvement after bevacizumab in patients with neurofibromatosis type 2. N Engl J Med 2009; 361(4):358–67.

42. Brackmann DE, Fayad JN, Slattery WH III, et al. Early proactive management of vestibular schwannomas in neurofibromatosis type 2. Neurosurgery 2001;49:274–80.

43. Gadre AK, Kwartler JA, Brackmann DE, et al. Middle fossa decompression of the internal auditory canal in acoustic neuroma surgery: a therapeutic alternative. Laryngoscope 1990;100(9):948–52.

The Endoscopic Approach to Vestibular Schwannomas and Posterolateral Skull Base Pathology

Daniel R. Pieper, MD[a,b,c],*

KEYWORDS

- Vestibular schwannoma • Acoustic neuroma • Endoscopy • Neuroendoscopy
- Surgical technique • Surgical technology

Key Abbreviations: ENDOSCOPIC APPROACH TO SKULL BASE SURGERY	
BAER	Brainstem auditory evoked responses
CPA	Cerebellopontine angle
CSF	Cerebrospinal fluid
HFS	Hemifacial spasm
IAC	Internal auditory canal
MVD	Microvascular decompressions
REZ	Root entry zone
TS	Transverse/sigmoid

The necessity of improved visualization during surgery with regard to clarity, magnification, and illumination has remained paramount in all aspects of surgery, but it is one of the most essential elements in skull base surgery. The idea of surgical endoscopy is not new. Max Nitze is credited with the first design of a surgical endoscope in 1879.[1] This initial invention, using a series of multiple lenses illuminated by a light at the tip, was developed to overcome the same obstacles surgeons still encounter: magnification and improved visualization in the depths of a surgical field. Doyen, in 1917, further developed this idea with the introduction of a crude endoscope used to visualize the cerebellopontine angle (CPA).[2] However, the primitive technology of lenses and light source at the time significantly limited this technology and it was quickly abandoned. With the microscope's superior illumination and magnification the idea of the endoscope was quietly dismissed.

[a] Michigan Head and Spine Institute, 26850 Providence Parkway, Suite 240, Novi, MI 48374, USA
[b] Oakland University/William Beaumont School of Medicine, Rochester, MI, USA
[c] Skull Base Surgery, William Beaumont Hospital, Royal Oak, MI, USA
* Keystone Medical Center, 46325 12 Mile Road, Suite 100, Novi, MI 48377.
E-mail address: Pieperd@usa.net

Otolaryngol Clin N Am 45 (2012) 439–454
doi:10.1016/j.otc.2011.12.011
0030-6665/12/$ – see front matter © 2012 Elsevier Inc. All rights reserved.

Because of this fundamental tenet, the introduction of the operating microscope was an essential advancement in neurosurgery in the latter part of the twentieth century. Surgical techniques and instruments were developed to build on the strengths and minimize the limitations of the operating microscope. Advancements in the field of microsurgery allowed the surgeon to compensate for the microscope's deficiencies by creating instruments and techniques that create linear corridors of visualization. These advancements, which provided accessibility to the posterolateral skull base, specifically the CPA, required either extensive removal of the temporal bone or mobilization and retraction of the cerebellum to provide a channel for the optics and the light source to adequately illuminate the surgical field (**Fig. 1**). Although the operating microscope provides significant improvement in visualization compared with surgical loupes and headlight, there are significant limitations to the microscope because of the location of the light source and optics outside of the surgical incision. Because the light source is located a distance from the surgical incision, a significant portion of the light is disbursed, and therefore unavailable for illumination of the deep recess of the CPA (**Fig. 2**A). Additionally, because light and optics travel in a straight line, illumination and visualization around corners is virtually impossible. As such, additional brain retraction or removal of bone is necessary to broaden the field of view, especially for surgery within the CPA.[3–5]

It was not until the 1970s that the surgical endoscope would once again emerge and gain wider acceptance in the field of surgery. The introduction of the endoscope to neurosurgery has been at a much slower pace compared with in general, otolaryngology, and orthopedic surgery. The major criticism of these early endoscopes was their bulkiness and poor resolution compared with the superiority of the operating microscope. As camera technology improved, the endoscope was introduced to neurosurgery for use in the ventricular system. The intraventricular procedures required that the endoscope be maintained in a relatively fixed position over the course of the procedure and therefore could be safely used by the addition of a rigid endoscope holder or a surgical assistant. The early results showing less tissue damage and enhanced visualization with faster patient recovery times fueled the interest of endoscopy within neurosurgery. However, it was not until the collaborative efforts between

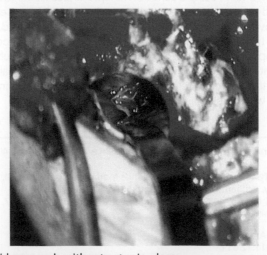

Fig. 1. Retrosigmoid approach with retractor in place.

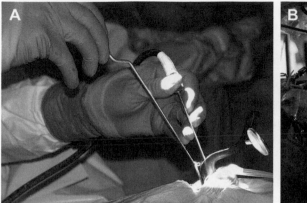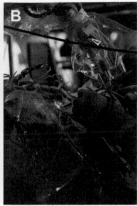

Fig. 2. (A) Microscope-assisted transsphenoidal approach. Note the amount of light disbursement. (B) Endoscopic approach to CPA. Note that the light source is entirely contained within the surgical field.

endoscopically trained otolaryngologists and neurosurgeons while accessing the pituitary fossa that the endoscope evolved into the world of skull base surgery.

In the 1990s the endoscope was reintroduced to the CPA, almost 80 years since Doyen had described his experience during a trigeminal neurectomy.[6–15] Since then a small but ever growing number of surgeons have reported their experiences using the endoscope as an adjunct to the surgical microscope and microsurgical techniques. Shahinian and colleagues in 2001 were the first to describe a fully endoscopic approach to the CPA.[16,17]

In 2005, our skull base team further developed this technique to access and treat several pathologies within the CPA extending through the incisura and foramen magnum superiorly and inferiorly, and lesions extending anteriorly into Meckel's cave, the internal auditory canal (IAC), and jugular foramen; posteriorly by the foramen of Luschka; and medially to access lesions involving the contralateral CPA. The major benefit of accessing the CPA through a fully endoscopic approach is the decreased tissue manipulation and retraction while simultaneously widening the field of view and obtaining a true 360-degree visualization of the structures of the CPA. Because the endoscope is a mere 4-mm diameter shaft, the approach around the cerebellar hemisphere can be obtained without the need for retractors, thereby obviating the need to sacrifice venous structures that would otherwise be at increased risk during cerebellar retraction (**Fig. 3**). The enhanced illumination, allowed by a focal, intradurally placed light source, and an unobstructed wide field of view from the endoscope allows unimpeded visualization from cranial nerve (CN) IV at the level of the incisura to the cervicomedullary junction through a cranial defect as small as 14 mm. However, as with the development of any new technique, significant obstacles were initially encountered. These primarily included stabilization of the endoscope, heat transmission from the light source, lack of endoscope-specific surgical instruments, and the ever-present learning curve.

TECHNICAL OBSTACLES IN ENDOSCOPY
Stabilization in Endoscopy

One of the earliest and most difficult technical obstacles was stabilization of the endoscope. In the early reports of endoscope-assisted approaches to the CPA, many

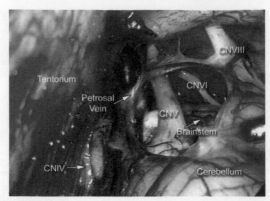

Fig. 3. Preservation of the petrosal vein during a trigeminal microvascular decompression.

authors describe manipulating the endoscope in one hand and working with the other hand. This significantly limits use of the endoscope. To fully use the endoscope in the approach, bimanual surgical technique is essential. Therefore, an effective strategy to stabilize the endoscope while using bimanual microsurgical technique had to be developed. Unlike the intraventricular approaches, visualization of the CPA requires constant changes to the field of view. Therefore, a rigid endoscope holder used in intraventricular procedures was not practical for procedures within the CPA. Additionally, because of the confined space during approaches to the CPA, the ability to use an assistant to stabilize the endoscope, as is typically done with transsphenoidal approaches, is not feasible. We were able to overcome this situation by using a pneumatically controlled multijointed, polyaxial arm (Mitaka Kohki, Tokyo, Japan). This arm works similarly to the operating microscope using a single button to release all of the joints, allowing for one-handed control of the endoscope and immediate and secure stabilization of the endoscope after the button is released, allowing the surgeon to carry out the procedure bimanually (Fig. 4).

Heat Transmission in Endoscopy

One of the major advantages of the endoscope is the enhanced illumination of the surgical field because the light is not disbursed as with the surgical microscope, but

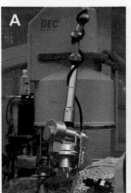
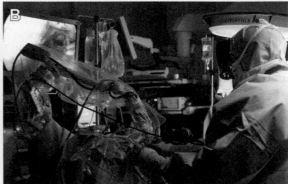

Fig. 4. (A) Pneumatic endoscope holder. (B) With the endoscope rigidly held, the surgeon can use bimanual surgical technique.

remains focused within the area of interest. However, this advantage is also a major disadvantage because the proximity of the xenon light to the structures within the CPA can become overheated. To overcome this problem we introduced a water-cooled sleeve to the outside of the endoscope (Medtronic, Xomed, Jacksonville, FL, USA) **(Fig. 5)**. A foot pedal is depressed periodically, which bathes the endoscope dissipating the heat generated from the light source allowing the procedure to continue unimpeded without removing the endoscope from the surgical field.

Surgical Instruments for Endoscopy

Instruments specifically designed for microsurgery are, in many cases, counterproductive for use in endoscopic procedures. This is not unique to neurosurgery but is well established and a necessary growing pain experienced by clinicians in other surgical specialties. The bayoneted and opposable grip instruments, specifically forceps, scissors, and bipolars, in most cases cannot be transferred from the microscope to the endoscopic procedure. To overcome this we surveyed instruments from the otolaryngology and sinus surgery sets to obtain perspective in designing straight-shafted pistol-grip forceps and scissors for use in these CPA endoscopic procedures **(Fig. 6)**. Because of the limited corridor to the CPA bounded by neural tissue posteriorly and petrous bone anteriorly, the trajectory for instruments is somewhat limited; therefore, each of these instruments has rotational capabilities to allow maneuverability in a 360-degree plane. The major instrument limitation encountered was the lack of a straight-shafted, rotational pistol-grip bipolar. Our initial attempts to use the bayoneted opposable bipolars from the microsurgical sets was unsuccessful because the tips kept scissoring and therefore could not be used reliably. Since our initial experience in 2005, such a bipolar is now developed that comes with three interchangeable tips, angled and straight (Karl Storz, Tuttlingen, Germany) **(Fig. 7)**. We also use a set of straight-shafted monitored microdissecting instruments **(Fig. 8)**. These instruments allow us to continually monitor cranial nerve activity while actively dissecting and resecting neoplasms within the CPA without changing instruments.

Learning Curve in Endoscopy

Most neurosurgeons have little if any formal training with endoscopy. As such, before beginning a neuroendoscopy practice, time must be spent familiarizing oneself with

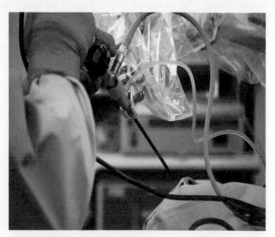

Fig. 5. Cooling sleeve connected to an irrigation source. The sleeve slides directly over the endoscope.

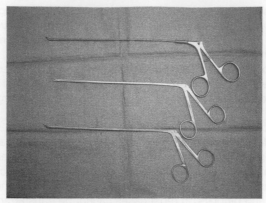

Fig. 6. Rotating pistol-grip endoscopic instruments.

the technique, the instruments, and manipulating the endoscope during surgery. Currently, most cameras provide a high-definition picture in two-dimensions. Therefore, the surgeon must learn to accommodate the loss of depth perception. This is easily overcome with practice, but is necessary to become proficient with endoscopy. Recent advances in camera technology may overcome this disadvantage in the near future, but until then this fundamental limitation is a major step in the learning curve.

Another significant learning obstacle is also one of the true advantages of the endoscope. The ability to use angled endoscopes provides the surgeon with a way to effectively look around corners without additional retraction or further drilling. I have found that the 30-degree endoscope is adequate for visualizing the IAC or Meckel's cave (**Fig. 9**). A significant learning curve exists for these angled endoscopes, and the greater the angle the greater chance for disorientation.

Patient Selection for Endoscopic Surgery

To create an adequate working corridor, especially to resect acoustic tumors, accessing the basilar cisterns is mandatory. This is never done blindly. The endoscope is directed along the superior-ventral aspect of the cerebellum until the arachnoid of the basilar cistern is visualized. The petrosal veins should be identified and preserved if possible (**Fig. 10**). After the arachnoid has been opened sharply, the egress of the cerebrospinal fluid (CSF) allows further relaxation of the cerebellar hemisphere and

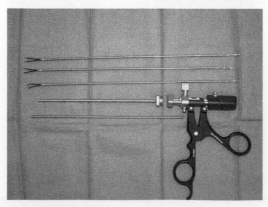

Fig. 7. Rotating pistol-grip bipolar set.

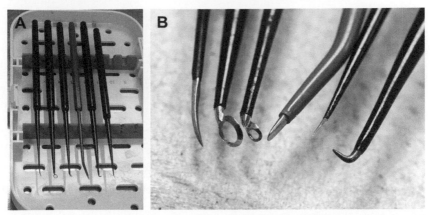

Fig. 8. (A) Monitoring endoscopic dissecting instruments. (B) Close-up view of the various dissecting tips.

a larger working corridor. Therefore, a contraindication of this approach is a tumor that has filled the prepontine cistern or involves significant mass effect elevating the posterior fossa pressure. In these cases a microscope-assisted approach is more prudent allowing the surgeon early access to the cisterna magna and ultimately providing a decrease in the intracranial pressure. We also limit the endoscopic approach to those tumors and pathologies where hearing is present and preservation is planned. In cases where hearing preservation is not a consideration we advocate a translabyrinthine approach, which in our experience offers the lowest risk to the facial nerve.

TECHNIQUE FOR ENDOSCOPIC SKULL BASE SURGERY

The following describes the technique for endoscopic skull base surgery.

- Anesthesia is typically positioned at the patient's feet to allow adequate room for placement of the monitors and sterile tables around the patent's head.
- The endoscope monitor should be positioned so that it is in a direct line of sight for the surgeon as he or she is working (**Fig. 11**). Placing the monitor out of the surgeon's line of sight can be extremely disorienting.

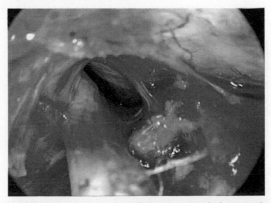

Fig. 9. View of the trigeminal nerve extending into Meckel cave through a 30-degree endoscope.

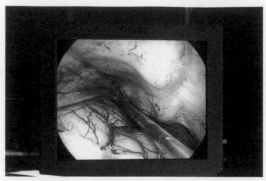

Fig. 10. Endoscopic view of the CPA. Identification of the petrosal vein and opening of the arachnoid layer of the prepontine cistern.

- The surgical nurse can be located to the surgeon's right or left based on preference, but positioned in such a way as the passing of instruments is unimpeded.
- We use intraoperative monitoring in all CPA cases. The ability for ease of communication between the electrophysiologist and anesthesia personnel is essential and must be considered in the room set-up.
- The patient is placed in a rigid headholder and the head turned toward the contralateral side to allow ease in accessing the postauricular region, being careful not to compromise the jugular veins. I emphasize this point of rigid head immobilization because we do not typically use paralytics during surgery of the CPA to effectively monitor the cranial nerves, especially CNVII.
- The patient's head is elevated approximately 30 degrees above the horizontal to allow gravity to assist with the exposure.[18]
- The hips and knees are slightly flexed so that the patient is in a comfortable semi-reclined position.
- The pneumatic endoscope holder is attached to the contralateral bedrail and is positioned to allow multiple trajectories for the endoscope.
- Monitoring electrodes are then placed to allow for the monitoring of cranial nerves and somotosensory evoked potentials as appropriate for the pathology of interest. A thorough discussion of intraoperative monitoring should take place with the anesthesiologist before intubation. This allows the anesthesia team to prepare should a monitored endotracheal tube be necessary and to allow preparation of the anesthetic agents and protocol to be reviewed to minimize contamination of the intraoperative monitoring techniques.

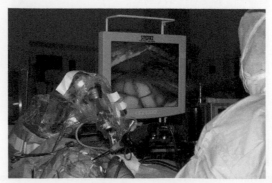

Fig. 11. Maintaining the monitor is essential.

- To minimize an unnecessarily large incision and bone removal, localization of the transverse-sigmoid junction (TS) should be performed before the incision. To determine the location of the TS, Day and colleagues[19] described two reliable superficial landmarks: a line drawn from the root of the zygoma to the inion, and a line drawn from the squamosal-parietomastoid suture junction to the tip of the mastoid, which is palpated along the posterior mastoid groove. The intersection of these two lines closely identifies the location of the TS.
- An oblique linear incision is then marked out centered on the TS.
- The incision is then infiltrated with epinephrine-enhanced local anesthetic.
- The area is then prepared with care to avoid contaminating the external auditory canal with any of the preparation solution because this interferes with intraoperative auditory monitoring.
- Before the incision, the patient is usually administered 1 to 2 g/kg of mannitol and gently hyperventilated to a $Paco_2$ of approximately 30 mm Hg unless contraindicated. We have found that using both of these modalities performed in advance significantly decreases the intracranial pressure, especially in obese patients, allowing the endoscope to easily cannulate the posterior fossa.
- A 2.5- to 3-cm incision is typically adequate to provide access; however, in cases where the patient is larger or more muscular or in instances where a larger craniectomy is planned to allow the use of surgical aspirators and endoscopic drills, the incision is tailored as needed. Although a perforator can be used to quickly access the dura at the level of the TS, we prefer to perform the craniectomy with standard fluted cutting and diamond burrs to minimize the risk to the TS. Rhoton[20] has described a method of placing the craniectomy 2 cm inferior to the asterion, two-thirds posterior, and one-third anterior to the occipitomastoid suture. This trajectory places the dural exposure just inferior to the TS.
- It is recommended that the drilling clearly identify and partially skeletonize the edges of the TS.
- In cases of microvascular decompressions (MVD) and neurectomies, a 14-mm craniectomy is adequate; however, in acoustic tumors we typically extend the craniectomy inferiorly along the sigmoid sinus another 5 to 10 mm to accommodate drills and aspirators easily (**Fig. 12**). If encountered, all exposed air cells of the mastoid must be thoroughly waxed to prevent postoperative CSF leaks.
- After the TS is adequately exposed, a curvilinear dural incision is made parallel to the TS. Care should be taken to leave an adequate dural cuff along the sinus edge to allow for ease of dural closure at the conclusion of the procedure.
- The endoscope is prepared to cannulate the posterior fossa and the camera adjusted to the correct orientation.

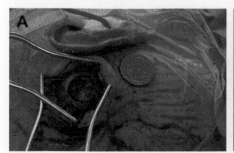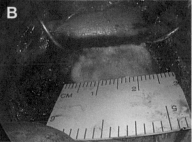

Fig. 12. (A) A 14-mm craniectomy for accessing the CPA. (B) The craniectomy can be extended to accommodate additional instruments, such as drills and surgical aspirators.

- A rigid 4-mm 0-degree endoscope is gradually introduced along the superior aspect between the cerebellar hemisphere and the tentorium, if accessing the interpeduncular cistern, or ventrally along the cerebellar hemisphere, if accessing the prepontine cistern.
- During the initial cannulation the endoscope is advanced in small increments to allow identification of the petrosal veins because these vascular structures are extremely varied in their location.
- After the petrosal veins are identified they are either mobilized or cauterized and transected to allow adequate visualization and access to the arachnoid membrane of the basilar cisterns.
- The arachnoid should be opened using sharp microsurgical technique to avoid unnecessary tension on the cranial nerves located in the vicinity. Opening the arachnoid membrane allows for the egress of CSF, which allows for additional cerebellar relaxation. At this point we generally identify CNIV through CNXI and the major vascular structures to minimize the risk of inadvertent injury.

One significant aspect that evolved over the course of the procedure's development was the discontinued use of brain retractors. Initially, we attempted to replicate the open microscope-assisted procedure to the endoscope. Therefore, we erroneously placed an intracranial retractor to enhance visualization and to minimize risk to the cerebellum during the introduction and removal of surgical instruments to the field. We quickly realized that the retractor significantly diminished surgical exposure and after the retractors were removed a significant increase in the working channel was achieved. Currently, we only use retractors when drilling the IAC to place a rigid barrier between the drill and the cerebellum.

TUMOR RESECTION

The following describes the technique for tumor resection.

- Before resecting the acoustic neuroma, the structures of the CNVII to CNVIII complex are identified. The cochlear nerve is typically identified along the inferior pole of the tumor and may be extremely splayed out along the tumor capsule (**Fig. 13**).
- At this point, the endoscope is advanced to the ventral aspect of the tumor to identify the facial nerve and nervus intermedius.

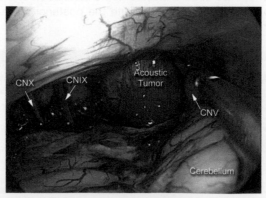

Fig. 13. Visualization of a left CPA acoustic neuroma. Note that the cochlear nerve is displaced and splayed over the inferior aspect of the tumor.

- Any vascular structures to the tumor should be coagulated and transected to further devascularize the tumor.
- Should bleeding be encountered, the endoscope should not be withdrawn because this precludes visualization and makes recannulation of the posterior fossa more difficult. Copious irrigation helps identify the source. Gentle pressure with hemostatic agents can be used. In cases of more profuse bleeding, identification of the source, gentle pressure, and bipolar cautery may be necessary.
- After the CNs are adequately identified, the porus acusticus is widened using a high-speed endoscopic drill (**Fig. 14**). Care is taken to avoid inadvertently entering to semicircular canals during drilling.
- At this point, the tumor capsule is opened sharply and the intracapsular contents are resected in a piecemeal fashion using either stimulating microdissectors or a surgical aspirator depending on the vascularity and consistency of the tumor (**Fig. 15**).
- Because these approaches are typically used for hearing preservation procedures, care is taken to begin the resection away from the cochlear nerve. As the tumor is debulked the tumor can be sharply dissected from the cochlear, facial, and intermedius nerves (**Fig. 16**).
- At the conclusion of the resection, the facial nerve is always stimulated at the root entry zone (REZ) (**Fig. 17**). A favorable facial nerve outcome closely parallels the ability to successfully stimulate at a threshold of 0.05 mA.

CLOSURE

The following describes the technique for closure.

- Before decannulating the endoscope from the posterior fossa, a Valsalva maneuver is performed.
- After it is verified that the surgical field is hemostatically dry, the endoscope is withdrawn.
- The dura is closed in a watertight fashion. In instances where a watertight closure cannot be achieved, synthetic dural substitutes, autologous fascia, muscle or fat, or dural sealants can be used.
- We routinely reconstruct the cranial defect either with autologous bone or hydroxyapatite cement.
- The skin is closed in layers and a mastoid dressing is used to prevent a subgaleal fluid collection.

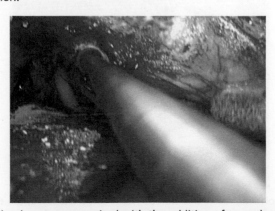

Fig. 14. Visualization is not compromised with the addition of an endoscopic drill.

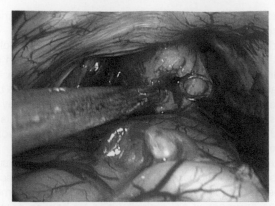

Fig. 15. The tumor is resected in a piecemeal fashion using stimulating dissectors. This allows for real-time continuous feedback of the facial nerve during the tumor resection.

OTHER INDICATIONS FOR THE ENDOSCOPIC APPROACH
Microvascular Decompression

Because MVDs typically involve relatively normal CPA anatomy without the deformation that accompanies neoplasms of the CPA (**Fig. 18**), these should be the surgeon's introduction to CPA endoscopy.

- After the CN of concern is identified, a thorough 360-degree inspection of the REZ should be performed before placement of any pledgets.
- After all offending vessels are identified, any venous structures should be treated first. Coagulation of the vein and transection allows greater manipulation of the arterial components with less risk of bleeding.
- The offending arteries should be thoroughly dissected away from the nerve and all arachnoid bands sharply cut. This allows mobility of the vessel and decreases the risk of inadvertent injury during placement of the pledgets.
- Should bleeding be encountered, the same steps described previously can be used.
- In the case of hemifacial spasm (HFS), a thorough inspection along the entire REZ, which typically extends inferiorly toward the foramen of Luschka, is

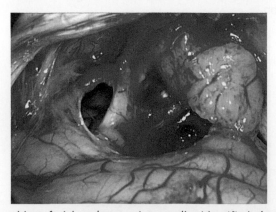

Fig. 16. With the cochlear, facial, and nervus intermedius identified, the tumor is dissected sharply to minimize injury.

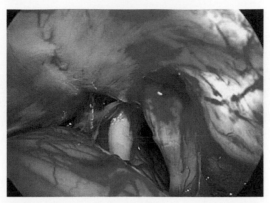

Fig. 17. After resection, a final brainstem auditory evoked responses and stimulation threshold of the facial nerve at the root entry zone are obtained before closure.

    necessary because failure to adequately decompress the entire REZ results in an incomplete resolution of the spasms.
- In MVD for HFS we typically perform pre- and post-MVD CNVII stimulation thresholds to evaluate the integrity of the nerve.
- A stimulation threshold at 0.05 mA is generally consistent with a favorable clinical facial nerve examination.

Vestibular Neurectomy

The resolution achieved with current high-definition cameras and monitors can exceed the resolution of most operating microscopes (**Fig. 19**). In vestibular neurectomies, this allows a greater delineation between the cochlear and vestibular components of CNVIII within the CPA. This provides for a more complete transection of vestibular fibers, while minimizing inadvertent injury to the cochlear nerve and its microvasculature. Continuous monitoring of brainstem auditory evoked responses is performed during the neurectomy to avoid injury to the cochlear nerve. As with the acoustic tumor resection procedure, before the neurectomy the facial nerve and nervus intermedius should be clearly identified to prevent inadvertent injury.

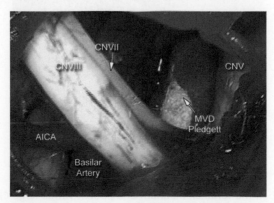

Fig. 18. Microvascular decompression for left-sided trigeminal neuralgia. AICA, anterior inferior cerebellar artery.

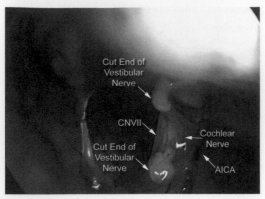

Fig. 19. Right-sided vestibular neurectomy.

CPA Cysts and Tumors

Because of the ability to use angled endoscopes (**Fig. 20**), visualization of cystic pathologies, such as epidermoid and arachnoid cysts, can be performed with minimal to no retraction while still adequately visualizing the extent of the lesion. This is especially effective for those tumors or cysts that cross the midline, extend into the foramen of Luschka, or extend above the incisura or below the foramen magnum. Similarly, accessing other cranial nerve neoplasms within the CPA even when they extend into Meckel's cave or the jugular foramen can be visualized using the angled endoscopes.

RESULTS OF ENDOSCOPIC SKULL BASE SURGERY

For the past 5 years we have performed 147 endoscopic posterolateral approaches. Of those, 37 have been performed for tumor resections, 23 specifically for acoustic tumors. The remaining 110 procedures were performed for CN MVDs and neurectomies. During this same period of time we have performed 543 open procedures, all for neoplasms of the CPA. This ratio is an important point of emphasis because endoscopy of the CPA is not intended to fully replace currently practiced open procedures.

There are significant contraindications for endoscopy. Additionally, it is our rationale that in cases where hearing preservation is not feasible, a translabyrinthine approach

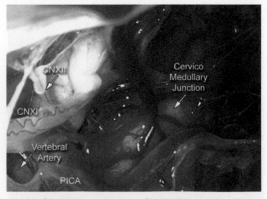

Fig. 20. View through the foramen magnum of a patient with a large CPA arachnoid cyst and a Chiari malformation. The cerebellar tonsils were elevated through the foramen magnum after the fenestration of the cyst.

offers a preferred option by reducing risk to the facial nerve. Tumors localized to the IAC with minimal involvement of the CPA are typically accessed by a middle fossa approach. Finally, we believe that a significant patient population is best treated with radiosurgery. Before any treatment, a multidisciplinary review is performed and the options fully discussed with the patient.

We elected to initially perform only MVDs as we introduced the endoscopic postero-lateral skull base approach to our practice. This was primarily because a comfort level with the technique was obtained; however, we quickly realized the deficiencies regarding the lack of appropriate surgical instrumentation. Much of the early work was to develop this instrumentation, specifically a functional bipolar forceps. It was not until the appropriate instrumentation was implemented before we began to expand to other CPA pathology. Therefore, the bulk of the neoplasms in our results were performed during the last 3 years.

Of the 37 tumors, we have had a clinically significant decline in hearing in three (8%) patients. All three of these cases occurred in acoustic tumors (13%). We have had one (0.6%) case of a facial nerve weakness (House-Brackman grade IV) in a facial nerve MVD for HFS. This patient fully recovered (House-Brackman grade I) within 6 months. There were no occurrences of facial nerve weakness in any of the acoustic neuroma patients. There was one case of a delayed CSF leak, which was surgically repaired. There were two wound infections that required removal of the hydroxyapatite cement.

Clinically, the operative time, hospital course, and return to work are substantially decreased compared with the open microscope-assisted technique. For nonneoplastic cases the procedure takes about 90 minutes. For acoustic tumors, the procedure typically requires about 120 to 180 minutes depending on the degree of IAC involvement. Postoperatively, most patients are in the hospital for 24 to 72 hours. Patients undergoing procedures that do not involve any manipulation or sacrifice of the vestibular nerve have a shorter length of stay, typically 24 hours for an MVD and up to 48 hours for a tumor resection. Patients with involvement of the vestibular nerve are typically admitted for at least 72 hours because of the postoperative vertigo. Those patients who do not experience any vertigo postoperatively may generally return to work within 2 weeks of surgery.

SUMMARY

Neuroendoscopy is an ever-evolving field. Technologic advancements have allowed the cost of the high-definition cameras and monitors to become financially accessible to most institutions. With further advancements within the field of three-dimensional endoscopic cameras, the learning curve will become less steep for those surgeons converting from a microscope-assisted background to the endoscope. The field of neuroendoscopy has made such rapid advancement that it has outpaced industry with regard to product development. As the field of surgeons interested in neuroendoscopy continues to populate, industry will become more fiscally interested in instrument development.

As with any new surgical technique, endoscopy of the CPA was initially met with a wide-degree of skepticism. The initial learning curve, especially with regard to instrument innovations, was time consuming but necessary. The scrutiny of a procedure's success is the degree to which it can be used by a significant population of the neurosurgical community, while simultaneously improving patient success. Our own results show that the improvement in patient outcomes, from a clinical and a cost-containment standpoint, support the continued use in this patient population.

REFERENCES

1. Mouton WG, Bessell JR, Maddern GJ. Looking back to the advent of modern endoscopy. 150th birthday of Maximilan Nitze. World J Surg 1998;22:1256–8.
2. Doyen E. Surgical therapeutics and operative techniques, vol. 1. London: Balliere, Tindall, and Cox; 1917. p. 599–602.
3. Andrews RJ, Bringas JR. A review of brain retraction and recommendations for minimizing intraoperative brain injury. Neurosurgery 1993;33(6):1052–64.
4. Fujimoto S, Kuyama H, Nishimoto K, et al. Effect of local retraction on local cerevral blood flow and neural function. Neurol Med Chir 1982;22:893–900.
5. Heros RC. Brain resection for exposure of deep extracerebral paraventricular lesions (technical note). Surg Neurol 1990;34:188–95.
6. Fries G, Perneczky A. Endoscope-assisted brain surgery. Part 2. Analysis of 380 procedures. Neurosurgery 1998;42:226–32.
7. Goksu N, Bayaz L, Kemalog Y. Endoscopy of the posterior fossa and dissection of acoustic neuroma. J Neurosurg 1999;91:776–80.
8. Jarrahy R, Berci G, Shahinian HK. Endoscope-assisted microvascular decompression of the trigeminal nerve. Otolaryngol Head Neck Surg 2000;123:218–23.
9. King WA, Wackym PA, Sen C, et al. Adjunctive use of endoscopy during posterior fossa surgery to treat cranial neuropathies. Neurosurgery 2001;49:108–16.
10. Magnan J, Chays A, Lepetre C, et al. Surgical perspectives of endoscopy of the cerebellopontine angle. Am J Otology 1994;15:366–70.
11. Miyazaki H, Deveze A, Magnan J. Neuro-otologic surgery through minimally invasive retrosigmoid approach: endoscope assisted microvascular decompression, vestibular neurectomy and tumor removal. Laryngoscope 2005;115:1612–7.
12. Rak R, Sekhar L, Stimac D, et al. Endoscope-assisted microsurgery for microvascular compression syndromes. Neurosurgery 2004;54:876–83.
13. Teo C, Nakaji P, Mobbs RJ. Endoscope-assisted microvascular decompression for trigeminal neuralgia: technical case report. Neurosurgery 2006;59(Suppl 2): ONSE489–90 [discussion: ONSE490].
14. Wackym PA, King WA, Barker FG, et al. Endoscope-assisted vestibular neurectomy. Laryngoscope 1998;108:1787–93.
15. Wackym PA, King WA, Poe DS, et al. Adjunctive use of endoscopy during acoustic neuroma surgery. Laryngoscope 1999;109:1193–201.
16. Eby JB, Cha ST, Shahinian HK. Fully endoscopic vascular decompression of the facial nerve for hemifacial spasm. Skull Base 2001;11:189–97.
17. Jarrahy R, Eby JB, Cha ST, et al. Fully endoscopic vascular decompression of the trigeminal nerve. Minim Invasive Neurosurg 2002;45:32–5.
18. Shevach I, Cohen M, Rappaport ZH. Patient positioning for the operative approach to midline intracerebral lesions: technical note. Neurosurgery 1992; 31:154–5.
19. Day JD, Kellogg JX, Tschabitscher M, et al. Surface and superficial anatomy of the posterolateral cranial base: significance for surgical planning and approach. Neurosurgery 1996;38(6):1079–84.
20. Rhoton A. Surface and superficial surgical anatomy of the posterolateral cranial base: significance for surgical planning and approach [comment]. Neurosurgery 1996;38:1083–4.

Management of Surgical Complications and Failures in Acoustic Neuroma Surgery

Selena E. Heman-Ackah, MD, MBA[a], John G. Golfinos, MD[b],
J. Thomas Roland Jr, MD[c],*

KEYWORDS

- Acoustic neuroma • Microsurgical resection • Complications
- Vestibular schwannoma

KEY POINTS

- Incomplete resection may be used in larger tumors to decrease the risk of certain complications.
- Expedient detection and management of cerebrospinal fluid leak is essential in decreasing the risk of further complications, including bacterial meningitis.
- The most common cranial nerve deficits encountered involve the cochlear and facial nerves.
- The highest rates of hearing preservation are reported with the middle fossa approach.
- Long-term facial nerve preservation is most affected by tumor size.
- Headache is most commonly associated with the retrosigmoid approach and can be diminished with meticulous closure technique.
- Seizure and intracranial hemorrhage are relatively uncommon complications associated with acoustic neuroma microsurgery.

Acoustic neuromas (ANs) or vestibular schwannomas (VSs) are relatively common benign tumors of Schwann cell origin that originate within or lateral to the Obersteiner-Redlich zone on the vestibular portion of the vestibulocochlear nerve. ANs account for approximately 6% of all intracranial tumors and 80% of all tumors of the cerebellopontine angle (CPA). Microsurgical resection is frequently used in the treatment. The surgical approach is governed mainly by preoperative hearing level,

Disclosures: The authors have nothing to disclose.
[a] Department of Otolaryngology, New York University, 462 First Avenue, New York, NY 10016, USA
[b] Departments of Neurosurgery and Otolaryngology, New York University, 530 First Avenue, Suite 8R, New York, NY 10016, USA
[c] Departments of Otolaryngology and Neurosurgery, New York University, 530 First Avenue, Suite 7Q, New York, NY 10016, USA
* Corresponding author.
E-mail address: john.roland@nyumc.org

Otolaryngol Clin N Am 45 (2012) 455–470
doi:10.1016/j.otc.2011.12.012
0030-6665/12/$ – see front matter © 2012 Elsevier Inc. All rights reserved.
oto.theclinics.com

tumor size, and tumor location. The middle fossa approach is used in patients with serviceable hearing (American Academy of Otolaryngology–Head and Neck Surgery hearing classification grade A or B and Gardner-Robertson scale grade 1 or 2) and intracanalicular lesions with less than 1 cm of CPA involvement. An extended middle fossa approach can be used for larger tumors. The retrosigmoid approach is used for patients with:

- Serviceable hearing
- Greater involvement of the CPA
- No lateral involvement within the internal auditory canal (IAC)
- Tumors medially positioned within the IAC.

These criteria vary from center to center.
The translabyrinthine approach is used in patients

- Without serviceable hearing
- With larger tumors for whom hearing preservation is not possible.

There is no size limitation associated with the translabyrinthine approach.

Over the past century the morbidity and mortality of AN resection has declined precipitously secondary to advances in microsurgical technique and perioperative care. However, as with any medical intervention, there exists the potential for complications to occur in association with AN microsurgery. Keen surgical technique is essential in preventing complications. In addition, early diagnosis and treatment are critical in the management of postsurgical complications of AN microsurgery to minimize sequelae.

INCOMPLETE RESECTION AND RECURRENCE

Because ANs are benign neoplasms, the risk of facial nerve injury, cochlear nerve injury, brainstem injury, and other complications must be weighed against the benefit of complete tumor resection. This risk/benefit conundrum presents itself most commonly when resecting larger ANs. Near-complete or subtotal tumor resection is used for several reasons. Near-complete AN resection most commonly is undertaken when there is a risk of neural injury in association with complete tumor resection. Conversely, subtotal tumor resection is undertaken in elderly or debilitated patients to minimize operative length and risk of morbidity. In either instance, microsurgical dissection is believed to compromise tumor blood supply, thereby inhibiting further tumor growth.

Within a review of 81 patients with large and giant ANs, subtotal tumor resection was performed in 5% of patients because of the patients' general health or was performed secondary to cerebellar herniation.[1] Similarly, in a review of 79 patients who underwent near-total and subtotal AN resection, a 10% rate of incomplete microsurgical AN resections was reported at the investigators' institution during the study period.[2] Within this cohort, a 3% regrowth rate was reported for patients who underwent near-total tumor resection and 32% regrowth rate for patients who underwent subtotal tumor resection with a mean time interval to detection of 3 years.[2] In a review of patients with large ANs, complete tumor resection was performed in 26% of patients, whereas 58% and 16% of patients underwent near-total and subtotal resection, respectively.[3] A 6% regrowth rate was reported within this cohort, which corroborates the results of other reports within the literature.[3,4]

Even with complete tumor resection, residual cell rests may remain adherent to intact or remnant nerves. Recurrence typically represents regrowth of these residual tumor rests. Mamikoglu and colleagues[1] reported a tumor recurrence rate of 1% after complete resection at 5-year follow-up. In a review of more than 1500 translabyrinthine approach microsurgical resections of AN, a 0.3% rate of recurrence was described.[5] Similarly, a review of 735 cases of complete tumor resection via the middle fossa approach revealed a 0.3% rate of tumor recurrence.[6] Residual and recurrent tumors typically remain asymptomatic until tumor regrowth is sizable (**Table 1**).

For this reason, patients are best followed up with serial magnetic resonance imaging (MRI). Fat suppression protocol MRI facilitates postoperative surveillance in patients who underwent reconstruction of operative defects with adipose tissue grafting.[5] Patients should be regularly monitored for evidence of tumor growth within at least the first 5 years postoperatively.

Subsequent Treatment of Tumor Regrowth

Within most patients, tumor regrowth does not occur. However, in the selected cohort of patients in whom regrowth is encountered, subsequent treatment is almost always necessary to control brainstem compression by tumor volume expansion. In the series by Bloch and colleagues,[2] all patients required subsequent treatment secondary to continued tumor growth. Fifty-nine percent of patients within the series by El-Keshlan and colleagues[4] required subsequent treatment.

Treatment options include repeating microsurgical resection and stereotactic radiosurgery. Repeating microsurgical resection has been associated with elevated rates of facial nerve injury.[7,8] Stereotactic radiosurgery for recurrence and regrowth has been

Table 1
Recurrence rates with incomplete and complete resection

Extent of Resection	Number of Patients	Percent with Resection	Recurrence and Time	Study
Subtotal	81	5%	—	Mamikoglu et al[1]
Complete	—	—	1% at 5 y	Mamikoglu et al[1]
Near total and subtotal	79	10%	3% regrowth for near total at 3 y 32% regrowth for subtotal at 3 y	Bloch et al[2]
Near total Subtotal Complete	—	58% 16% 26%	6% regrowth	Godefroy et al[3]
Translabyrinthine complete	1500	All	0.3%	Shelton[5]
Middle fossa complete	735	All	0.3%	Gjuric et al[6]

associated with facial nerve deficit rate of approximately 10%, trigeminal deficits of 4%, and a control rate of 94%.[9] The patient's age, functionality, medical comorbidities, and rate of tumor growth must be factored into the clinical decision making of the management of recurrence and regrowth.

CEREBROSPINAL FLUID LEAK

Cerebrospinal fluid (CSF) leak is the most commonly reported complication in association with AN microsurgery. CSF leak rates of 4% to 20% have been reported inassociation with middle fossa approach AN resection.[10,11] With the retrosigmoid approach, CSF leak rates of 3% to 12% have been reported.[12–15] CSF leak rates of 0% to 31% have been reported in association with the translabyrinthine approach.[1,3,14,16–19] However, a meta-analysis of more than 3351 procedures revealed no difference in CSF leak rates across approaches.[20] The only variable found to correlate with an increased rate of CSF leak was age, with a 5% increase rate of leaks in patients older than 50 years.[20] Similarly, a meta-analysis of 5964 patients who underwent AN resection revealed no difference in CSF leak rate across approaches.[16]

Controversial Relationship between Tumor Size and Rate of CSF Leak

The relationship between tumor size and the rate of CSF leak remains controversial. Large series by Slattery and colleagues,[21] Bryce and colleagues,[22] and Brennan and colleagues[14] revealed a correlation between larger tumor size and CSF leak. However, other reports challenge this notion.[20,23–25]

CSF Leak Routes

CSF leaks may occur via direct extension through the cutaneous incision or via air cell tracts to the middle ear and Eustachian tube. Multiple reviews have revealed a slight increased preponderance for CSF leak via air cell tracts as compared with direct incisional extension, with an average approximate 60% of CSF leaks having occurred via the mastoid air cells irrespective of surgical approach.[15,16,18]

CSF Closure Techniques

Various closure techniques have been used in an attempt to decrease the rate of CSF leak encountered after AN surgery, including:

- Autologous fascial grafts
- Artificial dural grafts
- Adipose tissue grafts
- Muscle grafts
- Fibrin glue.

In addition, various materials have been used to obliterate the air cell tracts, including:

- Bone wax
- Bone pate
- Hydroxyapatite granules
- Alloplastic glue
- Biomaterials.

Wu and colleagues[18] reported a decrease in CSF leak rate from 28.2% to 7.4% with a musculoperiosteal flap closure of translabyrinthine approach defects. They also noted a decrease in reoperation rate from 7.7% to 3.7% with this reconstructive technique.[18] However, the use of musculoperiosteal flaps limit the opportunity for fat saturation imaging in the postoperative follow-up of patients with AN, complicating the postoperative follow-up.[18] Fat grafting assists in the imaging follow-up of patients with AN. In addition, fat grafting has been found to decrease the rate of CSF leak from 5.7% to 2.2% when compared with muscle flap reconstruction.[26] With limited facial recess dissection, minimal dissection of the incus buttress, and packing of temporalis fascia around the incus to obstruct the mastoid antrum in addition to fat obliteration of the mastoid cavity, no CSF leaks were encountered in 61 patients after translabyrinthine approach AN resection.[17]

Graded Management of CSF Leak

When a CSF leak occurs, it may successfully be managed in a graded manner. The initial conservative management of CSF leaks may include head of bed elevation, bed rest, acetazolamide, and compressive dressing reapplication. If leak persists despite these measures, lumbar subarachnoid spinal fluid diversion drain may be placed to decrease intracranial pressure and allow for fluid siphoning from the CSF space. In most instances, lumbar drains are maintained for 3 to 5 days. If the lumbar drainage of CSF is unsuccessful in relieving leakage, reoperation is used. These procedures may include repeated obliteration of temporal bone cavity, obliteration of the Eustachian tube, repeated dural closure with or without muscle reinforcement, and oversewing the cutaneous incision.

In a review of 412 patients who underwent retrosigmoid approach posterior cranial fossa surgery, of whom 137 patients had AN, conservative management was successful in the treatment of those with CSF leak in 31% of patients, whereas 38% were successfully managed with lumbar subarachnoid spinal fluid diversion drain, and 31% required reoperation.[15] Surgical repair included Eustachian tube obliteration for CSF rhinorrhea and dural repair with muscle graft for incisional leaks.[15] Within a review of complications in 1687 patients who underwent AN surgery,[21]

- 53% of CSF leaks resolved with conservative management
- 16% resolved with lumbar drain
- 23% resolved after reoperation
- The additional patients underwent unspecified combined management.

The reported rates of success in the management of CSF leak with lumbar drain placement range from 31% to 83% in the recent literature, and reoperation rates have been reported to range from 21% to 61%.[14,15,18,20,27,28] The highest rates of reoperation have been reported with the translabyrinthine approach.[20] The successful management of CSF leaks is critical to prevent infection-related morbidity and mortality as seen with meningitis and brain abscess.

MENINGITIS

Meningitis is reportedly the second most common complication of AN microsurgery. The reported rates of meningitis after AN microsurgical resection range from 0.14% to 9.90%.[1,16,17,20,21,29,30] A meta-analysis of 13 studies including 2316 AN procedures revealed a meningitis rate of 3.7%.[21]

The presence of CSF leak increases the risk of meningitis in patients with AN after microsurgical resection. A meta-analysis of AN microsurgery revealed a statistically significant ($P<.0001$) increase in the incidence of meningitis in patients with CSF leak (14%) when compared with those without CSF leaks (2.5%).[16] Similarly, a review of 3000 patients who underwent AN resection revealed a meningitis rate of 21% in patients with CSF leak compared with no encountered episodes of meningitis in patients without CSF leaks.[20] In an analysis of patients with meningitis after AN resection, 82% of patients had a history of postoperative CSF leak.[22] For this reason, judicious management of CSF leaks as described earlier is of utmost importance.

Two forms of meningitis are encountered in postoperative patients after AN microsurgery: bacterial meningitis and chemical (aseptic) meningitis.

Bacterial meningitis typically presents with:

- Meningismus
- Severe headache
- Mental status changes
- Malaise
- High fever.

Analysis of CSF may reveal

- Leukocytosis
- Decreased glucose level
- Elevated protein level
- Positive gram stain
- Positive culture result.

A review of the literature regarding postoperative meningitis in patients who underwent craniotomy revealed *Staphylococcus* species, *Enterobacter*, and *Propionibacterium acnes* to be the most commonly encountered pathogens.[31] Bacterial meningitis, however, represented the minority of postoperative cases of meningitis.[29]

Most patients with postoperative meningitis after AN microsurgery present with chemical meningitis. Chemical meningitis, also known as aseptic meningitis, is believed to be the result of an inflammatory response to foreign substances within the subarachnoid space, namely, blood, hemoglobin, bilirubin, cotton wool lint, and bone dust. Animal studies support this assertion.[32]

In a review of 1146 patients who underwent CPA surgery, patients with bacterial meningitis confirmed by positive culture results accounted for only 22% of patients.[29] Presumed bacterial meningitis not confirmed by gram stain or culture results accounted for 22% of patients, whereas chemical meningitis accounted for 56% of patients.[29] In a review of patients with postoperative meningitis after posterior fossa craniotomy, 72% of patients presented with aseptic meningitis.[33] Chemical meningitis also typically presents with meningismus, headache, fever, and malaise.

A retrospective review of postoperative meningitis in patients after CPA surgery identified key clinical factors that are helpful in the differentiation of bacterial meningitis from chemical meningitis (**Table 2**).[29]

The management of postoperative meningitis in patients after microsurgical resection of ANs includes analgesics, corticosteroids, and antibiotics. Analgesics and corticosteroids are routinely used in the management of both bacterial and aseptic meningitis. Both analgesics and corticosteroids are instrumental in decreasing associated symptoms of headache and fever without deleterious side effects.[31,34] Empirically, patients are initiated on broad-spectrum antibiotics pending the return of gram stain and CSF cultures. Commonly, vancomycin and ceftriaxone are used for first-line empiric treatment.[31] Further use of antibiotics is dictated by culture and susceptibility results from CSF samples. Because most patients presenting with meningitis present with associated CSF leak, management of CSF leak as described earlier is essential in their management.

Table 2	
Key clinical factors in diagnosing bacterial versus chemical meningitis	
Bacterial Meningitis Predictors	**Chemical Meningitis Predictors**
CSF white blood cell count>6000 cells/mL	CSF white blood cell count<2000 cells/mL, mild CSF leukocytosis
CSF glucose level<20 mg/dL	Normal CSF glucose level
Elevated serum white blood cell count	Mildly elevated serum white blood cell count
Fever with temperature>102°F	Low-grade fever
Wound infections	—
Focal neurologic changes	—

Similar findings were reported by Ross and colleagues.[34]

DURAL SINUS THROMBOSIS

Dural sinus thrombosis is a less common complication of AN microsurgery. Rates of dural sinus thrombosis reported in the literature range from 0.1% to 4.6%.[21,35–37] In a review of 107 patients, the incidence of symptomatic dural sinus thromboses was reported to be 4.6% for suboccipital and translabyrinthine craniotomies.[35] Theories proposed to explain dural sinus thrombosis in AN microsurgery include:

- Retraction on the sinus intraoperatively
- Desiccation of the sinus during tumor resection
- Propagation of bone wax used for control of emissary veins.

A review of 161 patients who underwent retrosigmoid approach craniotomies for disease processes other than AN revealed a 4.3% incidence of sigmoid sinus thrombosis attributed to the use of bone wax.[36] Similarly, findings of sigmoid sinus thrombosis secondary to bone wax has been reported after retrosigmoid approach AN resection of AN.[37] Most commonly, transverse and sigmoid sinus involvement has been reported. Although many patients present asymptomatically, complaints of headache, visual obscuration, or blindness may occur.[36,37] On examination, increased intracranial pressure, papilledema, and active retinal hemorrhage may also be noted. The onset of symptoms may range from days to weeks after surgery. Within a series by Keiper and colleagues,[35] the onset ranged from 1 to 35 days postoperatively, with a mean onset of 15.6 days postoperatively. Computed topographic (CT) scan may be used as a screening tool for dural sinus thrombosis. However, magnetic resonance venogram (MRV) is a more definitive diagnostic tool. **Fig. 1** depicts the MRV and CT scans from a patient after retrosigmoid approach AN microsurgery who experienced thrombosis of the ipsilateral sigmoid sinus, lateral sinus, and jugular vein.

Management of dural sinus thrombosis may include:

- Steroids
- Volume repletion
- Anticoagulation
- Direct endovascular thrombolysis
- Carbonic anhydrase inhibitors
- Surgical thrombectomy.

The patient depicted in **Figs. 1** and **2** was managed with systemic anticoagulation alone. **Figs. 3** and **4** represent the posttreatment CT scan. Ventriculostomy or ventriculoperitoneal shunting for CSF diversion may sometimes be indicated for relief of

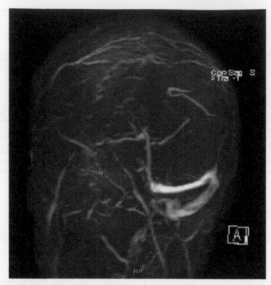

Fig. 1. Lateral sinus thrombosis (pretreatment). The MRV shows thrombosis of the right lateral sinuses within the anteroposterior view.

elevated intracranial pressure. However, in most cases in the absence of neurologic deterioration, dural sinus thromboses can be managed conservatively.[21,35]

CRANIAL NERVE DEFICITS
Cochlear Nerve

Hearing preservation in AN surgery may be accomplished by either the retrosigmoid approach or the middle fossa approach. Preservation of vascular supply to the cochlea and cochlear nerve is critical. Numerous factors affect the ability to preserve

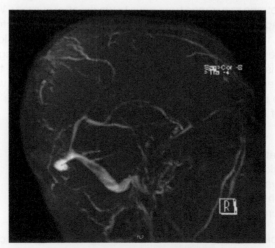

Fig. 2. Lateral sinus thrombosis (pretreatment). The MRV shows thrombosis of the right lateral sinuses within the lateral view.

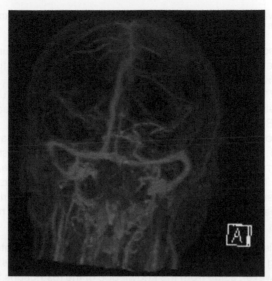

Fig. 3. Lateral sinus thrombosis (posttreatment). The MRV shows resolution of thrombosis previously noted within the right lateral sinuses within the anteroposterior view.

vascularity to the cochlea and reduce operative trauma to the nerve, thus affecting the success of hearing preservation. These factors include:[38]

- Tumor laterality within the IAC
- Tumor size
- Surgical approach
- Tumors located less than 3 mm from the fundus are associated with decreased rates of hearing preservation.[39]

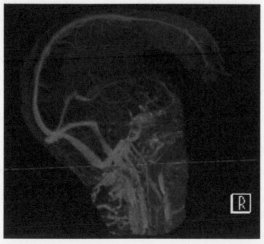

Fig. 4. Lateral sinus thrombosis (posttreatment). The MRV shows resolution of thrombosis of the right lateral sinuses within the lateral view.

Hearing preservation is best accomplished with smaller tumors and via the middle fossa approach.[38]

- Woodson and colleagues,[40] in a review of 156 patients who underwent middle fossa approach resection of AN, reported a hearing preservation rate of grade A or B in 93% of patients.
- A review of 119 patients with small to medium-sized ANs who underwent resection via a retrosigmoid approach revealed postoperative measurable hearing (grade A or B) in 30% of patients.[41]
- In a review comparing hearing preservation in the middle fossa approach with the retrosigmoid approach, grade A or B hearing was accomplished in 59.3% of patients via middle fossa approach versus 38.5% of patients via the retrosigmoid approach.[42] This report is most consistent with average reports in the literature; within most studies, middle fossa hearing preservation rates ranges from 50% to 70%, whereas retrosigmoid approach hearing preservation rates range from 30% to 40%.[38–44]

These data assist the neurotologist and neurosurgeon in preoperative counseling of patients regarding tumor resection approach and establishing realistic postoperative expectations. However, aside from the knowledge of the restrictions by approach, the awareness of advantages of each approach, and keen patient selection, there are no additional intraoperative or postoperative strategies that have been identified to positively influence cochlear nerve function and long-term hearing preservation. Intraoperative auditory brainstem response testing (ABR) and transient evoked otoacoustic emissions (TEOAE) are commonly used to monitor hearing during dissection and have been correlated with postoperative hearing outcome.[45,46] However, there are no data suggesting that intraoperative ABR or TEOAE positively influences postoperative hearing preservation.

Facial Nerve

During the microsurgical resection of AN, the facial nerve is also vulnerable. Tumor size has been found to have a large impact on facial nerve outcomes.

- Within a review of 119 patients with small to medium-sized ANs, facial nerve preservation (House-Brackmann grade≤II) 1 year postoperatively was accomplished in 96% of patients, with 91% graded as House-Brackmann grade 1.[41]
- A review of 77 patients with large and giant ANs revealed facial nerve function with House-Brackmann grade I or II in 45%.[1]
- In a review of 300 patients who underwent translabyrinthine approach AN resection, Tos and colleagues[25] reported complete preservation of facial nerve function in 87% of patients with tumor size 1 to 25 mm, 74% with tumor size 26 to 40 mm, and 42% with tumors larger than 40 mm.
- Complete facial paralysis was highest among the patients with tumors larger than 40 mm.[25]
- Similar findings were reported by Kaylie and colleagues.[47]

Surgical approach may be a factor in early postoperative facial nerve function, but long-term results seem to reveal no differences among surgical approaches.[47–49] Hillman and colleagues[42] compared the facial nerve results in patients after retrosigmoid and middle fossa approaches.

- Within the immediate postoperative period, complete facial nerve function was reported in 72% of patients who underwent middle fossa approach and 88% of those who underwent retrosigmoid approach.[42]

- At greater than 1-year follow-up, facial nerve function for both groups was similar (88% for middle fossa approach and 90% for retrosigmoid approach).[42]
- In addition, up to 41% of patients experience delayed facial paralysis or worsening of facial paresis in the immediate postoperative period.[38,50]

These findings support the assertion that facial nerve weakness after AN microsurgery largely represents neurapraxia related to surgical dissection, which often resolves with time.

Intraoperative Facial Nerve Monitoring

One factor has been identified that improves long-term facial nerve function outcomes: intraoperative facial nerve monitoring. The ability to stimulate the facial nerve at the brainstem with less than or equal to 0.2 mA has been correlated with a higher percentage (90%) of House-Brackmann grade I or II facial nerve function at 180 days postoperatively.[51] Other reports support this assertion.[50,52]

Eye Protection in Facial Nerve Complications

For patients with significant postoperative facial nerve deficits, meticulous eye care is essential. Patients should immediately be initiated on artificial tear and eye lubricant to maintain eye moisture. Patients should be instructed regarding eye protection, including eye shield or glasses or goggles, to prevent particulate matter form entering the eye in windy conditions. Early placement of gold weight may assist in corneal protection in patients with complete facial paralysis. With documented intraoperative sacrifice of the facial nerve or long-term facial paralysis, facial rehabilitation is necessary to decrease the debilitating sequelae of facial paralysis.

Facial Reanimation

To achieve facial reanimation in patients after facial nerve sacrifice, cable grafting or end-to-end anastomosis should be considered. Hypoglossal-facial transposition or orthodromic temporalis tendon transfer may be performed if the nerve endings cannot be reconnected. In a review comparing end-to-end anastomosis, cable grafting, and hypoglossal-facial transposition, end-to-end anastomosis was found to be superior in terms of facial nerve function followed by cable grafting.[53] In addition, static reanimation techniques, including facial sling and brow lift procedures, may be used.

Other Cranial Nerves Deficits

In addition to the cochlear nerve and facial nerve, deficiency in other cranial nerves may be encountered after AN microsurgical resection.

- In a review of 120 AN microsurgical procedures, a rate of trochlear nerve deficit was reported as 4.2%.[30]
- Tos and colleagues[25] reported a 0.9% rate of trigeminal nerve deficit secondary to AN microsurgery.
- Reported rates of abducens palsy range from 1.7% to 5.8%.[25,30]
- Vagal nerve deficits have been reported in 0.3% of patients.[25]
- Deficits in cranial nerves outside of the IAC are typically associated with larger ANs.[25,30]

HEADACHE

Headache is a commonly encountered complaint of patients after AN microsurgery; up to 65% patients report headache beyond the immediate postoperative period.[54–56]

Rates of postoperative headache vary by approach and are most commonly associated with the retrosigmoid approach.[54–56] In a meta-analysis of 1653 patients who underwent retrosigmoid, translabyrinthine, or middle fossa approach for resection of AN, long-term significant headache was reported in 36% of the patients who underwent retrosigmoid approach as compared with 16% and 1% of those who underwent translabyrinthine and middle fossa approaches, respectively.[55]

Headache within Immediate Postoperative Period

Headache within the immediate postoperative period may be caused by[38,55]

- Incisional pain
- Slight reduction in CSF pressure
- Dural irritation
- Dural stretch
- Spasm of nuchal musculature
- Irritating substances within the subarachnoid space.

Immediate postoperative headache may be reduced by minimizing retraction, decreasing tension of dural closure, and the use of lactated ringers for irrigation.[55] Prevention of desiccation of dural flaps may facilitate dural closure minimizing dural stretch and irritation.[38] In addition, placement of absorbable gelatin sponge (Gelfoam), telfa, or cottonoids during IAC drill out helps to prevent the collection of bone dust in the posterior fossa, which has been associated with postoperative headache and chemical meningitis.[38,55] Most often, headaches within the immediate postoperative period may be managed with acetaminophen and opioid analgesia.

Long-Term Headache

Long-term headache has most commonly been found to be associated with surgical technique and method of closure. With craniectomy, dural adhesion to nuchal musculature has been associated with dural stretch and headache.[55] Long-term headache has been correlated with decreased quality of life.[56] Therefore, methods of prevention should be used to decrease the risk of long-term postoperative headache.

- Prevention of bone dust contamination of the CSF space may be accomplished with materials commonly used for hemostasis or neural protection.
- Replacement of the bone flap or placement of adipose graft within the craniotomy defect has been associated with decreased rates of long-term postoperative headache.[56,57]
- Teo and Eljamel[57] reported a reduction in the rate of headache at 1-year follow-up from 12% to 1% with the replacement of bone flaps.

SEIZURE

Seizure is a less commonly encountered complication of AN microsurgery. It is most commonly associated with temporal lobe retraction in the middle fossa approach. Occasionally, violation of the temporal tegmental dura in the translabyrinthine approach can result in damage to the temporal cortex or temporal draining veins, resulting in seizure. In a review of 120 patients after AN microsurgical resection, a 6.6% rate of seizure was reported; 3.3% of patients experienced 1 seizure, and 3.3% of patients experienced multiple seizures requiring medication.[35] Slattery and colleagues[43] reported a 1.2% rate of seizure in their review of 162 patients. The minimal retraction necessary for safe operative exposure should be used to achieve safe AN resection.[58]

VASCULAR INJURY AND INTRACRANIAL HEMORRHAGE

With the advent of microsurgical technique and advances in perioperative care, rates of vascular injury, intracranial hemorrhage, parenchymal injury, and associated mortality have declined precipitously. Recently reported mortality rates in association with AN microsurgery are less than 2%.[21,25,30] Although the reported incidence is low, mortality seems to be associated with larger tumors.[59] Vascular fatalities are commonly associated with injury to the anterior inferior cerebellar artery.[59] Rates of postoperative intracranial hemorrhage range from approximately 0.8% to 1.7%.[21,25,30] Of note, hemorrhage may occur within the immediate postoperative period or in a delayed manner, 10 to 14 days postoperatively.[21] With clinical suspicion of intracranial hemorrhage, CT scan should be obtained urgently. Smaller, stable, delayed bleeds may be managed conservatively by observation.[21] However, in most cases, operative evaluation and control of hemorrhage are indicated. Early detection and evacuation of postoperative hemorrhage are essential.

SUMMARY

Despite the numerous advances in microsurgical technique and perioperative care in patients with AN, various complications may be encountered, including:

- CSF leak
- Meningitis
- Dural sinus thrombosis
- Cranial nerve deficits
- Headache
- Seizure
- Intracranial hemorrhage.

Important points to remember regarding complications of surgery for AN are as follows:

- Incomplete resection may be used in larger tumors to decrease the risk of certain complications.
- Expedient detection and management of CSF leak is essential in decreasing the risk of further complications, including bacterial meningitis.
- The most common cranial nerve deficits encountered involve the cochlear and facial nerves.
- The highest rates of hearing preservation are reported with the middle fossa approach.
- Long-term facial nerve preservation is most affected by tumor size.
- Headache is most commonly associated with the retrosigmoid approach and can be diminished with meticulous closure technique.
- Seizure and intracranial hemorrhage are relatively uncommon complications associated with AN microsurgery.

Awareness of the rates of complications and methods for prevention are essential in patient counseling and in optimizing patient outcomes. Patients need to understand that, although uncommon, complications of AN microsurgery include coma, death, stroke, paralysis, loss of hearing, facial nerve palsy, infection, bleeding, and spinal fluid leak. Although the risks of complication are low in experienced hands, the fully informed patient will be better prepared to deal with a complication should it occur.

REFERENCES

1. Mamikoglu B, Wiet RJ, Esquivel CR. Translabyrinthine approach for management of large and giant vestibular schwannomas. Otol Neurotol 2002;23:224–7.
2. Bloch DC, Oghalai JS, Jackler RK, et al. The fate of the tumor remnant after less-than-complete acoustic neuroma resection. Otolaryngol Head Neck Surg 2004;130:104–12.
3. Godefroy WP, van der Mey AG, de Bruine FT, et al. Surgery for large vestibular schwannoma: residual tumor and outcome. Otol Neurotol 2009;30:629–34.
4. El-Keshlan HK, Zeitoun H, Arts HA, et al. Recurrence of acoustic neuroma after incomplete resection. Am J Otol 2000;21:389–92.
5. Shelton C. Unilateral acoustic tumors: how often do they recur after translabyrinthine removal. Laryngoscope 1995;105:958–66.
6. Gjuric M, Wigand ME, Wolf SR. Enlarged middle fossa vestibular schwannoma surgery: experience with 735 cases. Otol Neurotol 2001;22:223–30.
7. Roche PH, Khalil M, Thomassin JM. Microsurgical removal of vestibular schwannomas after failed previous microsurgery. Prog Neurol Surg 2008;21:158–62.
8. Freeman SR, Ramsden RT, Saeed SR, et al. Revision surgery for residual or recurrent vestibular schwannoma. Otol Neurotol 2007;28:1076–82.
9. Pollock BE, Link MJ. Vestibular schwannoma radiosurgery after previous surgical resection or stereotactic radiosurgery. Prog Neurol Surg 2008;21:163–8.
10. Shelton C, Brackmann DE, House WF, et al. Middle fossa acoustic tumor surgery: results in 106 cases. Laryngoscope 1989;99:405–8.
11. Zanzaki J, Ogawa K, Tsuchihashi N, et al. Postoperative complications in acoustic neuroma surgery by the extended middle cranial fossa approach. Acta Otolaryngol Suppl 1991;487(Suppl):75–9.
12. Harner SG, Beatty CW, Bersold MJ. Retrosigmoid removal of acoustic neuroma: experience 1978-1988. Otolaryngol Head Neck Surg 1990;103:40–5.
13. Dutton JE, Ramsden RT, Lye RH, et al. Acoustic neuroma (schwannoma) surgery 1978-1990. J Laryngol Otol 1991;105:165–73.
14. Brennan JW, Rowed DW, Nedzelski JM, et al. Cerebrospinal fluid leak after acoustic neuroma surgery: influence of tumor size and surgical approach on incidence and response to treatment. J Neurosurg 2001;94:217–23.
15. Bayazit YA, Celenk F, Duzlu M, et al. Management of cerebrospinal fluid leak following retrosigmoid posterior cranial fossa surgery. ORL J Otorhinolaryngol Relat Spec 2009;71:329–33.
16. Selesnick SH, Liu JC, Jen A, et al. The incidence of cerebrospinal fluid leak after vestibular schwannoma surgery. Otol Neurotol 2004;25:387–93.
17. Goddard JC, Oliver ER, Lambert JR. Prevention of cerebrospinal fluid leak after translabyrinthine resection of vestibular schwannoma. Otol Neurotol 2010;31:473–7.
18. Wu H, Kalamarides M, El Garem H, et al. Comparison of different wound closure techniques in translabyrinthine acoustic neuroma surgery. Skull Base Surg 1999;9:239–42.
19. Merkus P, Taibah A, Sequino G, et al. Less than 1% cerebrospinal fluid leakage in 1,803 translabyrinthine vestibular schwannoma surgery cases. Otol Neurotol 2010;31:276–83.
20. Becker SS, Jackler RK, Pitts LH. Cerebrospinal fluid leak after acoustic neuroma surgery: a comparison of the translabyrinthine, middle fossa, and retrosigmoid approaches. Otol Neurotol 2003;24:107–12.
21. Slattery WH 3rd, Francis S, House KC. Perioperative morbidity of acoustic neuroma surgery. Otol Neurotol 2001;22:895–902.

22. Bryce GE, Nedzelski M, Rowed DW, et al. Cerebrospinal fluid leaks and meningitis in acoustic neuroma surgery. Otolaryngol Head Neck Surg 1991; 104:81–7.
23. Celikkanat SM, Saleh E, Khashaba A, et al. Cerebrospinal fluid leak after translabyrinthine acoustic neuroma surgery. Otolaryngol Head Neck Surg 1995;112: 654–8.
24. Gillman GS, Parnes LS. Acoustic neuroma management: a six-year review. J Otolaryngol 1995;24:191–7.
25. Tos M, Thomsen J, Harmsen A. Results of translabyrinthine removal of 300 acoustic neuroma related tumor size. Acta Otolaryngol Suppl 1988;452:38–51.
26. Ludemann WO, Stieglitz LH, Gerganov V, et al. Fat implant is superior to muscle implant in vestibular schwannoma surgery for the prevention of cerebrospinal fluid fistulae. Neurosurgery 2008;63:ONS38–43.
27. Fishman AJ, Marriana MS, Golfinos JG, et al. Prevention and management of cerebrospinal fluid leak following vestibular schwannoma surgery. Laryngoscope 2004;114:501–5.
28. Fishman AJ, Hoffman RA, Roland JT Jr, et al. Cerebrospinal fluid drainage in the management of CSF leak following acoustic neuroma surgery. Laryngoscope 1996;106:1002–4.
29. Sanchez GB, Kaylie DM, O'Malley MR, et al. Chemical meningitis following cerebellopontine angle tumor surgery. Otolaryngol Head Neck Surg 2008;138:368–73.
30. Sluyter S, Gramans K, Tulleken CA, et al. Analysis of results obtained in 120 patients with large acoustic neuromas surgically treated via the translabyrinthine-transtentorial approach. J Neurosurg 2001;94:61–6.
31. O'Malley MR, Haynes DS. Assessment and management of meningitis following cerebellopontine angle surgery. Curr Opin Otolaryngol Head Neck Surg 2008;16: 427–33.
32. Jackson IJ. Aseptic hemogenic meningitis: an experimental study of aseptic meningeal reactions due to blood and its breakdown products. Arch Neurol Psychiatry 1949;62:572–89.
33. Zarrouk V, Vassor I, Bert F, et al. Evaluation of the management of post-operative aseptic meningitis. Clin Infect Dis 2007;44:1555–9.
34. Ross D, Rosegay H, Pons V. Differentiation of aseptic and bacterial meningitis in postoperative neurosurgical patients. J Neurosurg 1988;69:669–74.
35. Keiper GL, Sherman JD, Tomsick TA, et al. Dural sinus thrombosis and pseudotumor cerebri: unexpected complications and suboccipital craniotomy and translabyrinthine craniectomy. J Neurosurg 1999;91:192–7.
36. Hadeishi H, Yasui N, Suzuki A. Mastoid canal and migrated bone wax in the sigmoid sinus: technical report. Neurosurgery 1995;36:1220–4.
37. Crocker M, Nesbitt A, Rich P, et al. Symptomatic venous sinus thrombosis following bone wax application to emissary veins. Br J Neurosurg 2008;22:798–800.
38. Bennet M, Haynes DS. Surgical approaches and complications in the removal of vestibular schwannoma. Otolaryngol Clin North Am 2007;40:589–609.
39. Colletti V, Fiorino F. Is the middle fossa approach the treatment of choice for intracanalicular vestibular schwannoma? Otolaryngol Head Neck Surg 2005;135: 459–66.
40. Woodson EA, Dempewolf RD, Gubbel SP, et al. Long-term hearing preservation after microsurgical excision of vestibular schwannoma. Otol Neurotol 2010;31: 1144–52.
41. Magnan J, Barbieri M, Mora R, et al. Retrosigmoid approach for small and medium-sized acoustic neuroma. Otol Neurotol 2002;23:141–5.

42. Hillman T, Chen DA, Arriaga MA, et al. Facial nerve function and hearing preservation acoustic tumor surgery. Otolaryngol Head Neck Surg 2010;142:115–9.

43. Slattery WH 3rd, Brackmann DE, Heiselberger W. Middle fossa approach for hearing preservation with acoustic neuromas. Am J Otol 1997;18:596–601.

44. Arts HA, Telian SA, El-Kashlan H, et al. Hearing preservation and facial nerve outcomes in vestibular schwannoma surgery: results using the middle cranial fossa approach. Otol Neurotol 2006;27:234–41.

45. Brackmann DE, Owens RM, Friedman RA, et al. Prognostic factors for hearing preservation in vestibular schwannoma surgery. Am J Otol 2000;21:417–24.

46. Kim AH, Edwards BM, Telian SA, et al. Transient evoked otoacoustic emissions pattern as a prognostic indicator for hearing preservation in acoustic neuroma surgery. Otol Neurotol 2006;27:372–9.

47. Kaylie DM, Gilbert E, Horgan MA, et al. Acoustic neuroma surgery outcomes. Otol Neurotol 2001;22:868–9.

48. Ho SY, Hudgens S, Wiet RJ. Comparison of postoperative facial nerve outcomes between translabyrinthine and retrosigmoid approaches in matched-pair patients. Laryngoscope 2003;113:2014–20.

49. Jacob A, Robinson LL Jr, Bortman JS, et al. Nerve of origin, tumor size, hearing preservation and facial nerve outcomes in 359 vestibular schwannoma resections at a tertiary care academic center. Laryngoscope 2007;117:2087–92.

50. Lalwani AK, Butt FY, Jackler RK, et al. Delayed onset facial nerve dysfunction following acoustic neuroma surgery. Am J Otol 1995;16:758–64.

51. Grayeli AB, Guindi S, Kalamarides M, et al. Four-channel electromyography of the facial nerve in vestibular schwannoma surgery: sensitivity and prognostic value for short-term facial function outcome. Otol Neurotol 2005;26:114–20.

52. Lin VY, Houlden D, Bethune A, et al. A novel method in predicting immediate postoperative facial nerve function post acoustic neuroma excision. Otol Neurotol 2006;27:1017–22.

53. Malik TH, Kelly G, Ahmed A, et al. A comparison of surgical techniques used in dynamic reanimation of the paralyzed face. Otol Neurotol 2005;26:284–91.

54. Ruckenstein MJ, Harris JP, Cueva RA, et al. Pain subsequent to resection of acoustic neuromas via suboccipital and translabyrinthine approaches. Am J Otol 1996;17:620–4.

55. Schaller B, Baumann A. Headache after removal of vestibular schwannoma via the retrosigmoid approach: a long-term follow-up study. Otolaryngol Head Neck Surg 2003;128:387–95.

56. Rameh C, Magnan J. Quality of life of patients following stage III–IV vestibular schwannoma surgery using the retrosigmoid and translabyrinthine approaches. Auris Nasus Larynx 2010;37:546–52.

57. Teo MK, Eljamel MS. Role of craniotomy repair in reducing postoperative headaches after a retrosigmoid approach. Neurosurgery 2010;67:1286–91.

58. Telischi FF, Landy H, Balkany TJ. Reducing temporal lobe retraction with middle fossa approach using a lumbar drain. Laryngoscope 1995;105(2):219–20.

59. Wiet RJ, Teixido M, Liang JG. Complications in acoustic neuroma surgery. Otolaryngol Clin North Am 1992;25:389–412.

Chemotherapy:
Present and Future

Anna R. Terry, MD, MPH[a], Scott R. Plotkin, MD, PhD[b],*

KEYWORDS

- Vestibular schwannoma • Neurofibromatosis type 2 • Growth factor inhibition
- Erlotinib • Bevacizumab

Key Abbreviations: Chemotherapy for Vestibular Schwannoma: Present and Future	
ADC	Apparent diffusion coefficient
CML	Chronic myelogenous leukemia
CNS	Central nervous system
HER	Human epidermal growth factor receptor
FSRT	Fractionated stereotactic radiotherapy
NF2	Neurofibromatosis type 2
PDGFR	Platelet derived growth factor receptors
VEGF	Vascular endothelial growth factor
VS	Vestibular schwannoma

Vestibular schwannomas (VS), also called acoustic neuromas, are among the most common benign tumors of the central nervous system (CNS). With an annual United States incidence rate of 0.99 per 100,000 person-years, they account for 62% of nerve sheath tumors and 5% of all primary brain and CNS tumors.[1] VS cause cranial nerve deficits, most commonly unilateral hearing loss, tinnitus, and trigeminal deficits (**Fig. 1**A). Patients are prone to damage of the facial nerve and further hearing loss as a result of treatment, with some surgical approaches sacrificing hearing to attain tumor control. Currently, there is no approved medical therapy for VS, and the mainstays of management are observation with serial imaging studies, surgery, or radiation when necessary.

Bilateral VS are the hallmark of neurofibromatosis type 2 (NF2), an autosomal-dominant tumor suppressor syndrome characterized by multiple schwannomas,

Disclosure: Dr Plotkin receives research support from PTC Therapeutics. Dr Terry has no conflicts of interest to disclose.
a Department of Neurosurgery, Massachusetts General Hospital, White 502, 55 Fruit Street, Boston, MA 02114, USA
b Department of Neurology and Cancer Center, Massachusetts General Hospital, Yawkey 9E, 55 Fruit Street, Boston, MA 02114, USA
* Corresponding author. Pappas Center for Neuro-Oncology, Massachusetts General Hospital, YAW 9E, 55 Fruit Street, Boston, MA 02114.
E-mail address: splotkin@partners.org

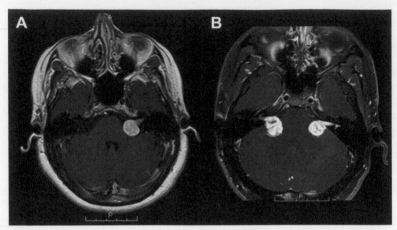

Fig. 1. Cranial MRIs of patients with (*A*) unilateral (sporadic) vestibular schwannoma and (*B*) bilateral vestibular schwannomas.

meningiomas, and ependymomas (see **Fig. 1**B). The incidence of NF2 is approximately 1 per 25,000 live births and accounts for 2% to 7% of patients with VS, depending on methodology.[2,3] Because of their location, bilaterality, and inexorable growth, NF2-related VS eventually lead to clinically meaningful hearing loss, cranial nerve deficits, and brainstem compression. Moreover, these patients often experience hearing loss as a result of surgery or radiation treatment.[4,5] Overall life expectancy in NF2 is greatly diminished, with older literature suggesting that 60% of patients die before age 44.[6] Indeed, disease-specific mortality in NF2 is greater than 90%, with nearly all deaths occurring as a direct result of tumor growth (causing brainstem compression and eventual hydrocephalus) or complications of treatment.[7,8]

In addition to the increased mortality of NF2, the bilateral nature of VS in this disorder leads to significant long-term morbidity and decreased quality of life caused by lower cranial nerve problems, including deafness, swallowing problems, facial diplegia, dysarthria, and aspiration pneumonia. Treatment-related morbidity is also higher in NF2-related VS, because of the bilateral nature of the problem and because nerve fibers are considered more likely to run through NF2-associated schwannomas, rather than lying on the surface as in sporadic VS.[9]

Given the morbidity and mortality of NF2-associated VS and the high risks of surgical treatment or radiation therapy, medical therapies that can slow or arrest tumor growth are urgently needed. Recently, a consensus conference recognized that rationally designed phase II clinical trials were a realistic short-term goal in treating NF2-related VS.[10] This article reviews the current standard therapies for VS, describes previous experience with chemotherapy, and delineates areas of current and future research.

STANDARD TREATMENTS FOR VS
Observation for VS

Progressive growth of tumors in the cerebellopontine angle carries a high rate of morbidity, with cranial nerve problems (including hearing loss), brainstem or cerebellar compression, and eventually hydrocephalus from compression of the fourth ventricle. However, the natural history of VS is unpredictable, especially for sporadic VS.

Tumors may grow at a steady rate, plateau at a certain size, or rarely even shrink. Additionally, tumors may recur after treatment. Given the increasing availability of cranial imaging and the high resolution now available in routine brain MRIs, diagnosis of small VS has now become commonplace.

Several studies have attempted to elucidate the natural history of VS.[11,12] The largest to date is a prospective evaluation of tumor growth data from more than 500 patients in the Danish national registry, followed for a median of 3.6 years.[12] During the follow-up period, 17% of tumors confined to the internal acoustic meatus grew, compared with 29% of extrameatal tumors. No relationship between tumor growth and patient gender or age could be determined. The same registry was used to assess changes in hearing over time in patients allocated to expectant management strategies.[13] Patients received annual audiologic and MRI examinations. At the outset of the study, 53% of patients had speech discrimination of greater than 70%; at the end of the 10-year observation period, this rate had fallen to 31%. Patients with hearing that was initially good maintained their hearing at higher rates than patients with impaired hearing at baseline.

These results seem to confirm that primary observation is justified for smaller, asymptomatic tumors. Indeed, a "watchful waiting" approach is common in clinical practice, particularly given the relatively slow growth of most VS and high risk of treatment-related morbidity including complete hearing loss. Larger, symptomatic tumors, or those with substantial cystic components, are often removed because they are more likely to cause morbidity related to progressive growth, and surgery becomes more challenging and risky with larger tumors. Thus, the chosen therapeutic approach may depend on the clinician's interpretation of the evidence for ongoing tumor growth. Consensus recommendations vary, but commonly use a tumor size threshold of 20 mm and a growth rate of greater than 2 mm per year (based on increase in the largest dimension) for recommendation of treatment. At this size, further growth may compromise cranial nerve function, and may also make future surgery more difficult. Additionally, an actively growing tumor is more likely to result in progressive hearing decline over time, especially if the tumor is already large at diagnosis.[14,15]

Surgery for VS

The decision to manage VS surgically is often straightforward for large, symptomatic tumors and those causing brainstem compression or hydrocephalus. However, surgery is frequently performed for smaller, asymptomatic tumors. The most compelling argument for surgery is the theoretical risk of progressive hearing deterioration over time.[13,16] Larger tumors are particularly problematic to manage conservatively. Based on what is known about the natural history of VS, progressive hearing loss is more likely with rapidly growing tumors, especially those that are large at baseline.[8,17] The morbidity of surgery increases with tumor size, because of the difficulties of exposure including cerebellar retraction and facial nerve damage. These issues arise frequently in surgical treatment of NF2-related VS, because they have a markedly faster growth rate than seen in sporadic VS and may present at a larger size.[18] Additionally, NF2 patients with bilateral VS may already have impaired hearing in one or both ears, raising the stakes for a high-risk surgery. Although hearing may stabilize with either surgery or radiation therapy, it usually does not improve.

As is the case for many complex, high-risk surgical procedures, outcomes for surgical treatment of VS are superior at larger institutions with more experienced, specialized surgeons. A retrospective cohort study of 2643 operations selected from a large national administrative database demonstrated a significant volume-outcome relationship for VS resection when adjusting for potential confounders such as age, gender, race, payor (type of insurance), geographic region, procedure timing, admission type and source, medical comorbidities, and NF status.[19] Postoperative complications including neurologic deficits, prolonged mechanical ventilation, facial nerve injury, and need for blood transfusion were less frequent at higher-volume hospitals or with higher-volume surgeons. Furthermore, length of stay was shorter, hospital charges were less, and perioperative mortality was reduced. The potentially high risks of short- and long-term morbidity from VS surgery and the relatively small number of tertiary care centers that have the requisite caseload and surgical experience to manage these risks further complicate the delivery of care for patients with VS, not all of whom have access to these settings.

Radiation Therapy for VS

Radiation is often used as adjuvant therapy for treatment of sporadic brain tumors. As the other mainstay of treatment for VS, radiation therapy can help avoid some of the morbidities associated with surgery. Although many larger VS are believed to be poor candidates for radiotherapy because of the concomitant risks of swelling near the brainstem, recent technical advances including fractionated radiation and radiosurgery have been used with some success to treat smaller tumors. However, outcomes for NF2-related VS are generally worse than those for sporadic VS.

In particular, fractionated stereotactic radiotherapy (FSRT) has been advocated to minimize the risk of hearing loss. A recent series of 106 patients treated with FSRT demonstrated excellent local tumor control (94% at 3 years and 93% at 5 years). Notably, the "useful" hearing preservation rate was 98% at 5 years in patients without NF2 but only 64% in patients with NF2.[20] The median irradiated tumor volume was small (3.9 cm^3), although the maximum tumor volume was greater than 30 cm^3. FSRT was generally well tolerated, with a low incidence of cranial neuropathies including radiation-induced toxicity to the trigeminal and facial nerve (<5%).

Another series of 190 previously untreated patients with unilateral VS examined the efficacy and complication rate of gamma knife radiosurgery. The 5-year tumor control rate, as defined by no requirement for surgical intervention, was 97%.[21] Patients had low rates of radiation-induced cranial neuropathies, although increasing marginal radiation dose did lead to higher rates of facial nerve weakness and decreased preservation of speech discrimination. Hearing-level preservation was 71% and preservation of speech discrimination was 91%, although the authors do not stratify by NF2 status; most patients in the sample had unilateral VS, which were more likely to be sporadic. As with surgery, hearing improvement was rare (7%), although many patients preserved their pretreatment hearing status.

In patients with smaller tumors, or in older patients with medical comorbidities, radiosurgery or FSRT may be an attractive alternative to neurosurgery, with lower rates of treatment-associated cranial neuropathies. Additionally, radiosurgery avoids problematic perioperative complications such as infection and cerebrospinal fluid leak. Patients successfully treated with radiotherapy may be able to avoid surgery in the future. However, for larger tumors, radiotherapy is often impractical or unsafe. In the NF2 population, the risk of secondary malignancy after radiation is a particular concern. These patients are usually younger than sporadic patients at the time of treatment (with more time to develop a malignancy) and have a genetic predisposition to tumor formation.[22]

MOLECULAR BIOLOGY IN VS

Given the high treatment-related morbidity of VS especially in NF2 patients, developing innovative and effective medical therapies is a high priority. For more than 10 years, development of promising chemotherapeutic agents has mainly focused on finding appropriate molecular targets based on the tumor's underlying biology. Drugs developed in this way have become the mainstay in treating breast cancer, chronic myelogenous leukemia, and other malignancies, with a resulting dramatic improvement in outcomes for some conditions. This section reviews the molecular biology of VS and describes its relevance to treatment; in addition, past and current uses of chemotherapeutic agents against VS are discussed and possible areas of future innovation are described.

NF2-related and sporadic VS demonstrate loss of the *NF2* gene product Merlin, a tumor-suppressor protein.[23,24] Merlin interacts with various receptor tyrosine kinases, including the human epidermal growth factor (HER) family, platelet-derived growth factor receptors (PDGFR), and c-KIT, thereby inhibiting their signaling. In human and *Drosophila* models, Merlin has been shown to control the surface availability of the HER-1/EGFR, HER-2, HER-3, and PDGF receptors.[25–28] Amplification of HER-1/EGFR, HER2, or PDGFR, an established mechanism of tumorigenesis in sporadic cancer, is not present in human VS specimens. Cultured *NF2*-deficient cells lack contact inhibition, an effect likely mediated by HER-1/EGFR signaling.[25] Overall, the loss of functional Merlin leads to dysregulation of a pathway associated with contact-dependent inhibition in normal Schwann cells, ultimately leading to tumorigenesis and continued growth of VS.

HER-2 signaling seems to be necessary for Schwann cell differentiation and proliferation, and activated HER-2 and HER-3 are abundantly expressed in sporadic and NF2-related VS. In an immunohistochemical analysis of 38 VS specimens, HER-2 was upregulated in 76% of sporadic and 94% of NF2-related VS.[29] Importantly, EGF ligand was upregulated in 100% of NF2-related VS, but not in sporadic VS. HER-1/EGFR expression levels correlated directly with VS tumor size and inversely with patient age. Similarly, PDGFRB is overexpressed in Schwannoma cells and, when stimulated by the ligand PDGF, has a mitogenic effect on tumor cells.[30]

Vascular endothelial growth factor (VEGF) is a mediator of angiogenesis and vascular permeability. Its activity is mediated by the receptor tyrosine kinases VEGFR1 and VEGFR2 and by the neuropilins NRP1 and NRP2. In the peripheral nervous system, semaphorins serve as negative regulators of the VEGF pathway and act through the neuropilin receptors.[31] VEGF and the receptor VEGFR1 have been detected in sporadic and NF2-associated schwannomas, with increased levels correlating with increased rates of tumor growth.[32,33] In a separate study, the expression pattern of VEGF and its receptors VEGFR2, NRP1, and NRP2 was determined in tissue samples from sporadic and NF-associated VS. VEGF was expressed in all VS and VEGFR2 in almost a third of tumor vessels.[34] Evidence from a transgenic mouse model shows that anti-VEGF agents bevacizumab and vandetanib can increase apoptosis, reduce tumor growth rate, and increase survival in rodents with intracranial schwannomas.[35] By using microscopy and whole-body imaging techniques, Wong and colleagues[35] demonstrated that these anti-VEGF agents decreased vessel permeability, thereby normalizing the vasculature of schwannoma xenografts in nude mice. The authors hypothesize that this occurs because the natural balance between VEGF and semaphorin 3 signaling is re-established. This antivascular effect may be the mechanism by which anti-VEGF therapies cause death of tumor cells and thereby delay progression.

These findings have spurred great interest in the development of targeted molecular therapies for the treatment of VS. According to a recent consensus conference, the HER family of receptors in particular is thought to furnish the most compelling target for rationally designed drug therapy.[10] HER-1/EGFR inhibitors, such as erlotinib, and the anti-VEGF agent bevacizumab have also been recently studied. Specific findings and current research are discussed later.

END POINTS FOR CLINICAL TRIALS

After a promising agent for a molecular target is identified, it must be tested in a well-designed clinical trial. One of the primary challenges in designing and conducting clinical trials is the choice of end points that are clinically appropriate, objectively measurable, and reproducible by other researchers. In the past, there has been a lack of consensus on end point standardization in the treatment of VS. In 2009, the authors' group at Massachusetts General Hospital (MGH) proposed a set of suggested response criteria to define end points for future phase II studies of anticancer drugs in VS.[2] By using objective and predefined criteria, important primary and secondary outcomes can be described (eg, time to tumor progression, hearing loss, or subjective symptoms) and related to patient prognostic factors, such as age, baseline tumor size, and tumor growth rate.

Hearing End Points

Hearing preservation is of crucial importance to patients, particularly those with NF2 who have bilateral tumors and frequently experience the loss of all usable hearing within their lifetimes as a result of tumor growth or treatment. Because most NF2 patients are diagnosed well after their acquisition of language, this hearing loss has a profound effect on their quality of life, social skills, and ability to function at home and in the workplace. Subjective measures of hearing, although they may be highly relevant to the patient's perceived symptoms and quality of life, are problematic for use as a primary outcome in a clinical trial.

Several methods have been suggested for the objective measure of changes in hearing, although no single method has been adopted for routine use in drug trials. The standard audiogram commonly incorporates the ability to detect sound (pure tone threshold) and speech discrimination (word recognition score based on standardized lists of words).[36] For example, the American Academy of Otolaryngology recommends testing pure tone thresholds at levels of 0.5, 1, 2, and 3 kHz, and testing speech discrimination scores at up to 40 dB above the speech discrimination threshold using a 50-word recorded list in the subject's native language.[37] A composite hearing scale, the Gardner-Robertson classification,[38] is sometimes used to report changes in hearing after treatment with open surgery or radiosurgery, combining pure tone threshold and word recognition into a four-level scale. However, this scale lacks sensitivity because of "floor effects" for those in lower categories (classes III, IV, and V), in which NF2 patients are more likely to fall. Time to hearing loss or failure has been proposed as an end point for clinical trials, but given the difficulty of assessing subjects with severely impaired hearing at baseline and the long follow-up times required, it may be impractical to use as a primary outcome.[2]

The authors suggest that maximum word recognition scores be used as the primary hearing end point in phase II clinical trials for anti-VS drugs. Word recognition affects basic communication more profoundly than does pure tone threshold. VS have a propensity to cause auditory nerve dysfunction because of direct pressure and secondary degeneration of the cochlea.[39] Indeed, hearing aids, although they decrease the pure tone threshold, are often of little benefit for patients with NF2 and bilateral VS, because sound amplification alone does not address the underlying auditory nerve dysfunction.

Finally, recent evidence on drug therapies for VS suggests that patients treated with targeted agents can experience measurable and clinically meaningful improvement in their hearing even in the absence of a radiographic response or with progressive disease as measured by MRI scan (discussed next). This may be caused by the amelioration of the auditory nerve dysfunction caused by tumor growth and tumor-associated edema. Intuitively, a clinically meaningful improvement in hearing is the most important outcome from the perspective of a patient agreeing to participate in a clinical trial, and probably the most objective and reliable way to achieve this is by measuring the word recognition score.

Radiographic End Points

Traditionally, changes in contrast enhancement on MRI or CT have been used to define objective radiographic tumor response to treatment. The neuro-oncology literature includes several novel modalities to measure radiographic response of malignant CNS tumors, including diffusion or perfusion changes in MRI imaging.[40] However, as with most benign CNS tumors, these methods have not been validated in either sporadic or NF2-related VS.

Historic methods of measuring tumor size and response, such as the 1981 World Health Organization criteria, revised in 2000 as the RECIST criteria,[41] and the Macdonald criteria for malignant glioma,[42] have all been used in the VS literature. Linear growth (based on largest tumor dimension) is often used as a treatment recommendation threshold, most commonly 2 mm per year.[12] However, NF2-related VS in particular are often larger and have a more irregular shape than sporadic VS, so linear dimension, whether unidimensional or bidimensional, is less likely to be an adequate surrogate for volume. More recently, and with the advent of higher-resolution MRI imaging, volumetric measurement has become the accepted method of defining radiographic response.[43] Using 3-mm axial slices through the internal auditory canal produces the greatest accuracy, with an intrarater coefficient of variation of less than 5% for tumors larger than 1 cm³.[43] In a recent paper on suggested response criteria, the authors suggest volumetric methods, with an objective radiographic response defined as a 20% or greater reduction in VS volume based on postcontrast T1-weighted MRI images collected with 3-mm or finer cuts through the internal auditory canal.[2]

Radiographic tumor response has been successfully used in phase II chemotherapy trials of various cancers. The underlying assumptions are that most chemotherapeutic drugs work by a cytotoxic mechanism, resulting in radiographic shrinkage, and that objective decrease in tumor size is related to other end points, such as overall survival or progression-free survival, that are clinically relevant to patients.[2] However, some agents are postulated to have cytostatic, rather than cytotoxic, effects, and may result in radiographic stabilization (or decrease in growth rate) rather than overt shrinkage. For sporadic VS, spontaneous involution occurs in approximately 8% of tumors, usually during a long period of observation given their slow growth rate. However, this rarely occurs in NF2-related tumors; in a recent analysis, only 3 (3.6%) of 84 tumors regressed by 2 mm or more during 9 months to 2 years of follow-up,[17] suggesting that any objective radiographic shrinkage of NF2-related schwannomas would be caused by drug activity and not by spontaneous involution.

It is well known that contrast enhancement may be misleading, reflecting radiation necrosis or "treatment effect" rather than tumor growth. In such cases, time to disease progression, rather than objective radiographic response, may be a more reliable indicator of the drug's clinical efficacy.[2] Indeed, progression-free survival at 6 months is now a frequently used primary end point in drug trials for recurrent malignant glioma.[44] Although histologically benign, given their problematic location and rapid growth, it is appropriate to consider NF2-related VS in a similar clinical category as malignant CNS tumors. In this setting, determination of progression-free survival at 12, 24, and 60 months would provide meaningful clinical information about drug activity for VS.

A final consideration relevant to NF2-related VS is the presence of multiple lesions. In principle, one target lesion (usually the largest or most symptomatic lesion) should be selected as the lesion of interest for assessing the primary end point of radiographic response. In NF2-related VS, this can be difficult because of the irregularity of the tumors, changes in previously treated tumors, and the presence of multiple or confluent tumors.

Tinnitus and Other End Points

In addition to the possible primary end points described previously, the design of future clinical trials should take into consideration subjective improvement in patient symptoms. Among the most bothersome of these symptoms is tinnitus. As with many subjective symptoms, there is no diagnostic test for tinnitus. Measurement of tinnitus is complicated by the fact that it is an extremely common symptom, with up to a third of the adult population reporting it at some point, although few individuals experience symptoms significant enough to affect their quality of life.[45] An individual's subjective emotional and psychologic responses to tinnitus can also affect its perceived severity, making an objective measurement more difficult.

Tinnitus can be a sensitive indicator of cochlear dysfunction. It can encompass the clinical spectrum from barely noticeable "white noise" to troublesome or even distressing whistling and ringing that can be heard despite loud background noise. In VS, as in Meniere's disease, it may correlate with hearing loss, although it may fluctuate less as hearing loss progresses. A clinical grading system for tinnitus has been proposed, assigning a value of 0 to 3, which incorporates degree of severity and continuity versus fluctuation.[46] More recently, a five-point severity grading scale (slight, mild, moderate, severe, and catastrophic) has been proposed,[47] but no one system has been accepted for general use in clinical trials. In their studies, the authors have used a grading scale along with the Tinnitus Reaction Questionnaire, which assesses the psychologic distress associated with tinnitus.[47]

Vertigo and balance problems are common in NF2 patients with bilateral VS, but are notoriously difficult to measure objectively. Although there is a well-validated objective scale for facial nerve palsy, the House-Brackmann scale,[48] facial nerve dysfunction is often a consequence of surgical treatment rather than of the natural history of the disease. The same is true of trigeminal nerve dysfunction. Therefore, these entities are unlikely to be used as primary clinical end points, although they certainly have a profound influence on the patient's overall quality of life.

CURRENT EXPERIENCE WITH TARGETED CHEMOTHERAPY

Targeted molecular therapy has been the primary goal of anticancer drug research for at least a decade. Before the introduction of targeted chemotherapeutic agents, experience with chemotherapy to treat VS was extremely limited. One small series noted stabilization of tumor growth and hearing loss in two patients treated with the classic cytotoxic drugs cyclophosphamide, doxorubicin, and dacarbazine,[49] although clinical end points were not prespecified. In principle, the benign histology of VS makes them relatively resistant to these cytotoxic agents, which are most effective in destroying the rapidly dividing cells of malignant tumors.

Basic research on the tumor biology of schwannomas has unveiled exciting potential targets for rational drug design in their treatment.[50,51] In vitro, treatment of NF2-deficient cells with HER-1/EGFR inhibitors can reduce cellular proliferation. The finding that overexpression of various growth factor receptors in sporadic VS correlate with higher growth rate[26] further spurred efforts to find drug therapies that could be used as molecular targeting agents for these tumors.

Erlotinib

Erlotinib is an oral HER-1/EGFR tyrosine kinase inhibitor that is approved for the treatment of non–small cell lung cancer and pancreatic cancer. It has been shown to inhibit the growth of VS xenografts in nude mice.[52] Several phase I and II studies in high-grade glioma suggest that this drug is well tolerated in patients with CNS neoplasms. Although erlotinib has been shown to cross the blood–brain barrier, it is not known whether the drug crosses the blood–nerve barrier, or whether such an intact barrier exists in VS.[53] Although a potentially promising targeted therapy for VS, phase II trials have yet to be performed.

The authors' group recently conducted a small retrospective study of erlotinib treatment in 11 patients with NF2 and progressive VS.[53] All patients were either considered poor candidates for surgery or radiation therapy, or had refused such treatment. Erlotinib was offered to these subjects on a compassionate-use basis. Follow-up testing included serial MRI scanning for volumetric analysis of tumors (at baseline and at clinical visits every 3 months) and audiologic evaluations of pure-tone thresholds and word recognition scores (discussed previously). Information on toxicity and side effects was also collected.

Although significant radiographic and hearing responses were not observed, three patients had prolonged stable disease or slowing of their tumor growth rate. Because these patients had a slower rate of tumor growth at baseline, this seems to support the observation that erlotinib likely exhibits a cytostatic rather than a cytotoxic effect on NF2-deficient cells. Contralateral VS were also examined for radiographic changes during treatment, and many of these shrank. One subject with extensive peripheral schwannomas showed a 26% reduction in total body tumor volume (Plotkin, unpublished data, 2010).

Erlotinib was well tolerated overall with the major side effects being rash and gastrointestinal side effects. Of note, two patients experienced corneal keratopathy, of particular importance in NF2 because of the vulnerability of the trigeminal and facial nerve with treatment of VS.[53]

Overall, although durable radiographic and hearing responses were not observed, there is evidence that treatment with HER-1/EGFR inhibitors may promote stable disease for longer periods of time, or reduce the growth rate of rapidly growing tumors. This would be particularly attractive to NF2 patients, who are more likely to experience significant morbidity with surgical or radiation treatment. Along with the presumed cytostatic effects of erlotinib, this suggests that time to disease progression may be a more reasonable clinical end point for future phase II trials of anti-EGFR agents.

Bevacziumab

Bevacizumab is a humanized anti-VEGF monoclonal antibody approved for the treatment of various cancers, often in combination with traditional chemotherapeutic drugs. It has recently been approved by the Food and Drug Administration to treat glioblastoma that has recurred after initial therapy. Its usual mode of administration is by intravenous infusion every 2 to 3 weeks.

In a recent study conducted by the authors' group, 10 consecutive patients with NF2 and progressive VS who were not candidates for standard surgical or radiation treatment were given bevacizumab and assessed for radiographic and hearing responses.[34] Patients were followed with serial MRI and clinic visits every 3 months. In addition to the volumetric methods described previously, the mean apparent diffusion coefficient (ADC) was examined to assess whether baseline tumor-associated vasogenic edema might correlate with tumor shrinkage. In addition, serial audiologic evaluations, including assessment of pure tone threshold and word recognition score, were performed. Overall, the medication was well tolerated, with the most notable side effects being elevated liver enzymes, proteinuria, and hypertension all (grade 1 or 2).

Tumors shrank with treatment in 9 of 10 patients, six of whom had a durable imaging response during the follow-up period. Before treatment, the median annual volumetric growth rate for the tumors of interest was 62%, and the median best response to treatment was a reduction of 26%.[34] Additionally, there was a strong correlation between the baseline ADC and the percent decrease in tumor volume at 3 months, underscoring the role of bevacizumab in normalizing the abnormally increased vascular permeability of tumor vessels and reducing intratumoral edema.[34,54]

Although three patients were not eligible for testing hearing response because of either a treatment-induced deafness or a near-normal baseline word recognition score, four of the remainder had a hearing response and two had stable hearing. Two patients experienced an especially dramatic improvement in their hearing, from 8% to 98% and from 34% to 78% word recognition, respectively.[34] Both of these patients regained what could be termed "useful hearing," allowing them to resume full employment. These responses were durable during the entire follow-up period of 16 months.

Finally, there is some evidence that bevacizumab resulted in clinical improvements not related to the primary outcomes, which are nonetheless important to overall quality of life. One patient with a large VS had intractable headaches and vomiting associated with brainstem compression, but experienced a dramatic improvement in his symptoms within 4 weeks of commencing treatment. Other patients reported subjective improvements in their baseline tinnitus.[34]

Five patients in the erlotinib study[53] were subsequently included in the bevacizumab study, because they had stopped erlotinib either because of treatment failure (tumor growth) or side effects. Four of these five patients achieved either a radiographic or hearing response with bevacizumab.[34] Thus, there is evidence that bevacizumab may have a more consistent and durable activity in this patient population.

A smaller clinical series from Germany (two patients) demonstrated similarly promising results, with radiographic regression of greater than 40% and a substantial improvement in hearing after 6 months of treatment.[55] Neither patient was a candidate for traditional therapies and both faced imminent hearing loss caused by tumor progression.

As a VEGF inhibitor, bevacizumab has been associated with vascular complications in larger trials, such as hypertension, hemorrhage, and vascular embolism. After a highly publicized adverse event in 1997, a fatal cerebral hemorrhage from an unrecognized brain metastasis in a 29-year-old patient with hepatocellular carcinoma,[56] the safety of bevacizumab for patients with central nervous system (CNS) metastatic disease was called into question and such patients were excluded from future trials. Several studies since that time have attempted to clarify the degree of hemorrhage risk with bevacizumab. A recent retrospective analysis of subjects enrolled in clinical trials demonstrated that patients with CNS metastases are at similar risk of hemorrhage, independent of bevacizumab therapy.[56] This was also true of patients with highly malignant recurrent glioblastoma, contributing to its eventual Food and Drug Administration approval for treatment of this condition.

Preliminary data suggest that bevacizumab induces not only radiographic tumor shrinkage but also an improvement in hearing, sometimes dramatically. Moreover, an effective medical therapy, even if it merely arrested tumor growth and led to modest improvements in hearing over time, could help patients avoid surgery for longer periods of time, thereby postponing treatment-related morbidity including the risk of increased hearing loss. Thus far, most patients treated with bevacizumab are not candidates for surgery or radiation, or have experienced tumor recurrence or progression after such therapy. Including patients at earlier stages of disease will help clarify the role of bevacizumab compared with accepted therapies.

Anti-VEGF agents have shown promising activity in preliminary studies. Indeed, they may be more effective in this patient population than in malignant disease, given the benign histology and overall slower growth rate of NF2-associated tumors including schwannomas. Larger multicenter clinical trials with longer follow-up periods are urgently needed to clarify the role of bevacizumab treatment and define its degree of efficacy. **Table 1** provides a summary of early evidence from studies with targeted therapies erlotinib and bevacizumab.

Table 1
Summary of studies with targeted chemotherapies for vestibular schwannoma

Agent and Study	Early Evidence and Conclusions
Erlotinib Plotkin et al, 2010[53]	Three of 11 patients had prolonged stable disease or slowing of tumor growth rate Radiographic changes: • Contralateral VS shrinkage in many • One had 26% reduction in total body tumor volume Early conclusions: • Treatment with EGFR inhibitors may promote stable disease for longer periods of time, or reduce the growth rate of rapidly growing tumors • NF2 patients could benefit most because they are more likely to experience significant morbidity with surgical or radiation treatment • Time to disease progression may be reasonable clinical end point for future phase II trials of anti-EGFR agents
Bevacizumab Plotkin et al, 2009[34]	• Nine of 10 patients had tumor shrinkage • Strong correlation between baseline ADC and percent decrease in tumor volume at 3 months • Four of seven had hearing response • Two of seven had stable hearing • Two patients experienced improvement in their hearing from 8% to 98% and from 34% to 78% • One patient with intractable headaches and vomiting experienced dramatic improvement in symptoms within 4 weeks of commencing treatment • Subjective improvements in tinnitus reported
German study Mautner et al, 2010[55] Plotkin et al, 2009[34] Mautner et al, 2010[55]	Two of two patients demonstrated: • Regression >40% • Substantial improvement in hearing after 6 months of treatment Early conclusions: • Treatment with bevacizumab can result in clinically significant hearing improvement and tumor shrinkage in some NF2 patients • Prospective clinical trials are underway to confirm these findings in a multicenter setting

ONGOING TRIALS

Previous experience with erlotinib (which inhibits tumor Schwann cell proliferation) and bevacizumab (which suppresses vascularization) has increased recognition of the potential of targeted molecular therapies not only for malignant tumors, but also for benign yet locally aggressive tumors, such as VS. Currently, a National Cancer Institute–approved phase II study is recruiting patients at MGH, National Cancer Institute, and Johns Hopkins, with a goal of clarifying the efficacy and biologic activity of bevacizumab in the treatment of VS. Several trials of other monoclonal antibodies have been proposed and are outlined briefly next.

PTC299

A planned phase II clinical trial of the oral anti-VEGF agent PTC299 is ongoing at the authors' institution (MGH/PTC Therapeutics/Department of Defense).[57] In animal models, PTC299 has been shown to decrease VEGF levels in the tumor and bloodstream and decrease the number of blood vessels associated with the tumor, thereby slowing tumor growth. Planned enrollment is 25 patients, with assessment of radiographic response (using the volumetric methods described previously) and hearing response (using word recognition tests). Secondary outcomes will include effects on pure tone thresholds, brainstem auditory evoked responses, subjective perception of tinnitus, circulating angiogenic factors, and assessment of side effects.

Lapatinib

A clinical trial of the anti-HER-1/HER-2 agent lapatinib is ongoing (New York University/GlaxoSmithKline).[58] Outcomes assessed will include volumetric analysis and perfusion on MRI, and formal audiogram every 3 months for 1 year. An example of a rationally designed clinical trial, this study was based on a recent immunohistochemistry study of specimens from patients with sporadic and NF2-related VS, which were screened for receptor tyrosine kinase activation.[59] Overexpression of EGFR family receptors and evidence of ERK1/2 downstream signaling was observed in these tumor specimens. Based on these findings, lapatinib was tested in vitro in a human schwannoma model, resulting in decreased Schwann cell proliferation.

Imatinib

Imatinib (Gleevec), the agent most successfully used to target the bcr-abl oncogene in chronic myelogenous leukemia, also inhibits c-KIT and PDGFR signaling. It has been demonstrated that sporadic and NF2-related VS have increased expression of PDGFR and c-KIT compared with normal Schwann cells.[60] In vitro, imatinib inihibited schwannoma proliferation, induced apoptosis, and reduced anchorage-independent growth.[57] Thus far, transgenic models are impractical to carry these findings forward to in vivo studies. However, the vast clinical experience with imatinib and its relatively low toxicity may justify an open-label trial in humans with progressive VS. Pilot studies of imatinib in NF1-related plexiform neurofibromas and malignant peripheral nerve sheath tumors are currently underway, although the drug has not yet been formally tested in VS.

SUMMARY

The unpredictable natural history of sporadic and NF2-related VS presents unique management dilemmas. In the past, these tumors have been managed solely with surgery or radiotherapy, with only a limited role for medical therapies. Given their problematic location near the brainstem and the high morbidity of surgical or radiation treatment, clinically effective medical therapies are urgently needed, particularly in NF2 where tumors are more likely to be larger and more aggressive.

The past few years have witnessed exciting new research into targeted molecular therapies for all cancers. Although in the recent past these agents have mostly been used to combat malignant disease, they may be uniquely well-suited to the benign histology and immunology of VS, especially those related to NF2. Anti-VEGF and anti-HER agents have shown particular promise in the treatment of progressive VS and are under active investigation. It is hoped that an effective drug treatment for VS, particularly in patients with NF2, will emerge over the next few years, providing safer, less invasive treatment options, preserving hearing, and enhancing overall quality of life for patients.

REFERENCES

1. Central Brain Tumor Registry of the United States. Statistical report: primary brain tumors in the United States, 2004-2006. 2010. Available at: http://www.cbtrus.org. Accessed January 9, 2010.
2. Plotkin S, Halpin C, Blakeley J, et al. Suggested response criteria for phase II antitumor drug studies for neurofibromatosis type 2 related vestibular schwannoma. J Neurooncol 2009;93(1):61–77.
3. Evans D, Moran A, King A, et al. Incidence of vestibular schwannoma and neurofibromatosis 2 in the North West of England over a 10-year period: higher incidence than previously thought. Otol Neurotol 2005;26(1):93–7.
4. Phi J, Kim D, Chung H, et al. Radiosurgical treatment of vestibular schwannomas in patients with neurofibromatosis type 2: tumor control and hearing preservation. Cancer 2009;115(2):390–8.
5. Samii M, Gerganov V, Samii A. Improved preservation of hearing and facial nerve function in vestibular schwannoma via the retrosigmoid approach in a series of 200 patients. J Neurosurg 2006;105(4):527–35.
6. Otsuka G, Saito K, Nagatani T, et al. Age at symptom onset and long-term survival in patients with neurofibromatosis type 2. J Neurosurg 2003;99(3): 480–3.
7. Baser M, Friedman J, Aeschliman D, et al. Predictors of the risk of mortality in neurofibromatosis 2. Am J Hum Genet 2002;71(4):715–23.
8. Baser M, Makariou E, Parry D. Predictors of vestibular schwannoma growth in patients with neurofibromatosis type 2. J Neurosurg 2002;96(2):217–22.
9. Hamada Y, Iwaki T, Fukui M, et al. A comparative study of embedded nerve tissue in six NF2-associated schwannomas and 17 nonassociated NF2 schwannomas. Surg Neurol 1997;48(4):395–400.
10. Evans D, Kalamarides M, Hunter-Schaedle K, et al. Consensus recommendations to accelerate clinical trials for neurofibromatosis type 2. Clin Cancer Res 2009; 15(16):5032–9.
11. Fisher L, Doherty J, Lev M, et al. Concordance of bilateral vestibular schwannoma growth and hearing changes in neurofibromatosis 2: neurofibromatosis 2 natural history consortium. Otol Neurotol 2009;30(6):835–41.
12. Stangerup S, Caye-Thomasen P, Tos M, et al. The natural history of vestibular schwannoma. Otol Neurotol 2006;27(4):547–52.
13. Stangerup S, Caye-Thomasen P, Tos M, et al. Change in hearing during "wait and scan" management of patients with vestibular schwannoma. J Laryngol Otol 2008;122(7):673–81.

14. Hajioff D, Raut V, Walsh R, et al. Conservative management of vestibular schwannomas: third review of a 10-year prospective study. Clin Otolaryngol 2008;33(3): 255–9.

15. Massick D, Welling D, Dodson E, et al. Tumor growth and audiometric change in vestibular schwannomas managed conservatively. Laryngoscope 2000;110(11): 1843–9.

16. Arts H, Telian S, El-Kashlan H, et al. Hearing preservation and facial nerve outcomes in vestibular schwannoma surgery: results using the middle cranial fossa approach. Otol Neurotol 2006;27(2):234–41.

17. Slattery W, Fisher L, Iqbal Z, et al. Vestibular schwannoma growth rates in neurofibromatosis type 2 natural history consortium subjects. Otol Neurotol 2004;25(5): 811–7.

18. Smouha E, Yoo M, Mohr K, et al. Conservative management of acoustic neuroma: a meta-analysis and proposed treatment algorithm. Laryngoscope 2005;115(3): 450–4.

19. Barker F, Carter B, Ojemann R, et al. Surgical excision of acoustic neuroma: patient outcome and provider caseload. Laryngoscope 2003;113(8):1332–43.

20. Combs S, Volk S, Schultz-Ertner D, et al. Management of acoustic neuromas with fractionated stereotactic radiotherapy (FSRT): long-term results in 106 patients treated in a single institution. Int J Radiat Oncol Biol Phys 2005;63(1): 75–81.

21. Flickinger J, Kondziolka D, Niranjan A, et al. Results of acoustic neuroma radiosurgery: an analysis of 5 years' experience using current methods. J Neurosurg 2001;94(1):1–6.

22. Evans DG, Birch JM, Ramsden RT, et al. Malignant transformation and new primary tumours after therapeutic radiation for benign disease: substantial risks in certain tumour prone syndromes. J Med Genet 2006;43(4):289–94.

23. Rouleau G, Merel P, Lutchman M, et al. Alteration in a new gene encoding a putative membrane organizing protein causes neurofibromatosis type 2. Nature 1993; 363(6429):515–21.

24. Twist E, Ruttledge M, Rousseau M, et al. The neurofibromatosis gene is inactivated in schwannomas. Hum Mol Genet 1994;3(1):147–51.

25. Curto M, Cole B, Lallemand D, et al. Contact dependent inhibition of EGFR signaling by NF2/merlin. J Cell Biol 2007;177(5):893–903.

26. O'Reilly B, Kishore A, Crowther J, et al. Correlation of growth factor receptor expression with clinical growth in vestibular schwannomas. Otol Neurotol 2004; 25(5):791–6.

27. Lallemand D, Manent J, Couvelard A, et al. Merlin regulates transmembrane receptor accumulation and signaling at the plasma membrane in primary mouse Schwann cells and in human schwannomas. Oncogene 2009;28(6):854–65.

28. Fraenzer JT, Pan H, Minimo L Jr, et al. Overexpression of the NF2 gene inhibits schwannoma cell proliferation through promoting PDGFR degradation. Int J Oncol 2003;23(6):1493–500.

29. Doherty J, Ongkeko W, Crawley B, et al. ErbB and Nrg: potential molecular targets for vestibular schwannoma pharmacotherapy. Otol Neurotol 2008;29(1): 50–7.

30. Ammoun S, Flaiz C, Ristic N, et al. Dissecting and targeting the growth factor-dependent and growth factor-independent extracellular signal-regulated kinase pathway in human schwannoma. Cancer Res 2008;68(13):5236–45.

31. Klagsbrun M, Takashima S, Mamluk R. The role of neuropilin in vascular and tumor biology. Adv Exp Med Biol 2002;515:33–48.

32. Cayé-Thomasen P, Werther K, Nalla A, et al. VEGF and VEGF receptor-1 concentration in vestibular schwannoma homogenates correlates to tumor growth rate. Otol Neurotol 2005;26(1):98–101.
33. Uesaka T, Shono T, Suzuki S, et al. Expression of VEGF and its receptor genes in intracranial schwannomas. J Neurooncol 2007;83(3):259–66.
34. Plotkin S, Stemmer-Rachamimov A, Barker F, et al. Hearing improvement after bevacizumab in patients with neurofibromatosis type 2. N Engl J Med 2009; 361(4):358–67.
35. Wong H, Lahdenranta J, Kamoun W, et al. Anti-vascular endothelial growth factor therapies as a novel therapeutic approach to treating neurofibromatosis-related tumors. Cancer Res 2010;70(9):3483–93.
36. Halpin C, Rauch S. Using audiometric thresholds and word recognition in a treatment study. Otol Neurotol 2006;27(1):110–6.
37. Committee on Hearing and Equilibrium Guidelines for the evaluation of hearing preservation in acoustic neuroma (vestibular schwannoma). American Academy of Otolaryngology-Head and Neck Surgery Foundation, Inc. Otolaryngol Head Neck Surg 1995;113(3):179–80.
38. Gardner G, Robertson J. Hearing preservation in unilateral acoustic neuroma surgery. Ann Otol Rhinol Laryngol 1988;97(1):55–66.
39. Mahmud MR, Khan AM, Nadol JB Jr. Histopathology of the inner ear in unoperated acoustic neuroma. Ann Otol Rhinol Laryngol 2003;112(11):979–86.
40. Gerstner E, Sorensen A, Jain R, et al. Advances in neuroimaging techniques for the evaluation of tumor growth, vascular permeability, and angiogenesis in gliomas. Curr Opin Neurol 2008;21(6):728–35.
41. Therasse P, Arbuck S, Eisenhauer E, et al. New guidelines to evaluate the response to treatment in solid tumors. European Organization for Research and Treatment of Cancer, National Cancer Institute of the United States, National Cancer Institute of Canada. J Natl Cancer Inst 2000;92(3):205–16.
42. Macdonald DR, Cascino TL, Schold SC Jr, et al. Response criteria for phase II studies of supratentorial malignant glioma. J Clin Oncol 1990;8(7): 1277–80.
43. Harris G, Plotkin S, Mccollin M, et al. Three-dimensional volumetrics for tracking vestibular schwannoma growth in neurofibromatosis type II. Neurosurgery 2008; 62(6):1314–9.
44. Lamborn K, Yung W, Chang S, et al. Progression-free survival: an important end point in evaluating therapy for recurrent high-grade gliomas. Neuro Oncol 2008; 10(2):162–70.
45. McCombe A, Baguley D, Coles R, et al. Guidelines for the grading of tinnitus severity: the results of a working group commissioned by the British Association of Otolaryngologists, Head and Neck Surgeons. Clin Otolaryngol Allied Sci 2001; 26(5):388–93.
46. Klockhoff I, Lindblom U. Meniére's disease and hydrochlorothiazide: a critical analysis of symptoms and therapeutic effects. Acta Otolaryngol 1967;63(4): 347–65.
47. Wilson PH, Henry J, Bowen M, et al. Tinnitus reaction questionnaire: psychometric properties of a measure of distress associated with tinnitus. J Speech Hear Res 1991;34(1):197–201.
48. House J, Brackmann D. Facial nerve grading system. Otolaryngol Head Neck Surg 1985;93(2):146–7.
49. Jahrsdoerfer R, Benjamin R. Chemotherapy of bilateral acoustic neuromas. Otolaryngol Head Neck Surg 1988;98(4):273–82.

50. Chang S, Lamborn K, Kuhn J, et al. Neurooncology clinical trial design for targeted therapies: lesions learned from the North American Brain Tumor Consortium. Neuro Oncol 2008;10(4):631–42.
51. Neff B, Welling D, Akhmametyeva E, et al. The molecular biology of vestibular schwannomas: dissecting the pathogenic process at the molecular level. Otol Neurotol 2006;27(6):197–208.
52. Clark J, Provenzano M, Diggelmann H, et al. The ErbB inhibitors trastuzumab and erlotinib inhibit growth of vestibular schwannoma xenografts in nude mice: a preliminary study. Otol Neurotol 2008;29(6):846–53.
53. Plotkin S, Halpin C, McKenna M, et al. Erlotinib for progressive vestibular schwannoma in neurofibromatosis 2 patients. Otol Neurotol 2010;31(7):1135–43.
54. Jain R. Normalization of tumor vasculature: an emerging concept in antiangiogenic therapy. Science 2005;307(5706):58–62.
55. Mautner V, Nguyen R, Kutta H, et al. Bevacizumab induces regression of vestibular schwannomas in patients with neurofibromatosis type 2. Neuro Oncol 2010; 12(1):14–8.
56. Besse B, Lasserre S, Compton P, et al. Bevacizumab safety in patients with central nervous system metastases. Clin Cancer Res 2010;16(1):269–78.
57. Clinical trial description. PTC299 for treatment of neurofibromatosis type 2. Available at: http://clinicaltrials.gov/ct2/show/NCT00911248?term=ptc299&rank=1. Accessed January 9, 2010.
58. Clinical trial description. Lapatinib study for children and adults with neurofibromatosis type 2 (NF2) and NF2-related tumors. Available at: http://clinicaltrials.gov/ct2/show/NCT00973739?term=lapatinib+vestibular+schwannoma&rank=2. Accessed January 9, 2010.
59. Ammoun S, Cunliffe C, Allen J, et al. ErbB/HER receptor activation and preclinical efficacy of lapatinib in vestibular schwannoma. Neuro Oncol 2010;12(8):834–43.
60. Mukherjee J, Kamnasaran D, Balasubramaniam A, et al. Human schwannomas express activated platelet-derived growth factor receptors and c-kit and are growth inhibited by Gleevec (Imatinib Mesylate). Cancer Res 2009;69(12): 5099–107.

Habilitation of Auditory and Vestibular Dysfunction

Hillary A. Snapp, AuD[a],*, Michael C. Schubert, PhD, PT[b]

KEYWORDS

- Vestibular schwannoma • Auditory dysfunction • Vestibular dysfunction
- Quality of life • Hearing rehabilitation

Key Abbreviations: HABILITATION OF AUDITORY AND VESTIBULAR DYSFUNCTION	
APHAB	Abbreviated Profile of Hearing Aid Benefit
BiCROS	Bilateral CROS
BAI	Bone-anchored implant
CPA	Cerebellopontine angle
CROS	Contralateral routing of signals
DVA	Dynamic visual acuity
GHABP	Glasgow Hearing Aid Benefit Profile
HSN	Head shaking–induced nystagmus
IAC	Internal auditory canal
rTMS	Repetitive transcranial magnetic stimulation
SCC	Semicircular canal
SNR	Signal-to-noise ratio
SSD	Single-sided deafness
SSQ	Speech, Spatial and Qualities of hearing scale
THI	Tinnitus Handicap Inventory
TRQ	Tinnitus Reaction Questionnaire
UHL	Unilateral hearing loss
VPT	Vestibular rehabilitation
VS	Vestibular schwannoma

Vestibular schwannomas (VS) are benign tumors arising from the Schwann cell of the vestibular nerve, often in the internal auditory canal (IAC). The incidence of VS has been estimated to be between 7 and 15 people per million,[1–4] and constitute about 80% of all tumors found in the cerebellopontine angle.[5,6] Along with the vestibulocochlear nerve (CN8), the IAC houses the facial nerve (CN7) and the internal auditory artery. Symptom presentation is usually related to where the tumor arises. If the tumor arises in the IAC, tinnitus and hearing loss are often the first symptoms. However, if the

[a] Department of Otolaryngology, University of Miami, 1120 Northwest 14th Street, Fifth Floor, Miami, FL 33136, USA
[b] Department of Otolaryngology Head and Neck Surgery, Johns Hopkins University, 601 North Caroline Street, Room 6245, Baltimore, MD 21287, USA
* Corresponding author.
E-mail address: hsnapp@med.miami.edu

Otolaryngol Clin N Am 45 (2012) 487–511
doi:10.1016/j.otc.2011.12.014
0030-6665/12/$ – see front matter © 2012 Elsevier Inc. All rights reserved.

oto.theclinics.com

growth occurs in the cerebellopontine angle (CPA), the tumor may become quite large before symptoms of hearing loss are revealed. Thus, although unilateral hearing loss (UHL) is often the initial sign of VS, the pathogenesis of the associated structures within the space can sometimes result in vestibular (ie, vertigo, imbalance), facial, or even vascular symptoms (ie, headaches, fatigue) as the driving force for an individual to seek medical attention.

Total hearing loss in the affected ear may be a significant handicap.[7] Abnormal vestibular function occurs in many patients but usually abates with central compensation. Hearing loss becomes a long-term disability, often requiring sustained intervention and management throughout the life of the patient. For those who do not have spontaneous vestibular compensation or are slow to compensate, vestibular rehabilitation, chemical labyrinthotomy with gentamycin, or tumor removal may be necessary.

AUDITORY HABILITATION
Hearing Loss

UHL is the most common symptom of patients with VS, followed by tinnitus and imbalance.[2,7] Often, whether from natural history, radiation, or surgery, the result is profound hearing loss.[8,9] The deficits associated with UHL have been well documented. These individuals experience reduced sound awareness, difficulty communicating in noise, and reduced ability to localize. The communication deficits experienced by individuals with severe to profound UHL may produce psychological, social, and vocational issues.

The auditory pathway consists of afferent fibers transmitting acoustic information regarding frequency, intensity, and timing of a sound source to the auditory cortex. The auditory fibers are tonotopically organized, allowing for preservation of frequency-specific cues that provide discrete information to higher-order auditory structures regarding pitch and loudness. Binaural hearing integrates the timing and intensity differences of acoustic signals arriving at each ear to interpret the spatial aspects of sound. This process enables the auditory system to efficiently separate and localize sounds, increase loudness, and improve sound quality. Hearing impairment from VS may occur at the cochlea, cochlear nerve, brainstem, or a combination of sites. Binaural cues such as interaural timing and level differences, binaural summation, and head-related transfer function play a critical role in localization and listening-in-noise ability. Although ipsilateral coding is maintained in the better hearing ear, for adults in complex listening environments, the loss of binaural cues can result in a considerable handicap.[10,11]

Clinical evaluation
The goals of auditory rehabilitation in the VS population are to:

1. Restore access to sound
2. Reduce the associated deficits caused by the hearing loss.

To provide the best form of rehabilitation, accurate assessment of these deficits must be made. A comprehensive evaluation is conducted of the integrity of the peripheral and central auditory systems to determine the degree of associated handicap.

Standard audiometric test battery The objectives are to:

1. Establish frequency specific residual hearing sensitivity for both ears
2. Confirm or deny the presence of a contributing conductive component
3. Assess word-recognition ability in quiet.

The resulting data provide the clinician with tangible hearing outcomes as a starting point for the counseling process. The patient on a watch-and-wait plan may have a notably different auditory profile from one who has undergone complete resection. It can be expected that the rehabilitation of these patients may differ substantially. Clinicians cannot anticipate an individual's success in real-world listening without establishing a more complete auditory profile that assesses individualized performance beyond that of the pure tone audiogram. Auditory processing capabilities can vary significantly by individual.

Speech in noise Compromised speech-in-noise ability is a primary deficit experienced by individuals with severe to profound UHL.[12] A good test battery should include speech-in-noise measures to evaluate each patient's signal-to-noise ratio (SNR) loss. Which is the increase in SNR ratio required to obtain 50% correct words, sentences, or words in sentences, compared with normal performance.[13] This component is important because not all patients will demonstrate the same degree of impairment in noise.[11,14] Taylor[14] demonstrated that individuals who presented with similar hearing loss configurations on pure tone audiometric testing could vary by more than 20 dB in performance on speech-in-noise measures. This finding is powerful evidence that an individual's performance in noise cannot be predicted on the pure tone audiogram alone. Real-world listening is far more complex and dynamic than what is represented in the standard audiogram. By including speech-in-noise measures in the evaluation process, the clinician is provided with individualized deficit-specific information regarding communication ability in complex listening environments. This information is not only valuable in determining appropriate intervention, but also functions as a counseling tool to assist the clinician in setting realistic expectations for the patient's communication needs.

Sound localization The ability to localize sounds becomes impaired in UHL patients because of the loss of interaural level and timing cues. Objective assessment of localization is not regularly incorporated into the clinical test battery. Current treatment options such as contralateral routing of signal (CROS) hearing aids (see later discussion) and bone-conduction implants continue to be limited in their ability to remediate the loss of localization.[15–20] Clinicians should take care to counsel patients in detail regarding expectations for localization after treatment.

Subjective measures Along with the auditory impairment, patients and their clinicians must consider the psychological, social, and vocational impact that may be contributing to the handicap. Subjective assessment of how the hearing loss is affecting the patient's quality of life is an important parameter in the determination of postoperative treatment options. A subjective questionnaire should be specific and should be selected based on the communication needs of the patient. Several measures exist in the literature and include the following:

The Abbreviated Profile of Hearing Aid Benefit (APHAB) is a widely used 24-item subjective outcome measure evaluating disability associated with hearing loss. Specifically it assesses ease of communication, reverberation, listening in background noise, and aversiveness to sound.[21] The APHAB is a popular tool, due to its usefulness for determining disability and the change in disability after treatment.

The Glasgow Profile of Hearing Aid Benefit (GPHAB) is an outcome measure that assesses auditory disability, handicap, hearing aid benefit, and hearing aid satisfaction using 4 specific listening and communication situations. In addition, the GPHAB allows patients to identify up to 4 additional situations for customized assessment.[22]

The Speech, Spatial and Qualities of hearing scale (SSQ) is a validated measure to assess impairment associated with binaural function. The 3 domains provide comprehensive information about listening to speech in complex environments, including localization, direction, and movement of sound, segregation of sounds, and ability to attend to multiple auditory inputs.[23] The SSQ is unique in that it allows for some assessment of localization. The deficit-specific questions of the SSQ make it an ideal tool for use in the VS population.[8,23]

Physical and cognitive contributors should also be considered prior to intervention.

Intervention

Appropriate intervention addresses the goals of the patient through compensation for the physiologic and subjective handicaps as indicated by outcome measures. Preoperative hearing loss can range from mild to profound. Most preoperative hearing losses can be successfully treated with traditional amplification as long as the hearing loss is not too severe and word-recognition ability remains intact. Despite good residual hearing across the low- to mid-frequency range, some preoperative VS patients present with unaidable high-frequency hearing loss. These patients can be considered for alternative amplification options such as frequency-compression and frequency-transposition hearing aids. These devices attempt to shift sound from the unaidable high-frequency region to a lower frequency to be interpreted by the ear. This option varies in success, and is sometimes rejected because of dissatisfaction with sound quality.

For those patients whose hearing loss progresses to the severe to profound UHL range, also referred to as single-sided deafness (SSD), a variety of options exist (**Table 1**). The treatment goal for these patients is to provide access to sound arriving at the affected ear, thereby compensating for the head-shadow effect. Patients with severe to profound UHL are not candidates for traditional amplification. These patients must consider options that use their better hearing ear to provide access to sound arriving from the SSD ear. The anticipated effect of this is restoration of sound awareness and improvement in listening-in-noise ability.

Options for these patients traditionally have been limited to CROS and bilateral CROS (BiCROS) amplifiers. The CROS system attempts to restore access to sound arriving from the affected side by collecting sound with a microphone placed on the SSD ear and transferring it via wired or wireless transmission to a receiver in the normal ear. However, obstacles such as the need to wear bilateral hearing aids, occlusion in the normal ear, and poor or unnatural sound quality have led to poor acceptance of these devices.[16] Historically, patients who rejected CROS amplifiers were left to rely entirely on their better hearing ear.

Other treatment options have focused on bone conduction as a means to transmit sound to the functioning cochlea. Some early attempts at this included the transcranial CROS and the bone-conduction hearing aid. The transcranial CROS attempted to stimulate the contralateral cochlea by sending an air-conduction signal via a high-power hearing aid in the nonfunctioning side. This device was not well accepted, due to reports of discomfort and poor sound quality. Although bone-conduction hearing aids tend to provide better sound quality and ease of listening, they have seen little use in the adult population because of physical discomfort and lack of aesthetic appeal.

In recent years treatment options have expanded to include alternative forms of bone-conduction stimulation to remediate profound UHL. Based on the same principles, improvements in technology have led to options that provide good sound quality, comfort, and aesthetic appeal. The TransEAR (Ear Technology Corporation, Johnson City, TN, USA) amplifier uses a bone conductor that is custom fitted to the medial bony portion of the ear canal, thereby sending the acoustic

Table 1
Treatment options for rehabilitation of severe to profound UHL

Treatment	Benefits	Limitations
CROS hearing aid	Noninvasive Relatively low cost Lifts head-shadow Can be trialed at minimal cost	Requires 2 hearing aids Occludes normal hearing ear Reports of unnatural sound quality Lack of aesthetic appeal

BiCROS hearing aid	Noninvasive
	Relatively low cost
	Lifts head-shadow
	Added gain for patients with
	  hearing loss in better ear
	Can be trialed at minimal cost
		Requires 2 hearing aids
		Reports of unnatural sound
		  quality
		Lack of aesthetic appeal

Transcranial CROS	Noninvasive
	Relatively low cost
	Can be trialed at minimal cost
		Less successful at lifting head
		  shadow
		Poor sound quality
		Discomfort due to high gain
		  levels

Bone-conduction
  hearing aid
	Noninvasive
	Relatively low cost
	Improved sound quality/ease
	  of listening
	Can be trialed at minimal cost
		Lack of aesthetic appeal
		Physical discomfort caused
		  by need to wear headband
		  for stimulation

TransEAR	Noninvasive
	Relatively low cost
	Improved sound quality/ease
	  of listening
	No need for device on better
	  hearing ear
		Limited published data on
		  performance in SSD
		  population
		Unable to trial in office

Bone-anchored implants	Lifts head-shadow: improved
	  performance compared
	  with CROS
	Can experience device
	  preoperatively through in-
	  office demonstrations
	Reports of improved sound
	  quality/ease of listening
	No need for device on better
	  hearing ear
	No physical discomfort
	Decreased feedback and
	  distortion issues
		Invasive
		Semipermanent
		High cost option
		Preoperative trial not feasible[a]

[a] Although some clinicians allow trials with a demonstration device at home, that is not the recommendation of the authors, whose opinion is that this often leads to misconception about device performance, due to lack of control regarding device placement, output levels, distortion, and feedback.

information through the skull via vibration to the functioning cochlea in the opposite ear. Sophono Inc (Boulder, CO, USA) has introduced a transcutaneous bone-conduction implant recently approved by the Food and Drug Administration. A dental bone conductor appliance has been developed by Sonitus Inc (San Mateo, CA, USA). As of this writing, percutaneous bone-anchored implants (BAIs) are approved and marketed in the United States by Cochlear Corp. (Denver, CO, USA) and Oticon Medical (Somerset, NJ, USA).

Recently BAIs have gained increased popularity as a treatment option for patients with profound UHL. As with the previously discussed options, BAIs (**Fig. 1**) collect sound arriving at the nonfunctioning ear and deliver it to the functioning cochlea by way of bone conduction. As an implant system, BAIs consist of an osseointegrated titanium fixture with a percutaneous abutment that is implanted into the mastoid bone behind the ear, which allows for direct bone conduction (**Fig. 2**) in contrast to transcutaneous stimulation by a bone-conduction hearing aid. A sound processor is attached to the implant externally and transmits sound via vibration of the skull to the functioning cochlea.

Quickly becoming the standard form of treatment, BAIs have met with some controversy because they require surgical intervention to remediate the hearing loss. The goals of BAIs for SSD are the same as those previously discussed for noninvasive options: to compensate for the head-shadow effect and restore sound awareness on the impaired side. As a result, clinicians are faced with the challenge of deciding whether the benefit received by a BAI warrants recommending a more invasive form of treatment. There is strong evidence that patients who receive a BAI for remediation of UHL experience improvement in both quality of life and listening-in-noise ability.[24–26] Furthermore, comparison studies have consistently reported improved performance and patient satisfaction with BAIs compared with the noninvasive CROS hearing aid.[17–19] Although there is considerable support for the use of BAIs over CROS, there has been some criticism regarding the quality of these studies.[27] At present, a critical mass of literature comparing the TransEAR amplifier with BAIs does not exist.

None of the listed treatment options restores true binaural hearing. The treatments are a means to provide access to sound arriving at the impaired ear. Benefits are limited, even in BAIs, and no objective evidence exists to support restoration of localization ability.[16–19,26] Degree of benefit varies by individual and must be thoroughly assessed before any treatment implementation. Counseling is an essential component of ensuring successful outcomes.

Selection process Selecting the appropriate treatment for the patient is a comprehensive process. It should be a collaborative effort that includes the patient, his or her communication partners, the surgeon, and other health care professionals involved in the medical management. A protocol based on known auditory deficits of the individual seeking treatment is essential for determining treatment options, candidacy, and expected outcomes. For those patients wishing to pursue a BAI, it is the clinician's responsibility to obtain as much information as possible to determine expected

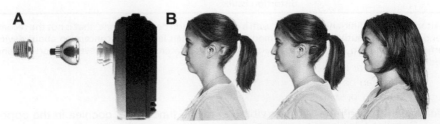

Fig. 1. Bone-anchored implant system. (*A*) Cochlear Baha implant system demonstrating the titanium fixture, abutment, and external processor. (*B*) View of postoperative implant/abutment, external processor fixed to abutment, and concealment by hair. (*Courtesy of* Cochlear Americas, Inc; with permission.)

Left   Right

Direct BC
from BAHA   AC normal
                                                                                way

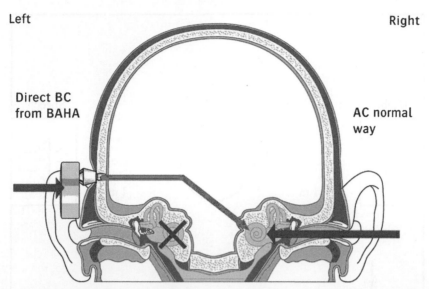

Fig. 2. Direct bone conduction through BAI system. A BAI collects sound from the affected side and delivers it to the functioning cochlea by direct stimulation of the skull. (*Courtesy of Cochlear Americas, Inc; with permission.*)

outcomes following surgery. The audiogram does not provide sufficient determination of candidacy; rather, it should be used as an indicator to identify those who may be a candidate. Candidacy should be determined by a comprehensive protocol evaluating the broad range of deficits and handicaps experienced by the patient.

- The evaluation process begins with comprehensive audiometry, including ear-specific word-recognition ability in quiet. The team reviews the hearing test and the expected auditory limitations associated with any hearing loss. The patient is then provided with information regarding all noninvasive alternative options, and a trial with a CROS hearing device is strongly encouraged.
- The next step is to assess speech-in-noise deficit using measures such as the Quick Speech-in-Noise Test (QuickSIN; Etymotic Research, Elk Grove Village, IL, USA),[13] the Bamford-Kowal-Bench Speech-in-Noise test (BKB-SIN; Etymotic Research),[28] or the Hearing in Noise Test (HINT; Maico, Eden Prairie, MN, USA).[29]
- Individuals with severe to profound UHL struggle the most with listening in noise (11), particularly when the signal of interest is arriving at the affected side and noise is masking the better hearing ear.[17–19] To assess binaural deficit related to the head shadow effect, testing should be conducted in the sound field with noise directed towards the better-hearing ear and speech stimuli towards the affected ear (**Fig. 3**).
  - This can be repeated with both the noise and speech presented at 0 degrees azimuth or with speech presented at 0° azimuth and noise directed at the better hearing ear.
- Baseline SNR loss is established for all conditions.
- Performance on speech-in-noise tasks is then reevaluated using the BAI bone-conductor demonstration device. The demonstration device is placed near the affected ear with the microphone directed toward the speaker.

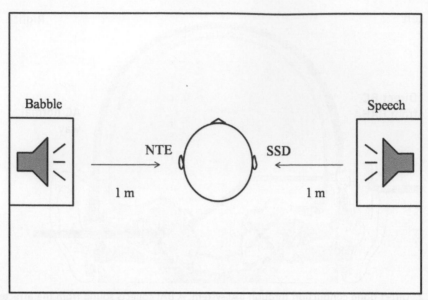

Fig. 3. Speech-in-Noise Test setup. Speech stimuli are directed toward the affected ear and babble noise is directed toward the better hearing ear.

- Performance is compared across varying conditions with the unaided baseline results, and potential benefit is predicted by overall improvement in adverse listening conditions.[30] This course of action not only provides the clinician with objective data regarding the expected performance with the implant following surgery, but also helps to establish realistic expectations for the patient. Tests such as the QuickSIN and BKB-SIN use a multitalker babble noise source, resulting in a highly relatable testing experience for patients. Speech-in-noise testing will frequently result in patient responses such as "this is the first time someone has really tested my hearing loss" or "this is exactly like the problem I have when I'm at a restaurant." Patients are able to experience the device by listening to it in-office and to appreciate the expected benefit using a simulated real-world listening environment, thus empowering both the clinician and the patient to make confident decisions regarding intervention.
- The same protocol (**Table 2**) can be applied using CROS hearing aids, and should be included in the selection process. Performance can be compared with baseline and BAI results.
- Time should be taken to demonstrate each device to the patient and review its function. The patient should be able to demonstrate the ability to manage the device, and this is even more crucial regarding the BAI, whereby the patient will be expected to manage the implant site as well as the external processor over a lifetime.

Once the evaluation process is complete, all of the data are reviewed with the patient to determine candidacy. No specific criteria exist for establishing the ideal candidate. Patients can present in a multitude of ways. The process is individual-specific and treatment decisions must be made with the patient. For example, consider the patient who demonstrates significant improvement on speech-in-noise testing, but displays very low handicap levels. Such a patient is not an optimal surgical

| Table 2 |
| Evaluation and verification treatment protocol for UHL |

Assessment of Candidacy

1. Basic comprehensive audiometric test battery
   a. Pure tone air and bone thresholds, speech recognition, immitance measures
   b. Ensure stable hearing, adequate residual hearing in better ear
2. Establish communication handicap/disability
   a. Use SSQ for assessment of localization/spatial deficits
3. Speech-in-noise testing in the sound field
   a. Establish SNR loss in unaided condition
   b. Reassess using demonstration devices when applicable (BAI, CROS)
   c. Speaker configuration
      i. Speech to affected ear, noise to better ear (270°/90° azimuth)
      ii. Speech to front, noise to better ear (0°/90° azimuth)
      iii. Speech and noise to front (0°/0° azimuth)
   d. Compare unaided to aided performance to predict benefit

Treatment Selection

1. Review single-sided deafness and potential auditory limitations
2. Review treatment options (see **Table 1**)
   a. Demonstrate devices to patients, report subjective benefit
3. Discuss benefits and limitations in relation to results of initial assessment

Fitting and Verification

1. Hearing aids
   a. Electroacoustic analyses
   b. Probe microphone measures
2. Bone-anchored implant
   a. Aided speech-in-noise testing in the sound field using previously described method
      i. Compare results to unaided and preintervention assessment results
   b. Aided loudness assessment using recorded speech at 55, 65, and 75 dBSPL
3. Device orientation
4. Validation of device benefit
   a. Hearing outcome measures
   b. Measures should be relevant the auditory deficits of the VS population

Management

1. Initial follow-up at 2–4 weeks
   a. Reassess hearing outcomes, fine tune as needed, verify speech-in-noise benefit
2. Long-term follow-up should be structured based on patient's communication needs and perceived handicap/disability
   a. Recommended minimum is 3 months, 6 months, and annually

candidate. Patients who present with very low handicap levels despite objective benefit often state postoperatively that they do not wear their devices often or that they do not perceive benefit from their device. Another patient may present with significant handicap but little to no benefit from aided speech-in-noise testing. This patient is likely to have unrealistic expectations and will be left frustrated and dissatisfied after surgery.

All of the aforementioned options are intended for patients who have normal to near-normal hearing in the better hearing ear. Indications for BAIs in this population have been limited to those persons who have less than 20 dB PTA in the better ear. However, many VS patients present with some degree of hearing loss in the better hearing ear. For these patients, particularly those with significant impairment, amplification of the better ear is required for adequate remediation of the hearing loss. This scenario has traditionally been addressed with bilateral CROS (BiCROS) amplification, and has recently been shown to have high satisfaction and acceptance rates.[31] Increasingly, BAIs also are being used in this complex patient population. A recent study by Wazen and colleagues[32] found that BAI patients with mild to moderate hearing loss in the better hearing ear showed improved performance on objective tests and that 91% reported improved quality of life. These findings are not without controversy, and it is noteworthy that these applications continue to be considered as outside the standard clinical guidelines. This fact underscores the importance of a comprehensive evaluation to determine candidacy. Conventional amplification may be considered for the better ear.

The evaluation and selection process uses a battery of objective and subjective tests to gather data for the clinician to use as a guideline in counseling the patient on the hearing loss, expectations, and options. Often, treatment is straightforward and patients find immediate success. However, for those patients who are faced with greater challenges such as reduced auditory processing ability, physical complications, cognitive factors, and so forth, motivation and realistic expectations will drive the outcome.

Fitting hearing devices Regardless of which treatment option is selected, fitting a device is a multistep process. The fitting protocol will vary slightly based on the intervention. During the fitting appointment, the device is programmed to the patient's residual hearing profile in the better hearing ear and to meet the listening needs of the patient. Adjustments may be made to increase patient comfort.

Key components to a successful fitting include:

- Ensuring that soft speech is audible
- Ensuring that loud sounds are within the level of patient comfort
- Maintaining clarity of speech.

Counseling patients on communication strategies and establishing realistic expectations with the patient and communication partners is a fundamental element of the fitting process. Care should be taken to ensure that device orientation, care, and maintenance are well understood.

The final step in the fitting process is device validation and verification. This step is an essential one in the process to determine whether the device is providing expected benefit and, in the case of hearing aids, meeting prescribed targets. Numerous options exist to assist the clinician in verification of performance, including, but not limited to, electroacoustic analyses, real ear measurements, functional gain testing, and speech-in-noise testing.

The accepted protocol for hearing-aid verification includes electroacoustic analyses and real ear measurements. BAIs are expected to be more difficult to verify objectively. At present, clinical tools for assessing frequency-specific output levels of implantable devices are lacking. A common means of validation/verification is testing threshold responses to narrow-band signals through the implant in the sound field. This method provides only limited information regarding device performance with soft sounds in a quiet environment.[33,34] Just as the pure tone audiogram is not an accurate representation of real-world listening abilities, functional gain measures are not an accurate representation of device performance and have long been criticized in the hearing-aid model.[33,34] The authors' recommendation is to repeat the previously described preoperative test protocol using speech-in-noise measures with the patient's implant system in place.[30] This action will validate whether the patient is receiving the listening-in-noise benefit predicted in the preoperative assessment. Speech-in-noise measures can also be used to evaluate performance at varying input levels. Such measures will help to verify soft-speech audibility and intelligibility, and identify whether loud speech is too loud or uncomfortable. Lack of objective measures to verify frequency and gain-specific output of implantable devices underscores the importance of a good clinical protocol to ensure success of a given treatment. The subsequent component of the validation process is postoperative and rehabilitative outcome measures such as the APHAB, GHABP, and SSQ previously discussed. It is recommended that at a minimum these are completed during the 2-week and 6-month follow-up appointments.

Management of rehabilitation of the VS patient Over time, patients are subject to changes in both their auditory profile and communication needs. Validation of user benefit and satisfaction is a fundamental component of ensuring successful long-term management of the VS patient, which is best achieved using subjective measures to determine each patient's individual needs. Much of the rehabilitation process relies on counseling. Simply empowering patients and their communication partners by enabling them to understand the auditory deficit instantly aids in the process of establishing realistic expectations. Following this, they can be successfully educated on how to optimize communication in their daily life. Global strategies are provided, but situation-specific strategies help each individual achieve success based on his or her personal communication needs.

Tinnitus

Tinnitus is the second most common complaint of patients with VS, and it has been estimated that approximately 70% of VS patients present with tinnitus.[27,35] Although tumor removal improves or even resolves tinnitus in many patients, it can also result in worsening of tinnitus.[35] In severe cases, tinnitus can be debilitating and can negatively affect quality of life.

Tinnitus is complex and difficult to treat. Historically, this has led many clinicians to avoid assessment and treatment of tinnitus during the rehabilitation process. However, given the prevalence of tinnitus in the VS population, it is the clinician's responsibility to assess the presence, severity, and psychosocial impact of tinnitus in these patients. Many patients report tinnitus, but what dictates its management is the degree to which it affects the patient's life. This extent can be determined by a thorough history and by using subjective measures such as the Tinnitus Handicap Inventory (THI) and the Tinnitus Reaction Questionnaire (TRQ). The THI is a validated tool for assessing the impact of tinnitus on daily living, and can be easily incorporated into the rehabilitation process.[36] The TRQ is used to assess the psychological distress associated with tinnitus, and can be used to assess changes over time.[37]

Several proposed treatment options are available for patients with tinnitus; however, reported results and success rates vary considerably.[38–40] The perception of tinnitus can provoke emotional reactions.[41] For this reason, many treatment options have included treating the emotional response rather than the tinnitus itself. A good treatment protocol addresses both the physiologic and psychological components of the disorder. For this reason it is essential to include subjective assessments as well as objective data. With the appropriate information many patients can be successfully remediated with counseling and/or cognitive behavioral therapy.[41] During the counseling process, patients should be provided with information regarding the origin of their tinnitus, its relationship to their VS, the emotional response to the tinnitus, coping strategies, lifestyle management, and treatment options. In many cases, simply informing the patient can result in reduced stress and anxiety, thereby reducing the negative response to the tinnitus. The goal of cognitive behavioral therapy is to reduce the negative associations to tinnitus by changing thought processes to alter the emotional response of the patient.[41]

Many current treatment protocols call for sound generators in the ipsilateral ear to either mask the tinnitus or facilitate habituation.[38,40] The application of this approach is limited in postsurgical treatment because of the profound hearing loss. As a result, treatment of tinnitus in the VS population is met with even greater challenges. Neuromonics (Neuromonics Inc, Bethlehem, PA, USA) tinnitus treatment (NTT)[42] suggests a contralateral protocol for the assessment and treatment of patients with unilateral severe to profound hearing loss. NTT uses an acoustic stimulation to promote desensitization by prescribing a broadband signal customized for each patient's audiometric profile combined with relaxing music that intermittently covers the patient's tinnitus perception.[42,43] As early as 1983, Tyler[41] suggested the possibility of masking tinnitus using the contralateral ear. Subsequent research, however, has been limited and warrants further study.

New approaches to managing tinnitus include repetitive transcranial magnetic stimulation (rTMS). rTMS stimulates the motor cortex using low-frequency magnetic pulses applied at the temporal lobe,[44] which is thought to produce an inhibitory effect on the tinnitus.[44] Although not readily available for clinical application, rTMS has shown promise in recent studies.[45,46] Khedr and colleagues[47] were able to demonstrate temporary reduction in tinnitus even when stimulation was at the contralateral temporal lobe. Given that rTMS acts at the cortical level rather than at the ear level by previously described devices, may prove it to be a viable option for the VS population.

Treatment of tinnitus should include a multidisciplinary approach involving physicians, audiologists, psychologists, and/or psychiatrists. In some patients the perception of tinnitus is so debilitating that it results in depression and anxiety. Signs or reports of extreme emotional distress should not be overlooked. Clinicians should familiarize themselves with severe emotional signs or reactions to tinnitus and should have a clear protocol in place indicating when to refer to a psychologist and/or psychiatrist as part of the multidisciplinary treatment plan.

Occasionally, auditory rehabilitation of patients with severe to profound UHL is complicated by the presence of debilitating tinnitus. Tinnitus is an extremely complex disorder that warrants comprehensive evaluation and management. The clinical assessment and treatment options related to patients with VS provided in this article should provide a practical overview to clinicians faced with the added challenge of tinnitus management. For further information, the reader is encouraged to consult other relevant articles.[15,37,40–42]

VESTIBULAR HABILITATION
Functional Anatomy and Physiology

Each labyrinth contains 3 semicircular canals and 2 otolith organs that detect head acceleration. The semicircular canals (horizontal, posterior, and superior) respond to angular acceleration and are roughly orthogonal to each other. Alignment of the semicircular canals (SCCs) in the temporal bone is such that each SCC has a contralateral coplanar mate. The posterior SCC forms a coplanar pair with the contralateral superior canal, and the horizontal SCCs are mated with each other. The coplanar pairs of the SCC exhibit a push-pull dynamic, which enables the secondary (central) neurons to detect head motion from either end organ. One end of each SCC is enlarged (the ampullated end) and contains the cupula, the sensory epithelium, and the sensory hair cell. The sensory hair cells house the kinocilia and stereocilia, which deflect based on endolymphatic flow. Their deflection causes either depolarization or hyperpolarization of the membrane potential, which will either excite or inhibit the afferent neuron. The horizontal SCC primarily detects horizontal head rotation; the superior SCC primarily detects pitch-down head rotation; and the posterior SCC primarily detects pitch-up head rotation.

The saccular and utricular end organs respond to linear acceleration and tilt. In the otolith end organs, sensory hair cells project into a gelatinous material that has calcium carbonate crystalline material (otoconia) embedded within. The otolith organs also have kinocilia and stereocilia as part of their sensory hair cells, which are also excited or inhibited depending on the direction of their deflection. Utricular excitation occurs during horizontal linear acceleration or static head tilt, and saccular excitation occurs during vertical linear acceleration.

The inferior vestibular nerve innervates the saccule and the posterior semicircular canals, whereas the superior vestibular nerve innervates the superior and horizontal semicircular canals as well as the utricle (**Fig. 4**). Recent data suggest most VS arise along the inferior vestibular nerve,[48,49] whereas older data reported that VS of the superior vestibular nerve were more common.[50,51] Occasionally, surgical removal of VS spares the superior or inferior vestibular nerve, with spared residual afferent

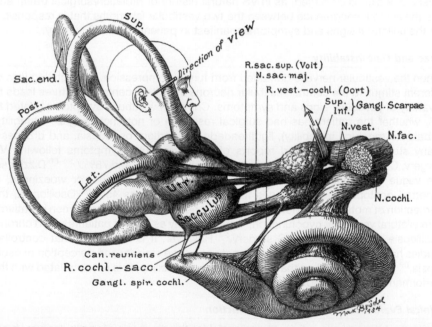

Fig. 4. Anatomy of the peripheral vestibular labyrinth. Structures include the utricle (Utr.), sacculus, superior (anterior) semicircular canal, posterior semicircular canal (inferior), and the lateral semicircular canal (horizontal). Note the superior vestibular nerve innervating the anterior and lateral semicircular canals as well as the utricle. The inferior vestibular nerve innervates the posterior semicircular canal and the saccule. The cell bodies of the vestibular nerves are located in Scarpa's ganglion (Gangl. Scarpae). (Picture provided courtesy of Cochlear™ Americas, © 2012 Cochlear Americas.)

function. This circumstance depends on tumor location and can be important for expectations regarding recovery. The superior and inferior divisions of the vestibular nerve travel together into the pontomedullary junction, where they bifurcate. Primary vestibular afferents from the superior division of the vestibular nerve synapse in the superior and medial vestibular nuclei, and the uvula, nodulus, flocculus, or fastigial nucleus of the cerebellum.[52–55] Primary vestibular afferents from the inferior branch synapse in the medial, lateral, or inferior vestibular nuclei, which, along with the superior vestibular nuclei and other subnuclei, comprise the vestibular nuclear complex.[56]

Secondary vestibular afferents relay signals from the vestibular nuclei to the extraocular motor nuclei, the spinal cord, and the flocculus of the cerebellum.[57] Although many vestibular reflexes are controlled by processes that exist primarily within the brainstem, extensive connections exist between the vestibular nuclei and the reticular formation,[58] thalamus,[59] cerebellum,[52] and the junction of the parietal and insular lobes. Connections with the vestibular cortex, thalamus, and reticular formation enable the vestibular system to contribute to the integration of arousal and conscious awareness of the body, and to discriminate between movement of self and the environment.[60,61] Connections with the cerebellum maintain calibration of the vestibulo-ocular reflex (VOR), contribute to posture during static and dynamic activities, and influence the coordination of limb movements.

In primates, primary vestibular afferents of the healthy vestibular system have a resting firing rate that is typically 70 to 100 spikes per second.[62,63] This rate means that the vestibular system is constantly sending afferent information to the brain, unless one side is damaged, as in VS natural history or radiation/surgical treatment. It is the acute incongruence between the two vestibular labyrinths that is responsible for the unilateral signs and symptoms manifest in patients after VS surgery.

Gaze and Gait Instability

When the vestibular nerve is damaged from tumor compression, the resulting loss of afferent stimuli to the central vestibular neurons and other central structures leads to a variety of vestibular signs and symptoms. Common vestibular symptoms related to VS, whether the patient has had surgical resection or not, include gaze instability, imbalance (postural instability), lightheadedness, vertigo, oscillopsia, and dizziness. Many studies have examined reports of such vestibular symptoms following VS surgery. Chronic reports of imbalance range between 31% and 78%.[7,64–66] Dizziness, the vague symptom used to describe lightheadedness, vertigo, or wooziness, is reported postoperatively in ranges from 4% to as high as 45%.[67] Oscillopsia, the perception of motion of the visual world during head movement, is common in patients with bilateral vestibular hypofunction,[68] and as many as 78% of patients report chronic oscillopsia symptoms after VS surgery.[24] However, it is interesting that controlled studies have not found any correlation between gaze stability and perception of oscillopsia,[69,70] thus suggesting that the perception of oscillopsia is not correlated with the performance of gaze stability.[71,72]

Clinical Evaluation of Vestibular Dysfunction

A review of the common clinical tests useful for the diagnosis of vestibular hypofunction is presented here. For extended information, the reader is encouraged to read a review by Schubert and Minor.[73]

Head-impulse test

The head-impulse (or head-thrust) test is widely accepted as a valid indication of semicircular canal function.[74–76] Each of the SCCs can be examined independently.[77]

- Patients are asked to visually fixate a near target (ie, examiner's nose) while their head is unpredictably and manually rotated using a small-amplitude (5°–15°), high-acceleration (3000–4000°/s^2) angular thrust. In healthy function, excitation of the vestibular afferents (via the applied head impulse) causes oculomotor muscle contraction to move the eyes in the direction opposite to the head movement and through the exact angle required to keep images stable on the fovea. In vestibular hypofunction, the eyes move less than the required amount, which can be observed by the examiner. In hypofunction, at the end of the head movement the eyes will not be looking at the intended near target. Instead a rapid, corrective saccade is made to bring the target back on the fovea. The appearance of these corrective saccades indicates vestibular hypofunction as evaluated by the head-impulse test.
- To measure function from the horizontal SCC mediated via the superior vestibular nerve, the head is manually rotated in the horizontal plane (**Fig. 5**). A simple method to measure function from the vertical SCC first rotates the head 45° to the side before imparting a pitch-head rotation. For example, to examine the left anterior and right posterior canal (coplanar mates), the head would first be placed at a 45° rightward rotation. From this static position, the head would

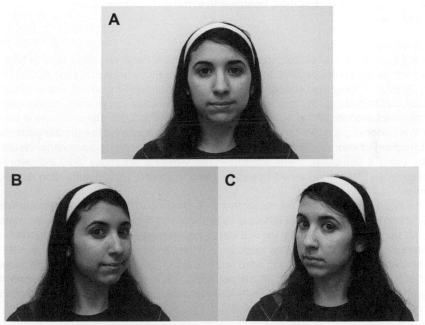

Fig. 5. Head-impulse test for the horizontal semicircular canal. The examiner applies the passive head-impulse test (HIT) to the patient, whose hands are not shown here. (A) The head is placed in a neck-neutral position and then rapidly moved to the left (B), which examines the left horizontal semicircular canal. The clinician should pause the head after the rotation and examine the eyes for a corrective saccade. Next, the head is slowly returned to center (A) and the right horizontal semicircular canal is examined with a rapid thrust rotation (C). For patients with cervical spine pathology, the clinician may choose to start with the head rotated to the side (as in B) and then rotate back to center (A), which in this example would examine the right horizontal semicircular canal. In this figure, the HIT is normal for each horizontal semicircular canal because the eyes have remained gazing forward.

then be quickly thrust downward (left anterior canal) and then separately upward (right posterior canal).

Head shaking–induced nystagmus

Nystagmus is an involuntary, repetitive back-and-forth motion of the eyes. Any nystagmus caused by vestibular pathology is composed of slow and fast eye-velocity rotations. The slow eye velocities are produced by the intact vestibular nerve, and the fast component is a resetting eye movement that brings the eyes close to the center of the oculomotor range.[78]

The head shaking–induced nystagmus (HSN) test is a useful tool to aid in the diagnosis of asymmetric peripheral vestibular input to central regions that mediate vestibular function. Typically a person with a unilateral loss of peripheral vestibular function will develop a horizontal HSN, with the quick phases of the nystagmus directed toward the healthy ear and the slow phases directed toward the hypofunctioning ear. Not all patients with a unilateral vestibular loss will have HSN.

- To complete the test, patients must have their vision blocked (eg, video infrared goggles).
- Next, the head is oscillated horizontally for 20 cycles at a frequency of 2 repetitions per second (2 Hz).
- On stopping the oscillation, people with symmetric peripheral vestibular input will not have HSN.

Dynamic visual acuity

Normal activities of daily life (such as running) can have head velocities of up to 550°/s, head accelerations of up to $6000°/s^2$, and high-frequency content of head motion from 2 to 20 Hz.[79,80] Only the vestibular system can detect head motion over this range of velocity, acceleration, and frequency. Gaze stability refers to the ability to see clearly during head motion, and is a behavioral measure of the VOR. Dynamic visual acuity (DVA) is becoming a more common tool to aid in the diagnosis of vestibular pathology and tracking of improvement in gaze instability.[69,81] DVA can be done either clinically or by using a computer.[82] The computerized versions are more valid indicators of hypofunction.[83] DVA done with passive head rotations can identify singular SCC lesions.[84]

The test is done by having subjects move their head actively or passively while attempting to identify flashing letters on a monitor or on a wall chart. The head motion should be greater than 100°/s (or ~2 Hz) to prevent other oculomotor systems from contributing to gaze stability. In healthy controls, head movement results in little or no change of visual acuity compared with keeping the head still. For patients with vestibular hypofunction, the VOR will not keep the eyes stable in space during the rapid head movements. This instability causes poor visual acuity during head motion in comparison with keeping the head still.

Static and dynamic balance

It is important to examine balance under static and dynamic conditions. Not only is this imperative to gauge function, it is also useful to assess the risk of a fall. Many tests exist for measures of static and dynamic balance. Because many patients after VS resection will have impaired balance, it is best to use those balance tests that have been validated in vestibular hypofunction. The best static measures of imbalance are those that attempt to isolate the unique sensory contributions for balance, namely vestibular afference, proprioception and vision. These sensory systems make up the primary balance effectors.

The modified clinical test for the sensory integration of balance is a quick, efficient means to measure static balance and determine the risk of a fall. This test asks patients to perform a Romberg test with eyes open then closed, standing on a firm then a foam surface. The foam surface offers a proprioceptive challenge. The test is therefore a battery of 4 separate, progressively more difficult tests that examine static balance with:

- Normal vision/normal proprioception: condition 1
- Absent vision/normal proprioception: condition 2
- Normal vision/altered proprioception: condition 3
- Absent vision/altered proprioception: condition 4.

Healthy controls should be able to stand for 30 seconds within 3 attempts for each of the 4 conditions. A recent study of United States adults aged 40 years and older (N = 5086) found the odds of falling increased as the time to failure decreased. Participants who failed in 20 to 29 seconds, 10 to 19 seconds, and fewer than 10 seconds had a 2.0-, 3.4-, and 3.6-fold increase in odds of falling, respectively.[85] Some other static tests that are more difficult include the tandem Romberg (standing heel to toe) and single-leg stance tests. Each static balance test is considered normal when balance is maintained for 30 seconds. **Table 3** lists of a few common tests of balance.

Vestibular Rehabilitation

Intervention evidence
Studies that investigate improvements of gaze and gait instability in patients after having VS resection are convincing. Compared with control groups, patients who performed customized vestibular rehabilitation have improved gaze stability[69] and improved static and dynamic balance.[86–88] The use of inhibitory amino acids (ie, baclofen) is known to cause inhibition between the bilateral vestibular nuclei, and is often provided as relief for related vestibular symptoms. Thus, it has been considered that patients who use baclofen and receive vestibular rehabilitation (VPT) may have a more complete recovery. However, the use of baclofen has not been found to improve static or dynamic balance measures beyond what customized vestibular rehabilitation could provide alone.[89]

The amount of retinal slip experienced during rehabilitation by subjects with VS resection seems to be critical to improvement. When post-VS patients were instructed to move their head as quickly as possible, with no apparent guidance concerning the amount of retinal slip experienced, no difference in imbalance was found compared with a group that had no head movement exercises.[90] However, when specific instructions are given for subjects to maintain fovea fixation of a target during the head rotation (vertical and horizontal), gaze stability improves[69,81] and subjective reports of dizziness[87,88] and disequilibrium lessen.[86] Those patients who are told to be active and are not specifically instructed to do vestibular rehabilitation exercises do not appear to recover as well.[87,88]

Intervention exercises
The optimal duration and repetition of these exercises are still unknown. However, studies that have shown benefit of a customized VPT program commonly advised patients to do the exercises between 3 and 5 times per day.[69,81,86–88] This repetition is supported by recent biomedical research suggesting that multiple time scales of learning exist, with different rates of both learning and forgetting. In addition, learning is influenced by the pattern of training, and rest periods seem to improve retention.

Table 3
Static and dynamic balance tests

Test	How to Do It	Interpretation	Expected Result
CTSIB	C1: Patient stands on firm surface feet together, arms across chest, eyes open C2: Patient stands on firm surface feet together, arms across chest, eyes closed C3: Patient stands on foam surface feet together, arms across chest, eyes open C4: Patient stands on foam surface feet together, arms across chest, eyes closed	Normal: mild sway, but ability to stand 30 s each condition Abnormal: fall, eyes open (when closed), patient takes a step/feet moved, arms become uncrossed	Acutely: C2–C4 commonly abnormal Chronic: C1–C3 normal, C4 may always be abnormal
Tandem Romberg	Stand heel to toe, arms crossed. Test often done with eyes open and closed	Normal: mild sway, but ability to stand 30 s Abnormal: fall, step/feet moved apart Age dependent, 30 s considered normal	Acutely: not able to stand in position Chronic: improved, may still be <30 s
Gait	Observe patient as he or she walks	None available	Acute: wide-based, slow, decreased arm swing and trunk rotation Compensated: normal
Turn head while walking	Ask patient to walk at normal speed and move head right or left every 3 s		Acute: side stepping, staggering, may not be able to keep balance Compensated: normal or mild sway

Abbreviations: CTSIB, clinical test for the sensory interaction on balance; C1–C4, conditions 1–4.

Table 4
Gaze stability exercises to improve retinal slip

Begin With	Progress To
Stand 10 ft from a 1-inch tall letter X placed at eye level. Keeping the target in focus, move your head left to right for 1 min. Move as quickly as you can, provided the target remains clear. Now do this with a vertical head rotation Hold 2 targets at arm's length from your head. Look with your eyes first, then turn your head toward the target. Attempt to do this for 1 min	Hold the letter at arm's length and eye level for 1 min, again taking caution to move as quickly as possible provided the target remains clear. Now do this with a vertical head rotation. This can be progressed using a busy background (checkerboard, venetian blinds) or while standing on foam Randomly place 6 or more targets (ie, letters A–F) on a wall. Start with A and progress to F using the same principle (eyes first followed by a head rotation, making sure the eyes remain fixed on the letter)
Hold one target at arm's length from your head. Close your eyes and turn your head away from the target, attempting to keep your eyes focused on the target. Open your eyes only after having turned your head	Progress to doing this standing, or decreasing base of support (bring feet together)

Each exercise is done for 1 minute, 5 times per day.

Learning is often uniquely paired with the environmental circumstances, suggesting that the therapy should involve different contexts. The cerebellum is essential for adaptation of most motor control systems, and data suggest that some normal function of specific lobes in the cerebellum is essential for learning.[91]

Gaze stability

Patients recovering from VS resection surgery should be instructed to perform gaze-stability exercises while an inpatient. These unique exercises task subjects to keep

Table 5
Examples of common balance exercises

Begin With	Progress To	Purpose
Stand with feet shoulder-width apart, arms across the chest, eyes closed for 15 s. Repeat 5 times	Bring feet closer together Stand on a compliant surface (ie, sofa cushion)	Enhances the use of vestibular input for balance by decreasing base of support and limiting proprioceptive input
Ankle sways. Stand with feet together and sway anterior/posterior and medial/lateral	Circle sways. Close eyes	Improves balance over limited base of support and teaches the patient to sway from the ankles: important postural function
Practice walking 5 forward steps, turning 180° then stopping	Make smaller turns	Challenges postural control
Walk and move your head side to side, up and down	Counting backward from 100 by threes	Uses distracting cognitive or motor demands to challenge balance

Each of the balance exercises should be performed 3 times a day for 1 to 2 minutes each repetition.

their eyes focused on a target (typically a letter) while they move their head horizontally and vertically for 1 minute.[81] It remains critical that the subjects are exposed to retinal slip. To achieve this, patients are instructed to move their head only as long as a target remains in focus. If the target begins to blur, the patients should be instructed to slow down their head velocity. This action is important because the brain can perceive a small amount of retinal slip (and thus drive adaptation) before visual acuity degrades.[92] **Table 4** lists some of the common vestibular adaptation gaze-stability exercises.

Gait stability

Static and dynamic balance exercises are equally important. These exercises reduce the risk of a fall. Static balance exercises are designed to improve the brain's ability to maintain a steady base of support. Dynamic balance exercises are designed to improve stability while moving. Important progressions that are more challenging should incorporate walking with head rotation, further requiring the brain to adjust to asymmetric vestibular input. Many variations of each type of exercise exist, and some typical examples are listed in **Table 5**.

SUMMARY

Removal of VS causes deficits in hearing, balance, and gaze stability. The resulting hearing loss eliminates the benefits of binaural listening that provide localization, loudness summation, and listening-in-noise ability. In the past, remediation of UHL was perceived as far too great a challenge for clinicians, and patients often went untreated. However, current treatment options have expanded to provide a wide range of possibilities for VS patients. Rehabilitation should no longer be limited to reliance on the better hearing ear, and modern treatment plans should include CROS, BiCROS, bone-conduction aids, and BAIs as options for all patients. Comprehensive auditory rehabilitation also includes tinnitus evaluation and management whenever necessary. For those VS patients with resulting vestibular deficits, symptoms can be debilitating, with a considerable impact on quality of life. The symptoms related to damage affecting the vestibular portion of the eighth cranial nerve are largely manageable with a return to activity and inclusion in a vestibular rehabilitation exercise program.

REFERENCES

1. Lin D, Hegarty JL, Fischbein NJ, et al. The prevalence of incidental acoustic neuroma. Arch Otolaryngol Head Neck Surg 2005;131:241–4.
2. Tos M, Stangerup S, Cayé-Thomasen P, et al. What is the real incidence of vestibular schwannoma? Arch Otolaryngol Head Neck Surg 2004;130:216–20.
3. Evans D, Gareth R, Moran A, et al. Incidence of vestibular schwannoma and neurofibromatosis 2 in the north west of England over a 10-year period: higher incidence than previously thought. Otol Neurotol 2005;26(1):93–7.
4. Stangerup SE, Tos M, Thomsen J, et al. True incidence of vestibular schwannoma? Neurosurgery 2010;67(5):1335–40.
5. Gal TJ, Shinn J, Huang B. Current epidemiology and management trends in acoustic neuroma. Otolaryngol Head Neck Surg 2010;142(5):677–81.
6. Anderson TD, Loevner LA, Bigelow DC, et al. Prevalence of unsuspected acoustic neuroma found by magnetic resonance imaging. Otolaryngol Head Neck Surg 2000;122:643–6.

7. Nicoucar K, Momjian S, Vader JP, et al. Surgery for large vestibular schwannomas: how patients and surgeons perceive quality of life. J Neurosurg 2006;105: 205–12.

8. Douglas SA, Yeung P, Daudia A, et al. Spatial hearing disability after acoustic neuroma removal. Laryngoscope 2007;117(9):1648–51.

9. Walsh RM, Bath AP, Bance ML, et al. The role of conservative management of vestibular schwannomas. Clin Otolaryngol 2000;25(1):28–39.

10. Anderson HT, Shroder SA, Bonding P. Unilateral deafness after acoustic neuroma surgery: subjective hearing handicap and the effectiveness of the bone-anchored hearing aid. Otol Neurotol 2006;27:809–14.

11. Welsh LW, Welsh JJ, Rosen LF, et al. Functional impairments due to unilateral deafness. Ann Otol Rhinol Laryngol 2004;113:987–93.

12. Giolas T, Wark D. Communication problems associated with unilateral hearing loss. J Speech Hear Disord 1967;41:336–43.

13. Killion MC, Niquette PA, Gudmundsen GI, et al. Development of a quick speech-in-noise test for measuring signal to-noise ratio loss in normal hearing and hearing impaired listeners. J Acoust Soc Am 2004;116(4):2395–405.

14. Taylor B. Speech-in-noise tests: how and why to include them in your basic test battery. Hear J 2003;56(1):40,42–46.

15. Newman CW, Sandridge SA, Jacobson GP. Psychometric adequacy of the tinnitus handicap inventory (THI) for evaluating treatment outcome. J Am Acad Audiol 1998;9:153–60.

16. Lin LM, Bowditch S, Anderson MJ, et al. Amplification in the rehabilitation of unilateral deafness: speech-in-noise and directional hearing effects with bone anchored hearing and contralateral routing of signal amplification. Otol Neurotol 2006;27(2):172–82.

17. Hol MK, Bosman AJ, Snik AF, et al. Bone-anchored hearing aids in unilateral inner ear deafness: an evaluation of audiometric and patient outcome measurements. Otol Neurotol 2005;26:999–1006.

18. Niparko JK, Cox KM, Lustig LR. Comparison of the bone anchored hearing aid implantable hearing device with contralateral routing of offside signal amplification rehabilitation of unilateral deafness. Otol Neurotol 2003;24:73–8.

19. Wazen JJ, Spitzer JB, Ghossaini SN, et al. Transcranial contralateral cochlear stimulation in unilateral deafness. Otolaryngol Head Neck Surg 2003;129(3): 248–54.

20. Wazen J, Ghossaini S, Spitzer J, et al. Localization by unilateral Baha users. Otolaryngol Head Neck Surg 2005;132(6):928–32.

21. Cox RM, Alexander GC. Abbreviate profile of hearing aid benefit. Ear Hear 1995; 16(2):149–243.

22. Gatehouse S. Glasgow Hearing Aid Benefit Profile: derivation and validation of a client-centered outcome measure for hearing aid services. J Am Acad Audiol 1999;10:80–101.

23. Gatehouse S, Noble W. The speech, spatial and qualities of hearing scale. Int J Audiol 2004;43(2):85–99.

24. Tufarelli D, Meli A, Alesii A, et al. Quality of life after acoustic neuroma surgery. Otol Neurotol 2006;27:403–9.

25. House JW, Kutz JW, Chung J, et al. Bone-anchored hearing aid subjective benefit for unilateral deafness. Laryngoscope 2010;120:601–7.

26. Newman CW, Sandridge SA, Wodzisz LM. Longitudinal benefit from and satisfaction with the Baha system for patients with acquired unilateral sensorineural hearing loss. Otol Neurotol 2008;28(8):1123–31.

27. Baguley DM, Bird J, Humphriss RL, et al. The evidence base for the application of contralateral bone anchored hearing aids in acquired unilateral sensorineural hearing loss in adults. Clin Otolaryngol 2006;31(1):6–14.

28. Etymotic Research, Inc. Bamford-Kowal-Bench Speech-in-Noise Test (Version 1.03) [audio CD]. Elk Grove Village (IL): Etymotic Research, Inc; 2005.

29. Nilsson M, Soli S, Sullivan J. Development of the Hearing in Noise Test for the measurement of speech reception thresholds in quiet and in noise. J Acoust Soc Am 1994;95:1085–99.

30. Snapp H, Fabry D, Telischi F, et al. A clinical protocol for predicting outcomes with an implantable prosthetic device (Baha) in patients with single-sided deafness. J Am Acad Audiol 2010;21(10):654–62.

31. Hill SL, Marcus A, Digges EN, et al. Assessment of patient satisfaction with various configurations of digital CROS and BiCROS hearing aids. Ear Nose Throat J 2006;85(7):427–30, 442.

32. Wazen JJ, Van Ess MJ, Alameda J, et al. The Baha system in patients with single-sided deafness and contralateral hearing loss. Otolaryngol Head Neck Surg 2010;142(4):554–9.

33. Seewald RC, Hudson SP, Gagne, et al. Comparison of two methods for estimating the sensation level of amplified speech. Ear Hear 1992;13(3):142–9.

34. Seewald RC, Moodie KS, Sinclair ST, et al. Traditional and theoretical approaches to selecting amplification for infants and young children. In: Bess FH, Gravel JS, editors. Amplification for children with auditory deficits. Nashville (TN): Bill Wilkerson Center Press; 1996. p. 161–91.

35. Kameda K, Shono T, Hashiguchi K, et al. Effect of tumor removal on tinnitus in patients with vestibular schwannoma. J Neurosurg 2010;112(1):152–7.

36. Newman CW, Jacobson GP, Spitzer JB. Development of the tinnitus handicap inventory. Arch Otolaryngol Head Neck Surg 1996;122(2):143–8.

37. Wilson PH, Henry J, Bowen M, et al. Tinnitus reaction questionnaire: psychometric properties of a measure of distress associated with tinnitus. J Speech Hear Res 1991;34:197–201.

38. Seidman MD, Standring RT, Dornhoffer JL. Tinnitus: current understanding and contemporary management. Curr Opin Otolaryngol Head Neck Surg 2010; 18(5):363–8.

39. Davis PB, Wilde RA, Steed LG, et al. Treatment of tinnitus with a customized acoustic neural stimulus: a controlled clinical study. Ear Nose Throat J 2008; 87(6):330–9.

40. Henry JA, Jastreboff MM, Jastreboff PJ, et al. Guide to conducting tinnitus retraining initial and follow-up interviews. J Rehabil Res Dev 2003;40(2):157–77.

41. Tyler R. Tinnitus treatment: clinical protocols. New York: Thieme; 2006. p. 1–22, 188–97.

42. Davis PB, Paki B, Hanley PJ. Neuromonics tinnitus treatment: third clinical trial. Ear Hear 2007;28(2):242–59.

43. Hanley PJ, Davis PB, Paki B, et al. Treatment of tinnitus with a customized, dynamic acoustic neural stimulus: clinical outcomes in general private practice. Ann Otol Rhinol Laryngol 2008;117(11):791–9.

44. Chen R, Classen J, Gerloff C, et al. Depression of motor cortex excitability by low-frequency transcranial magnetic stimulation. Neurology 1997;48: 1398–403.

45. Khedr EM, Rothwell JC, Ahmed MA, et al. Effect of daily repetitive transcranial magnetic stimulation for treatment of tinnitus: comparison of different stimulus frequencies. J Neurol Neurosurg Psychiatry 2008;79(2):212–5.

46. Smith JA, Mennemeier M, Bartel T, et al. Repetitive transcranial magnetic stimulation for tinnitus: a pilot study. Laryngoscope 2007;117(3):529–34.
47. Khedr EM, Rothwell JC, El-Atar A. One-year follow up of patients with chronic tinnitus treated with left temporoparietal rTMS. Eur J Neurol 2009; 16(3):404–8.
48. Jacob A, Robinson LL Jr, Bortman JS, et al. Nerve of origin, tumor size, hearing preservation, and facial nerve outcomes in 359 vestibular schwannoma resections at a tertiary care academic center. Laryngoscope 2007;117(12): 2087–92.
49. Khrais T, Romano GM. Nerve origin of vestibular schwannoma: a prospective study. J Laryngol Otol 2008;122(2):128–31.
50. Henschen F. Concerning the history and pathogenesis of cerebellopontine tumors. Arch Psychiatry 1915;56:21.
51. Clemis JD, Ballad WJ, Baggot PJ, et al. Relative frequency of inferior vestibular schwannoma. Arch Otolaryngol Head Neck Surg 1986;112:190–4.
52. Brodal A, Brodal P. Observations on the secondary vestibulocerebellar projections in the macaque monkey. Exp Brain Res 1985;58:62–74.
53. Furuya N, Kawano K, Shimazu H. Functional organization of vestibulofastigial projection in the horizontal semicircular canal system in the cat. Exp Brain Res 1975;24(1):75–87.
54. Korte GE, Mugnaini E. The cerebellar projection of the vestibular nerve in the cat. J Comp Neurol 1979;184:265–78.
55. Goldberg JM. Afferent diversity and the organization of central vestibular pathways. Exp Brain Res 2000;130:277–97.
56. Naito Y, Newman A, Lee WS, et al. Projections of the individual vestibular endorgans in the brain stem of the squirrel monkey. Hear Res 1995;87:141–55.
57. Highstein SM, Goldberg JM, Moschovakis AK, et al. Inputs from regularly and irregularly discharging vestibular nerve afferents to secondary neurons in the vestibular nuclei of the squirrel monkey. II: correlation with output pathways of secondary neurons. J Neurophysiol 1987;58:719–38.
58. Troiani D, Petrosini L, Zannoni B. Relations of single semicircular canals to the pontine reticular formation. Arch Ital Biol 1976;114:337–75.
59. Buttner U, Henn V. Thalamic unit activity in the alert monkey during natural vestibular stimulation. Brain Res 1976;103:127–32.
60. Dieterich M, Bense S, Stephan T, et al. fMRI signal increases and decreases in cortical areas during small-field optokinetic stimulation and central fixation. Exp Brain Res 2003;148:117–27.
61. Brandt T, Dieterich M. Vestibular syndromes in the roll plane: topographic diagnosis from brainstem to cortex. Ann Neurol 1994;36:337–47.
62. Goldberg JM, Fernandez C. Physiology of peripheral neurons innervating semicircular canals of the squirrel monkey, I: resting discharge and response to constant angular accelerations. J Neurophysiol 1971;34:635–60.
63. Lysakowski A, Minor LB, Fernandez C, et al. Physiological identification of morphologically distinct afferent classes innervating the cristae ampullares of the squirrel monkey. J Neurophysiol 1995;73:1270–81.
64. Wiegand DA, Fickel V. Acoustic neuroma—the patient's perspective: subjective assessment of symptoms, diagnosis, therapy, and outcome in 541 patients. Laryngoscope 1989;99:179–87.
65. Driscoll CL, Lynn SG, Harner SG, et al. Preoperative identification of patients at risk of developing persistent dysequilibrium after acoustic neuroma removal. Am J Otol 1998;19:491–5.

66. Darrouzet V, Martel J, Enee V, et al. Vestibular schwannoma surgery outcomes: our multidisciplinary experience in 400 cases over 17 years. Laryngoscope 2004;114:681–8.
67. Saman Y, Bamiou DE, Gleeson M. A contemporary review of balance dysfunction following vestibular schwannoma surgery. Laryngoscope 2009;119(11):2085–93.
68. Gillespie MB, Minor LB. Prognosis in bilateral vestibular hypofunction. Laryngoscope 1999;109(1):35–41.
69. Herdman SJ, Schubert MC, Das VE, et al. Recovery of dynamic visual acuity in unilateral vestibular hypofunction. Arch Otolaryngol Head Neck Surg 2003; 129(8):819–24.
70. Herdman SJ, Hall CD, Schubert MC, et al. Recovery of dynamic visual acuity in bilateral vestibular hypofunction. Arch Otolaryngol Head Neck Surg 2007;133(4): 383–9.
71. Grunfeld EA, Morland AB, Bronstein AM, et al. Adaptation to oscillopsia: a psychophysical and questionnaire investigation. Brain 2000;123(2):277–90.
72. Schubert MC, Herdman SJ, Tusa RJ. Vertical dynamic visual acuity in normal subjects and patients with vestibular hypofunction. Otol Neurotol 2002;23(3):372–7.
73. Schubert MC, Minor LB. Vestibulo-ocular physiology underlying vestibular hypofunction. Phys Ther 2004;84(4):373–85.
74. Harvey SA, Wood DJ, Feroah TR. Relationship of the head impulse test and head-shake nystagmus in reference to caloric testing. Am J Otol 1997;18:207–13.
75. Beynon GJ, Jani P, Baguley DM. A clinical evaluation of head impulse testing. Clin Otolaryngol 1998;23:117–22.
76. Schubert MC, Tusa RJ, Herdman SJ, et al. Optimizing the sensitivity of the head thrust test for identifying vestibular hypofunction. Phys Ther 2004a;84:151–8.
77. Cremer PD, Halmagyi GM, Aw ST, et al. Semicircular canal plane head impulses detect absent function of individual semicircular canals. Brain 1998;121:699–716.
78. Hain TC, Fetter M, Zee DS. Head-shaking nystagmus in patients with unilateral peripheral vestibular lesions. Am J Otolaryngol 1987;8:36–47.
79. Grossman GE, Leigh RJ, Abel LA, et al. Frequency and velocity of rotational head perturbations during locomotion. Exp Brain Res 1988;70:470–6.
80. Das VE, Zivotofsky AZ, DiScenna AO, et al. Head perturbations during walking while viewing a head-fixed target. Aviat Space Environ Med 1995;66:728–32.
81. Schubert MC, Migliaccio AA, Clendaniel RA, et al. Mechanism of dynamic visual acuity recovery with vestibular rehabilitation. Arch Phys Med Rehabil 2008;89(3): 500–7.
82. Dannenbaum E, Paquet N, Chilingaryan G, et al. Clinical evaluation of dynamic visual acuity in subjects with unilateral vestibular hypofunction. Otol Neurotol 2009;30(3):368–72.
83. Herdman SJ, Tusa RJ, Blatt P, et al. Computerized dynamic visual acuity test in the assessment of vestibular deficits. Am J Otol 1998;19(6):790–6.
84. Schubert MC, Migliaccio AA, Della Santina CC. Dynamic visual acuity during passive head thrusts in canal planes. J Assoc Res Otolaryngol 2006;7(4):329–38.
85. Agrawal Y, Carey JP, Hoffman HJ, et al. The modified Romberg balance test: normative data in U.S. adults. Otol Neurotol 2011;32(8):1309–11.
86. Herdman SJ, Clendaniel RA, Mattox DE, et al. Vestibular adaptation exercises and recovery: acute stage after acoustic neuroma resection. Otolaryngol Head Neck Surg 1995;113(1):77–87.
87. Enticott JC, O'leary SJ, Briggs RJ. Effects of vestibulo-ocular reflex exercises on vestibular compensation after vestibular schwannoma surgery. Otol Neurotol 2005;26(2):265–9.

88. Vereeck L, Wuyts FL, Truijen S, et al. The effect of early customized vestibular rehabilitation on balance after acoustic neuroma resection. Clin Rehabil 2008; 22:698–713.
89. De Valck CF, Vereeck L, Wuyts FL, et al. Failure of gamma-aminobutyrate acid-beta agonist baclofen to improve balance, gait, and postural control after vestibular schwannoma resection. Otol Neurotol 2009;30(3):350–5.
90. Cohen HS, Kimball KT, Jenkin HA. Factors affecting recovery after acoustic neuroma resection. Acta Otolaryngol 2002;122(8):841–50.
91. Schubert MC, Zee DS. Saccade and vestibular ocular motor adaptation. Restor Neurol Neurosci 2010;28(1):9–18.
92. Demer JL, Amjadi F. Dynamic visual acuity of normal subjects during vertical optotype and head motion. Invest Ophthalmol Vis Sci 1993;34(6):1894–906.

Habilitation of Facial Nerve Dysfunction After Resection of a Vestibular Schwannoma

Kelli L. Rudman, MD, John S. Rhee, MD, MPH*

KEYWORDS

- Facial nerve repair • Facial paralysis • Facial nerve algorithm
- Facial nerve substitution • Dynamic facial reconstruction
- Static facial reconstruction • Vestibular schwannoma • Acoustic neuroma

The incidence of facial nerve dysfunction after resection of vestibular schwannoma has significantly decreased with the widespread use of microsurgical techniques. Postoperative facial nerve weakness, however, is reported in 8% to 20% of patients in the immediate postoperative period.[1,2] The incidence is as high as 25% of patients when delayed postoperative paralysis is considered.[3] Facial nerve paralysis associated with resection of a vestibular schwannoma remains the most common indication for facial nerve habilitation. This overview presents common and emerging management options for facial habilitation after resection of vestibular schwannoma. Immediate and delayed nerve repair options, as well as adjunctive surgical, medical, and physical therapies for facial nerve dysfunction, are discussed. Two algorithms (**Figs. 1** and **2**) are provided as guides for the assessment and treatment of facial nerve paralysis after resection of vestibular schwannoma.

EARLY POSTOPERATIVE ASSESSMENT AND MANAGEMENT OF FACIAL PARALYSIS

Consultation for facial paralysis after resection of a vestibular schwannoma begins with obtaining the pertinent history, which includes determination of preoperative facial nerve function and inquisition regarding the functional and anatomic findings of the facial nerve during surgery; for example, whether increased stimulation thresholds were required with intraoperative electromyographic monitoring, whether the nerve was stretched, or whether the nerve was transected. If the nerve was transected, it is important to know if an anastomotic procedure was attempted. Examination of the patient provides clinical assessment of the facial nerve function. The

The authors have nothing to disclose.
Department of Otolaryngology and Communication Sciences, Medical College of Wisconsin, 9200 West Wisconsin Avenue, Milwaukee, WI 53226, USA
* Corresponding author.
E-mail address: jrhee@mcw.edu

Otolaryngol Clin N Am 45 (2012) 513–530
doi:10.1016/j.otc.2011.12.015
0030-6665/12/$ – see front matter © 2012 Elsevier Inc. All rights reserved.

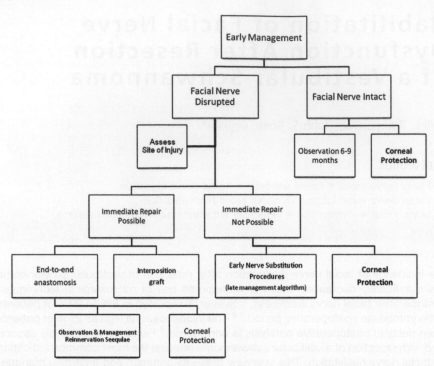

Fig. 1. Early postoperative management decisions in patients with facial paralysis after resection of a vestibular schwannoma.

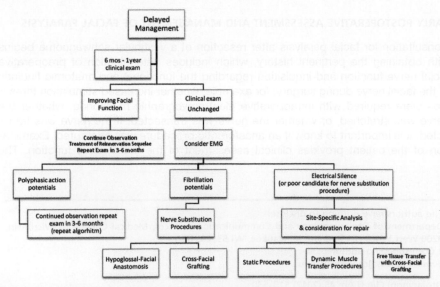

Fig. 2. Late postoperative management decisions in patients with facial paralysis after resection of a vestibular schwannoma.

House-Brackmann (HB) scoring system (**Table 1**) is the ideal facial nerve grading system for these patients.[4] The HB score should be documented at each visit. A complete cranial nerve examination must also be performed because other cranial nerve deficits (IX–XII), although uncommon, may alter management decisions. The ophthalmic division of the trigeminal nerve and the hypoglossal nerve are particularly important in this regard.

Early management decisions are based on clinical examination results and surgical details (see **Fig. 1**). If the facial nerve is disrupted during surgery, the gold standard for repair is primary end-to-end anastomosis or interposition grafting. When a truncated proximal facial nerve does not allow for primary repair, nerve substitution procedures may be considered early in the postoperative management (see **Fig. 2**). In some cases, nerve substitution procedures may be considered during the initial hospitalization. All of these patients require corneal protection.

If the facial nerve is anatomically intact at the end of surgery, the chance for regeneration is good, and provision of corneal protection is the most important treatment during the acute hospitalization and immediate future. These patients may be treated conservatively, with observation and delay of definitive treatment for 6 months to 1 year.

Immediate Facial Nerve Repair: Primary Anastomosis and Interposition Grafting

There is a disruption of the facial nerve in an estimated 2% to 10% of vestibular schwannoma resections.[5] When this occurs, the gold standard is to repair with

Table 1
House-Brackmann Grading Scale

Grade	Description	Characteristics
I	Normal	Normal facial function in all areas
II	Mild dysfunction	*Gross:* slight weakness noticeable on close inspection; may have very slight synkinesis *At rest:* normal symmetry and tone *Motion:* forehead, slight to moderate movement; eye, complete closure with minimal effort; mouth, slight asymmetry
III	Moderate dysfunction	*Gross:* obvious but not disfiguring difference between the 2 sides; noticeable but not severe synkinesis *At rest:* normal symmetry and tone *Motion:* forehead, slight to moderate movement; eye, complete closure with effort; mouth, slightly weak with maximal effort
IV	Moderately severe dysfunction	*Gross:* obvious weakness and or/disfiguring *At rest:* normal symmetry and tone *Motion:* forehead, none; eye, incomplete closure; mouth, asymmetric with maximum effort
V	Severe dysfunction	*Gross:* only barely perceptible motion *At rest:* asymmetry *Motion:* forehead, none; eye, incomplete closure; mouth, slight movement
VI	Total paralysis	No movement

primary end-to-end anastomosis or interposition nerve grafting. The repair of the facial nerve follows standard microsurgical techniques, with delicate and minimal nerve handling and tensionless approximation of the epineurium. The goal of exposing many neurotubules to one another is encouraged by freshening the nerve ends to angles of 45° before anastomosis.[6]

Primary end-to-end anastomosis of the intracranial facial nerve is possible when a proximal stump remains at the brainstem, and is much more difficult in the absence of a proximal stump because the nerve is not covered by epineurium at the brainstem and, therefore, is difficult to suture. Primary end-to-end anastomosis is advantageous to the patient because it addresses the deficit at the time of the initial surgery while possibly avoiding a second operation. In addition, primary repair avoids deficits from the use of a nerve graft for interposition. The main challenge in primary anastomosis involves obtaining a tensionless repair. Often, a tensionless repair necessitates facial nerve rerouting to provide additional length of the distal segment. The ability to perform rerouting and mobilization depends on the surgical approach used for resection and the surgeon's experience.[7]

Following a translabyrinthine approach:

- 5 to 10 mm of nerve can be mobilized by drilling out the nerve from the stylomastoid foramen and following it through to the internal auditory canal.
- Once the nerve is mobilized and repositioned, it may be sutured to the proximal stump.
- Because of the technical difficulty of suturing this anastomosis, fibrin glue has been described as an alternative for fixation of the nerve at the brainstem. Advocates of fibrin glue maintain that there is decreased neural trauma using glue rather than suture.[5,8,9]
- The tenuous anastomosis (with either suture or fibrin glue) is supported by packing. A variety of materials has been proposed as support, including abdominal fat, fascia, or acellular dermal matrix.[7,8,10]

In one case series reporting rerouting with anastomosis at the cerebellopontine angle, 15 of 18 patients achieved HB grade III or IV outcomes.[10]

When primary end-to-end anastomosis is not possible, interposition grafting is the next preferred option. Advantages for the patient are similar to end-to-end repair, except for donor nerve morbidity. Some investigators advocate the use of interposition grafting versus facial nerve rerouting because it is not as technically demanding. In addition, the blood supply of the distal facial nerve remains uninterrupted when using an interposition graft.[5,8] The main disadvantage of interposition grafting is that there are 2 anastomotic sites. The sural and great auricular nerves are the most commonly used donor nerves. Like primary end-to-end repair, the intracranial anastomotic sites should be surrounded with structural support. Multiple case series using interposition grafting between the intracranial facial nerve and the extratemporal facial nerve report HB scores better than III in 45% to 75% of patients at 1 year.[6,8,11]

Corneal Protection

Corneal protection is of paramount importance for patients with facial paralysis. The cornea is at risk secondary to paralytic lagophthalmos and lower lid laxity. The risk is increased when accompanied by a sensory deficit of the ophthalmic division of the trigeminal nerve. The inability to completely close the eye leaves the cornea exposed to foreign bodies and the risk of drying, and may lead to exposure keratitis, abrasions, ulcerations, and abscess formation. Devastating consequences to vision may occur, therefore immediate postoperative protection is essential. Conservative, nonsurgical options should be used in the immediate postoperative period until more definitive options are available. These interventions include frequent use of artificial tears, application of lubricating ophthalmic ointment, and application of an occlusive moisture chamber during sleep.[12]

When patients are at high risk for corneal injury, early surgical intervention should be considered. High-risk patients include those who:

- Lack Bell phenomena
- Have trigeminal sensory deficits
- Are unable to independently perform frequent eye care
- Are advanced in age
- Have a significant contralateral vision deficit.

Tarsorrhaphy and placement of an upper eyelid weight are the common early procedures performed. In high-risk patients, the treating physician should strongly consider surgical intervention for corneal protection before the patient's discharge from the initial hospitalization.

Tarsorrhaphy
Tarsorrhaphy involves partially sewing the eyelids together and is a reversible, technically simple procedure that was the standard of care for corneal protection for many years. It remains an option for temporary protection. However, because tarsorrhaphy results in poor cosmetic outcomes and deficits in the visual field, it is reserved for patients with the highest risk of exposure keratitis, those who have failed other options, or those with corneal sensory deficits.

Placement of an upper eyelid weight
Placement of an upper eyelid weight, most commonly a gold weight, is the first-line surgical treatment for paralytic lagophthalmos. Gold weights are well tolerated by patients and can easily be removed if facial function returns. Prefabricated gold weights from 0.6 to 1.8 g are available.

- To choose the appropriately sized weight, a sample weight is taped to the upper eyelid, centered over the medial limbus, while the patient is in an upright position.
- The weight remains in place for 15 minutes to allow the patient to adapt and make size adjustments.
- The largest weight that produces eyelid closure with only slight lid ptosis is chosen.
- Placement of an upper eyelid weight can be performed under local anesthesia.

Although widely used, gold-weight placement does carry some risks:

- Implant extrusion is the most commonly reported undesired outcome. The literature demonstrates a wide range of implant extrusion from 1% to 45%.[13,14]
- Gold allergy is reported in 3% to 9% of the population.
- Local inflammation
- Implant bulging
- Postoperative infection.

Recently, thin-profile platinum weights have been described as an alternative to gold. The platinum weights are 11% smaller than the gold counterparts because of platinum's greater density, and allergy to platinum has not been described. Thin-profile platinum weights are implanted using the same surgical procedure as gold weights. Silver and colleagues[15] described their experience with 100 patients who underwent placement of platinum weights; all patients had adequate closure of the eye and only 6% experienced complications, with a 2.9% incidence of extrusion and 2% incidence of local tissue thickening.

The lower eyelid may also need to be addressed to provide adequate corneal protection in patients with facial paralysis. The orbicularis oculi muscle contributes to the integrity and tension of the medial and lateral canthal ligaments. Patients with paralytic lower lid deficits often present with paralytic ectropion, punctal displacement, and epiphora. Older patients with preoperative lower lid laxity and patients who do not undergo reinnervation procedures are at the highest risk. There are several procedures to address the lower lid, including tightening procedures such as the Bick procedure, lateral tarsal strip, medial canthoplasty, and mid-lid wedge resection. Lower lid elevation procedures include augmentation of the inferior tarsus with cartilage grafts or palate mucosa.

Because multiple surgical options are available and the lower lid anatomy is complex, a thorough examination is required before planning the repair.

- Normally, the lower lid should sit at the height of the lower limbus or above. A snap test performed by pulling the lower lid down and then allowing it to rebound may ascertain whether excessive laxity is present. A normal lower lid rebounds in 1 to 2 seconds, and a delayed retraction signifies loss of elasticity.
- Another helpful examination maneuver is a lateral traction test; this simulates a lid-tightening procedure. If the lateral traction test shows excessive punctum displacement (>2 mm), a medial canthoplasty should be considered.[16]

Most commonly, the authors prefer the Bick procedure or lateral tarsal strip in primary cases.

- The Bick procedure involves resecting a lateral wedge of the lower lid, developing a tongue of tarsus, and resuturing the lower lid to the lateral orbital rim (Fig. 3).[17]
- The lateral tarsal strip procedure involves performing an inferior lateral cantholysis to free the lower lid. The inferior lateral tarsus is exposed and sutured to the lateral orbital rim.
- Vagefi and Anderson[18] described a modification to the standard lateral tarsal strip that includes the addition of a mini-tarsorrhaphy whereby the lower and upper tarsus are denuded and sutured together to create a sharp canthal angle and prevent upper eyelid overhang.[16] This mini-tarsorrhaphy modification is not reversible and should not be performed in patients who may have nerve recovery.

Despite the careful preoperative examination and surgical execution, a significant percentage of patients have recurrence of lower lid laxity and require reoperation.

If a patient is not at high risk for corneal injury, periocular procedures may be performed electively. The decision to perform periocular reanimation procedures is dictated by:

- Patient symptoms
- Adherence to eye-lubricating regimens
- Patient-specific anatomic issues
- Timetable of anticipated facial nerve recovery.

Periocular procedures are often performed as an adjunct during a nerve substitution operation, dynamic muscle transposition, or static procedures.

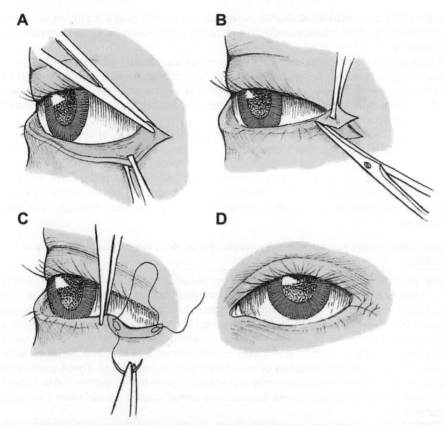

Fig. 3. Bick procedure. (*A–D*) The operative steps performed in a Bick procedure for lower lid ectropion repair. (*From* Wackym PA, Rhee JS. Facial paralysis. In: Snow JB, Wackym PA, editors. Ballenger's otorhinolaryngology. Shelton (CT): People's Medical Publishing House; 2009. p. 408. Copyright © 2009 BC Decker Inc; with permission.)

DELAYED POSTOPERATIVE ASSESSMENT AND MANAGEMENT

In patients who have complete facial paralysis in the presence of an intact facial nerve at the conclusion of resection, observation for 6 months to 1 year is recommended. This time allows opportunity for the regeneration of facial nerve at the expected 1 mm per day. Physical examination findings with or without facial electromyography (EMG) will dictate management decisions at the time of follow-up (see **Fig. 2**). If any degree of facial movement is detected, continued observation is recommended because improved function is likely anticipated.

If there is no detectable facial muscle tone, facial EMG can be a helpful diagnostic tool. There are 3 outcomes of the EMG:

1. Polyphasic action potentials
2. Fibrillation
3. Electrical silence.

If the EMG shows polyphasic action potentials, neural regeneration is anticipated and nerve substitution procedures are not indicated at this time. The patient may continue to be observed with repeat physical examination in 3 months.

If the EMG demonstrates fibrillation potentials, motor end plates are intact, but there is no evidence of neural regeneration, and nerve substitution procedures should be considered.

When a patient presents with late facial paralysis (usually >2 years), EMG may demonstrate electrical silence, and this indicates nonviable motor end plates. When this occurs, nerve substitution procedures should not be performed and free innervated muscle transfer, dynamic muscle transpositions, or static procedures should be considered.

Although the algorithms (see **Figs. 1** and **2**) presented are meant to guide management decisions, treatment of facial paralysis is complex, and patients may require a combination of procedures to obtain optimal outcomes. A review of nerve substitution procedures, dynamic muscle transpositions, and static procedures follows. Adjunctive therapies for further optimization and management of these patients, including the use of botulinum toxin injections and physical therapy, are also discussed.

Nerve Substitution Procedures: Hypoglossal-Facial Anastomosis and Cross-Facial Grafting

When primary repair of the facial nerve is not possible, nerve substitution operations offer the patient the best outcome to restore meaningful movement and tone. The most commonly used nerve substitution procedures are hypoglossal-facial anastomosis (XII–VII) or cross-facial (VII–VII) grafting. Prerequisites for nerve substitution procedures include the presence of an intact proximal donor nerve, an intact distal facial nerve, and viable motor end plates as determined by EMG. Preoperative counseling includes a clear discussion of realistic surgical expectations. These operations do not restore mimetic voluntary facial movement, but do have the potential to restore tone and symmetry at rest as well as providing some voluntary facial movement with rehabilitation.

The XII-VII substitution operations produce the most consistent results, with approximately 90% of patients demonstrating improved tone and symmetry.[19] Three main techniques exist for XII-VII substitution procedures:

1. Complete hypoglossal-facial nerve anastomosis
2. Partial hypoglossal-facial nerve anastomosis
3. Jump or interposition grafting between the hypoglossal and facial nerves.

Complete hypoglossal-facial nerve anastomosis

- The most proximal aspect of the facial nerve is identified at the stylomastoid foramen, and the nerve is dissected away from the parotid up to the main trunk at the pes anserinus.
- The hypoglossal nerve is divided distal to the descendens hypoglossi takeoff and then mobilized medial to the digastric muscle.
- A tensionless anastomosis is performed to the proximal facial nerve (**Fig. 4**).

The main disadvantage to end-to-end anastomosis is the sacrifice of the ipsilateral hypoglossal nerve, which leads to hemitongue atrophy. The findings of a recent meta-analysis of hypoglossal-facial anastomosis demonstrated a resulting difficulty with speech in 10% to 60% of patients and swallowing in 20% to 46% of patients.[19] If a patient has concomitant lower cranial nerve deficiencies (IX and X), postoperative hypoglossal dysfunction may exacerbate the deficits and lead to increased difficulty with speech and swallowing.

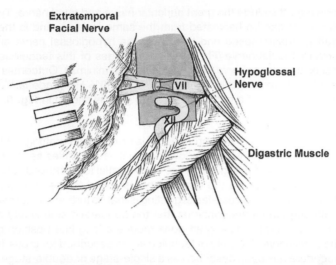

Fig. 4. Hypoglossal-facial substitution procedure. The hypoglossal nerve is mobilized medial to the digastric muscle and sutured to the proximal facial nerve. (*From* Wackym PA, Rhee JS. Facial paralysis. In: Snow JB, Wackym PA, editors. Ballenger's otorhinolaryngology. Shelton (CT): People's Medical Publishing House; 2009. p. 408. Copyright © 2009 BC Decker Inc; with permission.)

Partial hypoglossal-facial nerve anastomosis and jump graft
Because of the postoperative hypoglossal deficits, alternatives such as partial end-to-side hypoglossal-facial anastomosis and interposition jump grafts have been developed. Although these techniques can also be associated with some degree of tongue atrophy, clinically significant negative outcomes on speech and swallowing have not been described.[19] In these techniques, the hypoglossal nerve is not fully transected at the site of the anastomosis; rather, a small wedge that is no more than one-half of the diameter of the nerve is used. The facial nerve or interposition graft is sutured via an end-to-side anastomosis to the hypoglossal nerve.

Partial hypoglossal-facial nerve anastomosis
The partial hypoglossal-facial anastomosis is an attractive technique because only 1 anastomosis is performed and the power source, the hypoglossal nerve, is directly connected to the facial nerve. The primary difficulty with end-to-side hypoglossal-facial anastomosis is the mobilization of the nerves to approximate one another, and often the facial nerve requires mobilization. The intratemporal segment of the facial nerve may be mobilized from the stylomastoid foramen through the mastoid segment with the goal of mobilizing enough proximal facial nerve to suture it to the hypoglossal nerve proximal to the takeoff of the descendens hypoglossi.[20,21] A modification that has been described is to combine a parotid release procedure with the intratemporal mobilization to provide an additional 3 to 5 mm of facial nerve.[22] The end-to-side hypoglossal-facial anastomosis has produced satisfactory facial function without hemitongue atrophy.[21,22]

Jump graft
The interposition jump graft is an attractive alternative because, similar to the partial end-to-side anastomosis, it also avoids difficulties in speech and swallowing. The procedure is also performed without retrieval of the facial nerve from the mastoid.

Options for nerve graft include the great auricular nerve and sural nerve. Typically the great auricular nerve can be harvested from the same incision, and is the preferred graft. The graft is anastomosed end-to-side to the hypoglossal nerve and end-to-end to the proximal facial nerve (**Fig. 5**). Disadvantages of this technique include 2 anastomotic sites and donor nerve morbidity (although minimal). Outcomes are similar to hypoglossal-facial anastomosis, with greater than 80% HB grade III.[19,23] A representative successful case of a partial XII-VII jump graft is shown in **Fig. 6**.

Cross-facial grafting

An alternative to hypoglossal-facial procedures is cross-facial grafting, which may be considered in those patients who have lower cranial neuropathies secondary to their resection. In theory, cross-facial grafting has the potential for improved volitional coordination of movement because the donor nerve is linked to the contralateral facial cortex. Another advantage of cross-facial grafting is that no further cranial nerve deficits are created, although there are concerns that the nonparetic side would experience some weakness. The cross-facial graft does require a long interposition graft, most commonly the sural nerve. A variety of techniques are described for cross-facial grafting.[24] The procedure has been described as a single-stage or double-stage operation. In the double-stage operation, the initial surgery involves harvesting the graft, performing the anastomosis to the donor nerve, and cross-facial placement of the graft. Nerve regrowth through the graft is allowed for at least 4 months and, once established, a second operation is performed to anastomose the graft to the affected facial nerve.

Historically, the cross-facial graft has had some disappointing results.[24] One disadvantage for patients with vestibular schwannoma is the length of time before clinical results are appreciated from this technique. Often, nerve substitution procedures are not considered until 6 to 9 months after surgery and if a 2-stage technique is performed, another 6 months passes before the final stage of the substitution procedure.

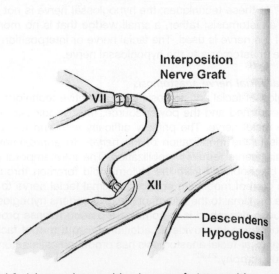

Fig. 5. Hypoglossal-facial nerve interposition jump graft. Interposition grafting is performed between the partially transected hypoglossal nerve to the proximal facial nerve. (*From* Wackym PA, Rhee JS. Facial paralysis. In: Snow JB, Wackym PA, editors. Ballenger's otorhinolaryngology. Shelton (CT): People's Medical Publishing House; 2009. p. 408. Copyright © 2009 BC Decker Inc; with permission.)

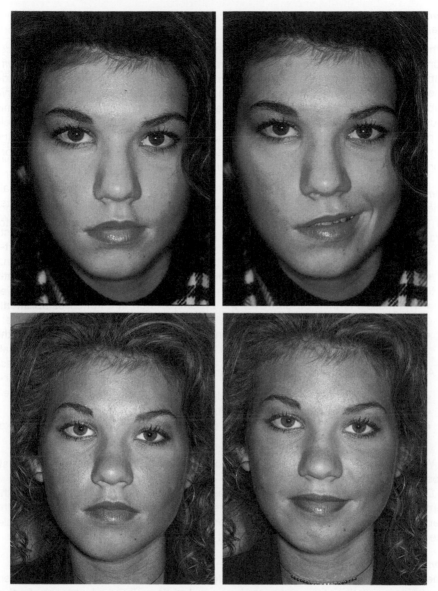

Fig. 6. Preoperative and postoperative photographs of a patient who underwent hypoglossal-facial interposition grafting. The patient underwent resection of a vestibular schwannoma and had complete right facial paralysis. (*Top right and left*) Preoperative photographs of the patient at rest and smiling. (*Bottom right and left*) Postoperative photographs taken 2 years after interposition grafting. A gold weight was also placed in the right upper eyelid.

This is followed by another 6-month to 2-year waiting period for facial movement, which brings into question the possibility of significant muscle atrophy and nonviable motor end plates. Recently, cross-facial nerve grafting has become an important tool in combination with free-muscle transfer.

Dynamic Muscle Transposition Procedures: Temporalis Muscle and Tendon Transposition

When patients are not candidates for, or are not interested in, nerve substitution procedures, dynamic muscle transposition can provide reanimation of the mouth with improved facial symmetry and volitional movement. Regional muscle transposition should also be considered in patients with long-term facial paralysis in whom nerve substitution procedures are contraindicated or have failed. The theory of dynamic muscle transfer is to transpose functional, innervated, and vascularized skeletal muscle to provide desired facial movements. The most commonly transposed muscles are the temporalis, masseter, and digastric muscles. The following discussion focuses on more commonly used techniques of the temporalis muscle and tendon transposition.

Temporalis muscle transposition

The temporalis muscle is fan shaped, arises from the temporal fossa, extends inferior to the anterior border of the mandibular ramus, and is innervated by the motor branches of the mandibular division of the trigeminal nerve. In the operation:

- The muscle is exposed
- The middle third is harvested from above the temporal line down to the zygomatic arch
- The muscle is then passed over the zygomatic arch through a subcutaneous tunnel to the oral commissure
- An incision is made at the oral commissure and the muscle is sutured at the modiolus.

A modification to this procedure includes:

- Further anchoring the fascia at the upper and lower vermillion borders[25]
- The muscle is sutured to pull the philtrum and lower lip back to midline
- Initially, overcorrection to expose the upper canine is preferred because relaxation will occur over 3 to 6 weeks.

With appropriate therapy, the patient should be smiling by the fourth to sixth postoperative week.

Disadvantages of the temporalis transposition include a possible depression in the temporal area as well as noticeable bulge over the zygomatic arch. Although the depression in the temporal area can be corrected by rotation of the residual muscle, the bulge over the zygoma is more difficult to correct.

Temporalis tendon transfer

The orthodromic temporalis tendon transfer is a more recent technique that offers dynamic reanimation of the oral commissure and midface.[26] The advantages of orthodromic temporalis tendon transfer over traditional temporalis transposition include orthodromic muscle contraction and improved vector of pull at the oral commissure. It also avoids midfacial bulkiness that may occur from temporalis transpositions. In this procedure:

- The tendon is removed from the coronoid process, then reinserted at the oral commissure.
- The operation may be performed via a preauricular transzygomatic approach or a transbuccal approach to access the coronoid process.
- Often the coronoid is transected at its neck, and the tendon, attached to the coronoid, is mobilized through a subcutaneous tunnel to a melolabial incision.

- The coronoid segment is then dissected from the tendon, and the tendon is secured to the modiolus and deep dermis in a slightly overcorrected position.
- The patient is immobilized for 1 week and then should resume facial retraining and physical therapy, which is especially important with this technique so that postoperative trismus does not develop.

The patient should begin to learn a temporal smile 2 weeks after surgery, and clinically noticeable recovery may occur in 4 to 6 weeks.

Free-Muscle Transfer: Gracilis Transfer with Cross-Facial Nerve Grafting

Free-muscle transfer is another option for patients with long-term facial paralysis, and is considered in patients with a greater than 2-year history of paralysis with unlikely functional motor end plates. Free-muscle transfer combined with cross-facial grafting provides an option for improved smile symmetry and midfacial tone. Much of the literature on free-muscle transfer relates to patients with posttraumatic or congenital facial paralysis; however, the application is relevant to patients with paralysis secondary to resection of a vestibular schwannoma. Many techniques have been developed for free-muscle transfer and include transfer of the pectoralis minor, latissimus dorsi, serratus anterior, extensor digitorum brevis, and extensor hallucis. The most commonly described transfer is the gracilis muscle.

The gracilis is a favorable candidate for free-muscle transfer to the face because of its size, shape, length, reliable vascular supply, and long single motor nerve.[27] Although use of the gracilis muscle is well established for facial reanimation, debate continues over the operative details. Single-stage and double-stage procedures have been described. Multiple donor nerves have also been described as candidates, such as the contralateral facial nerve, with or without sural nerve interposition grafting, or the ipsilateral motor nerve to the masseter.

Long-term results with free-muscle transfer are difficult to compare secondary to the variety of techniques: single-stage versus 2-stage, choice of transferred free muscle, and choice of donor neural input, as well as patients' demographic variables and surgeon-specific variables. Terzis and Olivares[28] recently reported the long-term outcomes of 24 patients treated with free-muscle transfer. All patients treated had improved smile scores at 2 years and continued their improvement in scores during prolonged follow-up.

Static Procedures for the Midface: Facial Sling and Multivector Suture

Although nerve substitution and dynamic procedures have become the preferred long-term treatment options, static suspension procedures remain important options for selected patients. These procedures are especially useful in patients who are not candidates for nerve substitution or dynamic procedures; for example, poor surgical candidates for the dynamic procedures due to medical comorbidities or those who have failed previous reanimation surgeries. These procedures may also be used as an adjunct while waiting for the return of facial function. Static procedures may be used to address specific facial areas of deficit, such as nasal vestibular stenosis and brow ptosis, or to restore nasolabial fold.

Facial sling
Midfacial asymmetry addressed by facial slings has been well described. Many materials may be used to create a sling, including:

- Autogenous material, such as palmaris longus or fascia lata tendon
- Alloplastic materials, such as expanded polytetrafluoroethylene (Gore-Tex; Gore and Associates, Newark, NJ, USA)

- Biomaterials, such as human acellular dermal matrix (Alloderm; LifeCell Corp., The Woodlands, TX, USA)
- Porcine dermal collagen (ENDURAGen; Tissue Science Laboratories plc, Aldershot, UK).

The use of polytetrafluoroethylene has been frequently reported because it is an easy material to work with, has no donor site morbidity, and is easily reversible. There is a small risk of extrusion and infection with the use of alloplasts. The basic surgical steps in facial sling placement are very similar to temporalis transposition. A tunnel is created from zygomatic arch to the orbicularis oris and lateral edges of the vermillion border of the upper and lower lip, and the sling is positioned and secured. As with the temporalis transposition, there should be slight overcorrection of the nasolabial fold and the corner of the mouth as relaxation is expected.[29]

Multivector suture technique
A multivector suture technique has also been introduced for nasolabial fold asymmetry. Multivector suture techniques have been described as in-office procedures performed with local anesthesia and with excellent patient tolerance. The principle is the same as for the static sling:

- Prolene sutures on a long Keith needle are threaded through a subcutaneous tunnel from the lateral orbital rim or temporal incision to small stab incisions within the neo-nasolabial fold at the nasal ala, midfold region, and oral commissure.
- To secure the suture and reduce the risk of suture migration, the suture material is threaded through polytetrafluoroethylene pledgets or harvested temporalis fascia pledgets.
- Each suture may be tightened or loosened as needed to create the multivector pull before securing.
- Often, only the incisions at the lateral orbital rim or temporal region require closure, whereas the stab incisions at the neo-nasolabial fold can be approximated with Steri-Strips.

Another reported advantage of this technique is the ability to easily correct laxity or stretch complication while in the office.[29,30]

Adjunctive Therapies for Facial Paralysis: Botulinum Toxin and Neuromuscular Retraining

Botulinum toxin has become a useful adjunct in the treatment of facial paralysis and facial nerve regeneration. Botulinum toxin may be used to treat the unaffected side for treatment of relative hyperkinesis or treatment of ipsilateral synkinesis. Botulinum toxin binds presynaptically and inhibits the release of acetylcholine, leading to a neuromuscular blocking effect. The effects of the toxin are usually realized 24 to 72 hours after injection but may take up to 1 week, and effects last 2 to 5 months. Adverse effects are rare and are typically related to the local effects of injection causing local hematoma or infection. Allergy to botulinum toxin has also been described, but is rare.

Facial symmetry

Facial symmetry may be improved by treating relative hyperkinesis of the unaffected side of the face. The unaffected side often appears to function with relative hyperkinesis, which causes the paralyzed side of the face to pull. This is especially noticeable when patients smile and, in some cases, may be noticeable at rest. Characteristic findings of relative hyperkinesis include deviation of the nasal tip and an unbalanced smile. Options to treat relative hyperkinesis include selective myotomy, myectomy, or

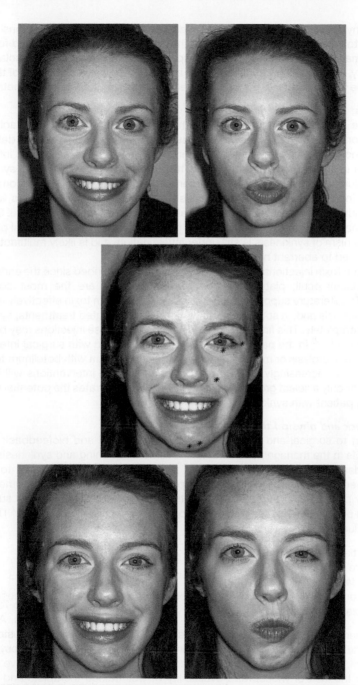

Fig. 7. A patient treated with botulinum toxin for synkinesis. (*Top left and right*) Oral-ocular synkinesis is demonstrated when patient smiles and puckers lips. (*Middle*) Planned injection sites to the orbicularis oculi, zygomaticus muscle, and mentalis muscle. (*Bottom left and right*) Postinjection results with decreased synkinetic movements.

neurectomy, as well as botulinum toxin injections. Botulinum toxin injections for relative hypertonicity are performed to target the nasolabial fold, lower lip, and forehead. The zygomaticus major and levator labii superioris are injected to treat nasolabial fold asymmetry. The depressor anguli oris may be injected to treat asymmetry of the lower lip, and the frontalis muscle may be injected for improved forehead symmetry.[30–34]

Synkinesis

One of the most troublesome problems that occurs after spontaneous facial nerve recovery or after reinnervation procedures is synkinesis. Synkinesis is defined as the presence of an unintentional motion in one area of the face during intentional movement in another area of the face.[35] The most common is oculo-oral synkinesis, which occurs when the patient has unintentional movement of the oral commissure when closing the eye. Oral-oculo synkinesis is also common, and occurs when the patient voluntarily moves his or her mouth and has unintentional eye closure. Synkinesis is estimated to occur in 15% to 50% of patients who recover from facial paralysis. The mechanism of synkinesis is still under investigation, and is likely multifactorial but in part related to aberrant neural regeneration.

Botulinum toxin injections for synkinesis have been described since the early 1990s. The orbicularis oculi, platysma, and mentalis muscles are the most commonly injected. The literature supports that low doses of botulinum toxin effectively eliminate ocular synkinesis and, in some patients who undergo repeated treatments, synkinesis resolves completely. This finding supports a theory that these injections may break the synkinetic cycle.[35] In the past, synkinesis has been treated with surgical intervention via selective neurolysis or myectomy. However, as treatment with botulinum toxin has evolved and is increasingly the standard of care, surgical interventions will likely be reserved for only a select group of patients. **Fig. 7** demonstrates the potential injection sites for a patient with synkinesis.

Biofeedback and physical therapy

In addition to surgical and medical intervention, physical and biofeedback therapy share a role in the management of facial movement retraining and synkinesis. Often, EMG guidance and a mirror are used to provide feedback for patients to identify and then reduce synkinetic movements or produce meaningful facial movements.[35,36] A recently published large retrospective study that included 160 patients supported the role of physical therapy as part of comprehensive facial rehabilitation.[37] The treatments included the following:

- Soft tissue mobilization (massage)
- Active assistive exercises
- Avoidance of mass movement
- Neuromuscular retraining with a mirror and/or EMG to control synkinesis
- Relaxation/meditation.

After therapy, the patients demonstrated significant improvement in their facial grading scale scores, with improved meaningful movement and decreased synkinesis and spasm. The main limitation for broad-spectrum adaptation of adjunctive physical therapy is the lack of widespread availability of well-trained therapists and the less than compelling demonstration of clinically significant improved outcomes.

SUMMARY OF FACIAL PARALYSIS TREATMENT

Treatment for facial paralysis after resection of a vestibular schwannoma is complex. The algorithms (see **Figs. 1** and **2**) provided and the accompanying discussion offer a foundation for developing an individualized plan for a patient. Options for facial nerve habilitation are constantly evolving, with the ultimate goal of restoring complete facial symmetry and movement still on the horizon.

REFERENCES

1. Hastan D, Vandenbroucke JP, van der Mey AG. A meta-analysis of surgical treatment for vestibular schwannoma: is hospital volume related to preservation of facial function? Otol Neurotol 2009;30(7):975–80.
2. Catalano PJ, Post KD, Sen C, et al. Preoperative facial nerve studies predict paresis following cerebellopontine angle surgery. Am J Otol 1996;17(3):446–51.
3. Magliulo G, D'Amico R, Di Cello P. Delayed facial palsy after vestibular schwannoma resection: clinical data and prognosis. J Otolaryngol 2003;32(6):400–4.
4. House JW, Brackmann DE. Facial nerve grading system. Otolaryngol Head Neck Surg 1985;93(2):146–7.
5. Bacciu A, Falcioni M, Pasanisi E, et al. Intracranial facial nerve grafting after removal of vestibular schwannoma. Am J Otolaryngol 2009;30(2):83–8.
6. Gidley PW, Gantz BJ, Rubinstein JT. Facial nerve grafts: from cerebellopontine angle and beyond. Am J Otol 1999;20(6):781–8.
7. Parhizkar N, Hiltzik DH, Selesnick SH. Facial nerve rerouting in skull base surgery. Otolaryngol Clin North Am 2005;38(4):685–710, ix.
8. Fisch U, Dobie RA, Gmur A, et al. Intracranial facial nerve anastomosis. Am J Otol 1987;8(1):23–9.
9. Sanna M, Jain Y, Falcioni M, et al. Facial nerve grafting in the cerebellopontine angle. Laryngoscope 2004;114(4):782–5.
10. Luetje CM, Whittaker CK. The benefits of VII-VII neuroanastomosis in acoustic tumor surgery. Laryngoscope 1991;101(12 Pt 1):1273–5.
11. Stephanian E, Sekhar LN, Janecka IP, et al. Facial nerve repair by interposition nerve graft: results in 22 patients. Neurosurgery 1992;31(1):73–6 [discussion: 77].
12. Rahman I, Sadiq SA. Ophthalmic management of facial nerve palsy: a review. Surv Ophthalmol 2007;52(2):121–44.
13. May M. Gold weight and wire spring implants as alternatives to tarsorrhaphy. Arch Otolaryngol Head Neck Surg 1987;113(6):656–60.
14. Schrom T, Wernecke K, Thelen A, et al. Results after lidloading with rigid gold weights–a meta-analysis. Laryngorhinootologie 2007;86(2):117–23.
15. Silver AL, Lindsay RW, Cheney ML, et al. Thin-profile platinum eyelid weighting: a superior option in the paralyzed eye. Plast Reconstr Surg 2009;123(6):1697–703.
16. Fedok FG, Ferraro RE. Restoration of lower eyelid support in facial paralysis. Facial Plast Surg 2000;16(4):337–43.
17. Leone CR Jr. Repair of ectropion using the Bick procedure. Am J Ophthalmol 1970;70(2):233–5.
18. Vagefi MR, Anderson RL. The lateral tarsal strip mini-tarsorrhaphy procedure. Arch Facial Plast Surg 2009;11(2):136–9.
19. Yetiser S, Karapinar U. Hypoglossal-facial nerve anastomosis: a meta-analytic study. Ann Otol Rhinol Laryngol 2007;116(7):542–9.
20. Atlas MD, Lowinger DS. A new technique for hypoglossal-facial nerve repair. Laryngoscope 1997;107(7):984–91.
21. Sawamura Y, Abe H. Hypoglossal-facial nerve side-to-end anastomosis for preservation of hypoglossal function: results of delayed treatment with a new technique. J Neurosurg 1997;86(2):203–6.

22. Roland JT Jr, Lin K, Klausner LM, et al. Direct facial-to-hypoglossal neurorrhaphy with parotid release. Skull Base 2006;16(2):101–8.
23. Hammerschlag PE. Facial reanimation with jump interpositional graft hypoglossal facial anastomosis and hypoglossal facial anastomosis: evolution in management of facial paralysis. Laryngoscope 1999;109(2 Pt 2 Suppl 90):1–23.
24. Lee EI, Hurvitz KA, Evans GR, et al. Cross-facial nerve graft: past and present. J Plast Reconstr Aesthet Surg 2008;61(3):250–6.
25. Boahene KD. Dynamic muscle transfer in facial reanimation. Facial Plast Surg 2008;24(2):204–10.
26. Byrne PJ, Kim M, Boahene K, et al. Temporalis tendon transfer as part of a comprehensive approach to facial reanimation. Arch Facial Plast Surg 2007; 9(4):234–41.
27. Chuang DC. Free tissue transfer for the treatment of facial paralysis. Facial Plast Surg 2008;24(2):194–203.
28. Terzis JK, Olivares FS. Long-term outcomes of free-muscle transfer for smile restoration in adults. Plast Reconstr Surg 2009;123(3):877–88.
29. Liu YM, Sherris DA. Static procedures for the management of the midface and lower face. Facial Plast Surg 2008;24(2):211–5.
30. Hadlock TA, Greenfield LJ, Wernick-Robinson M, et al. Multimodality approach to management of the paralyzed face. Laryngoscope 2006;116(8):1385–9.
31. Lindsay RW, Edwards C, Smitson C, et al. A systematic algorithm for the management of lower lip asymmetry. Am J Otolaryngol 2011;32(1):1–7.
32. Mehta RP, Hadlock TA. Botulinum toxin and quality of life in patients with facial paralysis. Arch Facial Plast Surg 2008;10(2):84–7.
33. Bikhazi NB, Maas CS. Refinement in the rehabilitation of the paralyzed face using botulinum toxin. Otolaryngol Head Neck Surg 1997;117(4):303–7.
34. de Maio M, Bento RF. Botulinum toxin in facial palsy: an effective treatment for contralateral hyperkinesis. Plast Reconstr Surg 2007;120(4):917–27 [discussion: 928].
35. Husseman J, Mehta RP. Management of synkinesis. Facial Plast Surg 2008;24(2): 242–9.
36. Cronin GW, Steenerson RL. The effectiveness of neuromuscular facial retraining combined with electromyography in facial paralysis rehabilitation. Otolaryngol Head Neck Surg 2003;128(4):534–8.
37. Lindsay RW, Robinson M, Hadlock TA. Comprehensive facial rehabilitation improves function in people with facial paralysis: a 5-year experience at the Massachusetts Eye and Ear Infirmary. Phys Ther 2010;90(3):391–7.

Importance of Local Support Groups for Acoustic Neuroma and Neurofibromatosis Patients

Judy B. Vitucci

KEYWORDS

• Support groups • Local support groups • Acoustic neuroma • Neurofibromatosis

Local support groups are a vital extension of the support network for acoustic neuroma patients. For many people, the local group is the only place where they can make personal contact with other patients who have gone through a similar experience.

ACOUSTIC NEUROMA SUPPORT GROUPS

Acoustic neuromas are relatively rare, and most newly diagnosed patients feel very much alone. Providing contact with other patients provides education, support, and comfort.

The local support groups provide an opportunity for networking on all issues relevant to acoustic neuroma patients. The groups assist with social and personal support for all acoustic neuroma patients, including newly diagnosed, watch-and-wait, and previously treated acoustic neuroma patients and their family members. They provide the opportunity for personal connection and encouragement and are helpful for individuals facing the challenges of an acoustic neuroma, giving them an opportunity to learn new ways to handle challenges, cope with changes, and maintain new behaviors. A small tip goes a long way to make a patient feel normal again. Additionally, support groups provide the opportunity for education on pre- and post-treatment issues affecting acoustic neuroma patients with guest speakers from the health care profession.

BENEFITS OF SUPPORT GROUPS FOR THE ACOUSTIC NEUROMA PATIENT
Communication

Acoustic neuroma patients and family members are able to communicate with each other in a nurturing, nonjudgmental environment with others who have shared a common acoustic neuroma experience. The open format allows participants to feel some degree of anonymity and to participate as they are comfortable. For

Acoustic Neuroma Association, 600 Peachtree Parkway, Suite 108, Cumming, GA 30041, USA
E-mail address: director@ANAUSA.org

Otolaryngol Clin N Am 45 (2012) 531–535
doi:10.1016/j.otc.2011.12.016
0030-6665/12/$ – see front matter © 2012 Elsevier Inc. All rights reserved.
oto.theclinics.com

some people, simply attending meetings and listening to the experiences of others can be helpful.

Sharing Information

For those who have experienced an acoustic neuroma, the value of sharing tips about everything from facial, eye, balance, headache, hearing, and tinnitus issues is invaluable. The sharing of information includes how to deal with specific problems, overcoming handicaps, and the ability to live with handicaps for a lifetime for some. The participants have an understanding incomparable to anyone else.

Education

Guest speakers from the health care profession are often a part of the local support group meetings. These medical professionals are able to present detailed information about various aspects of acoustic neuroma treatment and issues and address questions in a personal environment. For acoustic neuroma local support group meetings, guest speakers cover subjects such as treatment options, balance, facial issues, tinnitus, and hearing issues and devices.

Emotional Support

Since the acoustic neuroma patients have walked in their shoes, they can provide the important emotional support so necessary for some acoustic neuroma patients. Family members sometimes cannot fully understand the burden that acoustic neuroma patients must live with every day. The group helps patients develop realistic expectations and adjust to changing life situations, reassuring others that better times lie ahead. The healing power of groups is well documented and assists attendees by providing the mutual support that attendees provide one another.

Group Dynamics

All groups are unique yet ultimately behave similarly. Group leaders try hard not to focus on negativity at meetings and remember that everyone shares a commonality and can learn from each other. Occasionally, when a difficult person attends a meeting, it is important to recognize that this difficulty may be caused by fear. Information, support, networking with others, and reassurance can help to alleviate this fear, as well as emphasizing the positive. Groups help acoustic neuroma patients develop realistic expectations, with an understanding that sometimes things will not be exactly as they used to be. Much time is spent making connections and building relationships.

Testimonials for Acoustic Neuroma Support Group Members

The following testimonials are from acoustic neuroma association (ANA) members describing the positive impact received from attending a local support group meeting.

"We have faced a common trauma, coping with an acoustic neuroma. Face-to-face group meetings give the opportunity to be with others who truly understand. By sharing how we have coped and been helped by receiving medical information from professionals who may be new to us, we can restore ourselves by the strength furnished by a caring community."

— Ginny Fickel Ehr, ANA Founder

"I remember how desperately I wanted to be able to talk with someone. I feel one of the many benefits provided by our group, is its ability to provide encouragement and compassion for the newly diagnosed."

— Greg from Washington, D.C.

"I have found all the meetings that I have attended to be very informative and have made several friends. I have found it best to talk with individuals who have just started their AN journey and share my successful outcome."
— *Joe from New Jersey*

"My greatest reward from attending this group is watching newly diagnosed patients attend a meeting and having the opportunity to meet a variety of people with many treatment types as they weigh all their options. I see the hope in their eyes appear as they learn we have all survived, and life after an AN (acoustic neuroma) is possible."
—*Joan from Florida*

"I had great support from my family and friends, but they could not understand my concerns, thoughts, and feelings. I never knew anyone who had any type of brain tumor, so it seemed, at times, that I was going through this alone. Coming to the support group allowed me to meet people who also had a vestibular schwannoma. Even though our conditions may differ, it is a great feeling to relate to others."
—*Jennifer from Florida*

"The group gave me hope and made me realize that I wasn't alone. There were many others out there who shared similar problems to mine, and we were bonded on that basis. Together, we can make a difference for others who are newly diagnosed and those who have difficulty dealing with their present reality."
— *Carol from Florida*

"It has been very meaningful for us to share and learn from others who can truly understand the daily challenges we all face with acoustic neuroma. We are constantly seeking out solutions to make our lives better. We are reminded at each meeting that there is life after acoustic neuroma!"
— *Gail and Elaine from Michigan*

INFORMATION FOLLOWING ON NF INCORPORATED IS ADAPTED FROM THEIR WEBSITE: http://www.nfnetwork.org/
Neurofibromatosis

NF Incorporated provides information and support specifically for neurofibromatosis 2 (NF2). When someone contacts the national office, a package with NF2 information is distributed. The name is then forwarded to the national NF2 representative. NF Incorporated organizers realized there are not sufficient numbers of NF2 individuals in any 1 chapter. Yet NF2 individuals have specific needs, and a national NF2 representative was established in order to give voice to these needs.

Online

Local groups may have no other NF2 members and, as many NF2 individuals are deaf, communication can be difficult. The local NF support groups cannot provide the support that a person diagnosed with a rare disorder requires. Several strong local neurofibromatosis organizations established a national neurofibromatosis organization to still retain autonomy within the local groups while allowing for national and international collaboration. An NF2 representative tells everyone about www.nf2crew.org, which is an online support group specifically for NF2 individuals and their loved ones.

Research

NF Incorporated supports research with symposiums for clinicians and scientists to present and discuss the latest breakthroughs and with grants for specialists in the field. The group has helped to facilitate research translating basic science of chemical actions on these tumors into medications for human clinical trials.

Communication

With several hundred members worldwide, this group provides information, experience, and support that can only be gained from others who share and have gone through many of the problems experienced by patients with NF2. Even if a member is deaf, the ease of communication within this group provides a supportive environment for the patient's needs.

Education

NF Incorporated members understand the isolation of deafness and/or dealing with a rare disorder; thus the organization has supported NF2 gatherings in Nevada and Ohio, which professionals attend at times to give presentations and answer questions. Although these events are primarily social, they offer the rare opportunity for anyone with NF2, regardless of the stage of the disorder, to meet face to face with others who understand.

The neurofibromatosis organization produces patient packets available for the asking that contain, in part

- The book, "Understanding Neurofibromatosis," an introduction for patients and parents
- Glossary of terms
- Information on the NF2 crew, helpful resources, insurance coverage, DNA testing, cochlear implants, and more.

The packets are available by mail or electronic download from the NF Incorporated Web site.

Testimonials from Neurofibromatosis Support Group Members

The following statements are from NF2 Incorporated members describing the positive impact received from being involved with local and national neurofibromatosis support groups.

"Right from the beginning, what helped us cope immensely was our involvement with our local NF (neurofibromatosis) organization, NF Inc. Midwest. When Rachel was younger, we hosted several plant sales at our home, raising money for research and NF awareness in our community. As a result of these plant sales, we met other NF-affected families, and we started a local support group. We have made friendships and have stayed well informed by being connected to NF Inc. Midwest. I have met adults with NF who are leading normal lives, who are married, work, and are happy. This has always given me hope for my daughter's future."

— Liz and Rachel

"I have seen NF (neurofibromatosis) from every perspective imaginable—as a patient, a parent, and a family member. The devastation this disease has wreaked on our family is significant. ... I have been involved with NF groups for over 25 years, and we have come so far; the research has progressed so much. We are on the verge of major breakthroughs, and this is so exciting to me when I know where we were, when doctors had barely heard of NF, and now we are at the stage of clinical trials, and more and more research is being done, and more and more good, solid information is being published for families, and support groups are being formed so people are not alone anymore."

— Beverly

CONTACT FOR SUPPORT GROUPS

Acoustic Neuroma Association, 600 Peachtree Parkway, Suite 108, Cumming, GA 30041. Phone: 1-877-200-8211 or 770-205-8211. Fax: 1-877-202-0239 or 770-205-0239, http://www.ANAUSA.org. info@ANAUSA.org.

Neurofibromatosis, Incorporated, Post Office Box 66884, Chicago, Illinois 60666. Phone: 1-800-942-6825. http://www.nfnetwork.org.

Index

Note: Page numbers of article titles are in **boldface** type.

A

Age at diagnosis, 259, 260
Algorithms, decision-making, 346
Anesthesia, 377
Approaches, early surgical, 375–376
Asymptomatic tumors, 274
Audiogram, pure tone, 275
Audiologic evaluation, 275
Audiometry, behavioral, 285
Auditory and vestibular dysfunction, habilitation of, **487–511**
Auditory assessment, intraoperative, 288–289
    postoperative, 289
Auditory brainstem response testing, 275–276
    stacked, 276–277
Auditory evaluation, preoperative, intraoperative, and postoperative, **285–290**
Auditory habilitation, hearing loss and, 488–498

B

Balance, static and dynamic, 502–503, 504
Balance exercises, 505, 506
Bevacziumab, 479–481
Bick procedure, 518, 519
Biofeedback therapy, for facial paralysis, 528
Bleeding, potential sources of, 411, 412
Bone-anchored implants, percutaneous, 491–492, 493
Botulinum toxin, for facial paralysis, 526
Brainstem and direct eight-nerve intraoperative monitoring, 288–289
Brainstem response, auditory, 286

C

Cerebrospinal fluid leak, 412, 432, 458–459
Chemotherapy, ongoing trials, 482
    present and future, **471–486**
    targeted, 478–481
Clinical and diagnostic evaluation, **269–284**
Clinical evaluation, 272–274
Clinical progression of patients, 269–271
Clinical trials, hearing end points for, 476
    radiographic end points for, 477–478
Cochlea factor, stereotactic radiosurgery in, 358–359
Cochlear nerve, tumor resection and, 462–464
Compression of surrounding structures, 308

Otolaryngol Clin N Am 45 (2012) 537–543
doi:10.1016/S0030-6665(12)00012-6
0030-6665/12/$ – see front matter © 2012 Elsevier Inc. All rights reserved.
oto.theclinics.com

Moving?

Make sure your subscription moves with you!

To notify us of your new address, find your **Clinics Account Number** (located on your mailing label above your name), and contact customer service at:

Email: journalscustomerservice-usa@elsevier.com

800-654-2452 (subscribers in the U.S. & Canada)
314-447-8871 (subscribers outside of the U.S. & Canada)

Fax number: 314-447-8029

Elsevier Health Sciences Division
Subscription Customer Service
3251 Riverport Lane
Maryland Heights, MO 63043

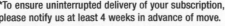

*To ensure uninterrupted delivery of your subscription, please notify us at least 4 weeks in advance of move.

ELSEVIER

Printed and bound by CPI Group (UK) Ltd, Croydon, CR0 4YY

03/10/2024

01040459-0011